Veterinary Mycotherapy and Medicinal Mushrooms

Veterinary Mycotherapy and Medicinal Mushrooms

J. A. Harper

OMG
MUSHROOMS

CONTENTS

www.omgmushrooms.com
contactus@omgmushrooms.com

NATIONAL LIBRARY OF AUSTRALIA

A catalogue record for this book is available from the National Library of Australia

ISBN: 9781764458634
EISBN: 9781921883941

First Edition
National Library of Australia Pre-publication Data
A cataloguing record for this book is available from the National Library of Australia.
Author: Harper, Julie-Ann
Title: Veterinary Mycotherapy and Medicinal Mushrooms
Sub-Title: An Evidence-Informed Guide to Functional and Medicinal Fungi in Veterinary Care

Disclaimer
This publication is provided for educational and informational purposes only. While every effort has been made to ensure accuracy at the time of printing, scientific understanding evolves and the authors, editors and publisher do not guarantee that all content reflects the most current developments.

Nothing in this book constitutes veterinary advice, medical instruction or professional guidance. Readers must exercise independent clinical and professional judgement. Any use, application or interpretation of the material is undertaken entirely at the reader's own risk.

The authors, editors and publisher disclaim all liability, including for negligence, for any loss, damage, injury or adverse outcome arising from reliance on any information contained within this text. This includes, without limitation, the use or misuse of mushrooms, extracts, supplements, cultivation methods or therapeutic approaches described herein. Always seek advice from a registered veterinarian regarding the health, treatment and wellbeing of animals.

Reference to specific products, extracts, cultivation techniques or suppliers does not imply endorsement, and omission does not imply inadequacy. All trademarks and product names mentioned are the property of their respective owners and are used solely for identification purposes.

Research limitations and interpretation
Many studies referenced in this book involve laboratory models, rodent studies or early-stage veterinary research. Results may not directly translate to individual animals or specific clinical situations. However, emerging findings provide promising insights that may inform future veterinary applications as research expands. The inclusion of research findings does not imply established therapeutic equivalence, safety or efficacy in all species, but reflects the growing scientific interest in this field.

No warranty statement
This publication is provided on an "as is" basis, without warranties of any kind, express or implied. While the authors and publisher have taken care to compile accurate, well-researched and current information, no representation is made regarding fitness for purpose, completeness or suitability of the material for any particular application. Readers are encouraged to use the content as a foundation for further inquiry, professional discussion and evidence-informed decision-making.

The material in this book may be cited for academic or professional purposes with appropriate acknowledgment of the authors and publisher.

Message to the Reader

Why I wrote this book – and what it is (and is not)

For many years I have had the privilege of knowing a number of integrative veterinarians – individuals whose compassion, clinical skill and breadth of vision continually remind me what true animal-centred care looks like. Their ability to bridge conventional medicine with complementary, evidence-informed therapies has profoundly influenced my own understanding of what is possible in modern veterinary practice. I hold deep respect for all veterinary professionals, yet it is integrative veterinarians who opened the door to conversations that felt both courageous and necessary: conversations about nutrition, immunity, chronic disease, ageing, and the therapeutic potential of mushrooms and their natural compounds – agents that have supported life for millennia.

My journey through Mycotherapy began in human health, where I quickly encountered a familiar tension: the longstanding divide between Western biomedical frameworks and traditional or Eastern medicinal systems. Mushrooms, it seemed, were often dismissed as too simple to be powerful, or too ancient to be relevant. Yet the science told a different story. As I studied, practised and eventually witnessed the effects first-hand, it became clear that functional mushrooms were neither fringe nor fanciful, they were historically significant, biologically complex and deeply relevant to modern health challenges. The world is now waking up to this, but the veterinary space still faces the same scepticism that delayed progress in human care.

Animals, however, have taught me one profound truth: they do not participate in placebo. They do not decide whether a therapy 'should' work. They simply respond – physiologically, behaviourally, metabolically – when something supports their system. Time and again, I witnessed improvements in animals that could not be attributed to belief or expectation, only to biology. This clarity has been one of the greatest motivators for writing this book. Where humans may second-guess or underestimate a therapy, animals often reveal its true therapeutic value.

Functional mushrooms are not new. They have been part of the medical landscape for decades, even if this history often goes unrecognised. Penicillin emerged from a fungal metabolite. Cyclosporine, the drug that transformed organ transplantation, was derived from a soil fungus. Lentinan, a clinically studied β-glucan from Shiitake, has been used in oncology protocols. Paclitaxel (Taxol), one of the most important anti-cancer agents ever developed, is produced through a fungal endophyte. Polysaccharide-K (PSK) and polysaccharopeptide (PSP) – both derived from *Trametes versicolor* – have been incorporated into synthetic and semi-synthetic cancer protocols for decades in parts of Asia. These are not anecdotes – they are reminders that fungi have already shaped the foundations of modern medicine.

Yet despite this legacy, the world of functional mushroom products has become crowded, confusing and, at times, deeply misleading. My work in this field has shown me how much misinformation exists around extraction, quality, sourcing and potency. Too many products labelled as 'medicinal' rely on myceliated and freeze-dried grain, low-grade powders, inferior tinctures, alcohol-based extractions or marketing statements unsupported by science.

In the veterinary sector, where precision and safety matter deeply, such compromises risk doing a disservice to both animals and clinicians. This is why I have centred this guide around whole-mushroom, fruiting-body-only, solvent-free extraction (sub-critical water extraction) – methods that preserve the complete biochemical matrix of the mushroom. SCWE retains the natural prebiotic fibre and the full spectrum of small but clinically relevant compounds – including polyphenols, terpenoids, sterols, peptides and antioxidant molecules – rather than focusing solely on β-glucans. These whole-food extracts more faithfully reflect how mushrooms function in nature and honour the evidence that supports their therapeutic potential.

I wrote this book to offer clarity in a field where clarity is urgently needed. It is not designed to replace clinical judgement, nor to suggest that mushrooms are a cure-all. What it *is* designed to do is provide veterinarians with a transparent, evidence-aligned resource that demystifies functional mushrooms and places them within a credible clinical framework. My hope is that the pages ahead will encourage more integrative veterinarians – and the wider profession – to explore Mycotherapy with both curiosity and confidence.

If this book ignites even one meaningful shift in how functional nutrition and mushroom therapeutics are understood for companion and performance animals, then every hour spent compiling, researching and refining it will have been worthwhile.

If you remain unconvinced about the place of mushrooms in animal wellness, the facts that follow may spark the curiosity needed to turn the page.

Amazing Facts About the World of Mushrooms

- The largest and oldest known living organism on Earth is a honey mushroom in Oregon that spans over 2,400 acres and is thousands of years old.
- Polypore mushrooms were found in the belongings of Ötzi the Iceman, dated to 3300 BC.
- Ancient rock art from Tassili, Algeria (7000 BC) depicts shamans carrying mushrooms in ceremonial scenes.
- In Ancient Egypt, mushrooms were reserved for pharaohs because they were believed to confer immortality.
- The Romans called mushrooms the food of the gods.
- Mushrooms have been used as both food and medicine for thousands of years across every major civilisation.
- Some cultures stored mushrooms in honey, a natural preservative still used today.
- Mushrooms have their own biological kingdom and are more closely related to animals than to plants.
- Fungi appeared on land an estimated 2.4 billion years ago, long before plants at 700 million years.
- Fungi exist everywhere, from the stratosphere to more than a mile underground.
- Some mushrooms glow in the dark through natural bioluminescence.
- Only about 4 to 7 percent of fungi on Earth have been formally identified, leaving millions of species still undiscovered.
- Without fungi breaking down organic matter, Earth would be buried under layers of dead plants and animals.

- Mycorrhizal fungi form vast underground networks, connecting over 90 percent of plants in the so-called wood-wide web.
- Plants use fungal networks to trade nutrients, share resources and warn each other of pests.
- Oyster mushrooms can break down petroleum and help clean oil spills in a process known as mycoremediation.
- Certain fungi can degrade plastics, pesticides and even toxic chemicals, turning them into harmless compounds.
- Mycelium can be grown into eco-friendly materials that replace plastic, leather and packaging foam.
- Scientists are developing mycelium building bricks that are strong, fire resistant and fully biodegradable.
- Slime moulds can solve mazes, optimise transport routes and adapt to changing environments, behaving like natural biological computers.
- Some mushrooms, such as Amanita muscaria, are linked to ancient winter-solstice traditions and may have inspired aspects of the Santa Claus story.
- Fungal alkaloids may have been used in ancient Greek initiation rites known as the Eleusinian Mysteries.
- Clinical research on psilocybin mushrooms is showing promising results for treatment-resistant depression, PTSD and addiction.
- NASA is studying fungi for growing self-repairing habitats and producing oxygen on Mars.
- Fungi are being studied for their ability to break down sterile planetary material and create the first layers of living soil, an essential step for supporting life beyond Earth.

TERMINOLOGY NOTE: Throughout this guide, both the terms **'functional mushrooms'** and **'medicinal mushrooms'** are used intentionally. In veterinary nutrition, 'functional mushrooms' is commonly adopted to describe species that provide physiological benefits beyond basic nutrition. Within Mycotherapy, traditional medical systems and emerging integrative research, these same species are often described as 'medicinal mushrooms' due to their long-recognised bioactive properties.

Because **Sub-Critical Water Extraction (SCWE)** preserves the full biochemical matrix of the fruiting body, bridging nutritional and therapeutic domains, the use of both terms reflects the dual nature of these extracts. This guide therefore employs each term, acknowledging their distinct histories while maintaining clarity for veterinary professionals and readers from diverse clinical and nutritional backgrounds.

SECTION ONE

PREFACE

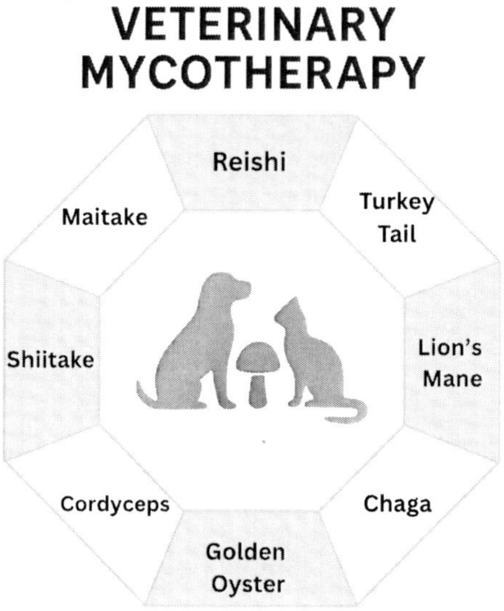

Mycotherapy – the therapeutic use of medicinal or functional mushrooms – is an emerging discipline within veterinary practice, and for that reason this guide is not presented as a comprehensive text. Rather, it is intended as a science-based starting point: a foundation that brings together current research, practical insights and early evidence in a field that is expanding rapidly.

While the literature on functional mushrooms in human health is substantial, animal-specific research remains comparatively limited. Much of what is presently understood in veterinary contexts is drawn from in vitro studies, translational research, practitioner experience and the many thousands of anecdotal case reports shared by integrative veterinarians and animal carers worldwide.

As more controlled, species-specific studies become available, the collective understanding of how medicinal mushrooms support animal health will continue to deepen – strengthening the evidence base that guides safe, effective and responsible mycotherapeutic practice.

The development of this guide has been shaped by the perspective of a Mycotherapist who also works directly in the cultivation of functional mushrooms. This dual involvement – from understanding fungal biology at the point of growth through to their clinical application – has informed a deeper appreciation of extraction integrity, fruiting-body chemistry and the relevance of whole-mushroom preparations in animal health. The content reflects extensive research into animal physiology, safety considerations and species-appropriate applications of functional mushrooms. Throughout its preparation, input was sought from integrative veterinarians whose clinical insights and professional feedback ensured the material aligns with real-world practice and contemporary veterinary principles. Their contributions have been central to grounding this work in both scientific evidence and practical relevance.

Integrative veterinarians have played a pivotal role in bringing medicinal mushrooms into the veterinary spotlight. Their willingness to explore emerging research, apply clinical reasoning and share observations from practice has advanced the field significantly. Their collaborative spirit continues to drive the evolution of Mycotherapy, helping translate early research into meaningful, species-appropriate insights. Their contributions are acknowledged with deep respect, as they remain essential to the ongoing refinement and ethical application of this emerging discipline.

> *Interest in functional mushrooms within the veterinary world is rising. A 2023 practitioner insight report from the U.S.- based Integrative Veterinary Medical Association (IVMA) noted that more than 40 % of integrative practitioners now include at least one medicinal mushroom in their clinical protocols, with immune support, oncology, cognitive decline and gut health being the most common applications.* Globally, functional mushroom use in pets has grown at an estimated 7-10 % annually over the past five years, reflecting increased consumer demand for natural, evidence-aligned adjuncts to conventional care. Although formal veterinary research still lags behind this interest, the momentum is undeniable - and it signals a growing need for high-quality education, transparent sourcing and scientifically grounded formulations. *IVMA Practitioner Insight Report, 2023*

As interest in functional mushrooms grows, so too does the importance of quality. The therapeutic potential of a mushroom is determined not only by species and dose, but by how it is grown, processed and extracted. Fruiting-body integrity, absence of grain-based fillers and extraction methods that preserve the full spectrum of bioactive compounds all play a critical role in clinical outcomes. Sub-critical water extraction (SCWE) - the method used in OMG Mushrooms formulations - is increasingly recognised for its ability to retain polysaccharides, triterpenes, antioxidants and heat-sensitive compounds in their natural ratios, providing practitioners with a more reliable and potent whole-mushroom extract. As veterinary interest rises, ensuring that research and practice are informed by high-quality materials is essential for meaningful, reproducible results.

This guide reflects that commitment. It is offered in the spirit of shared learning and continuous improvement, and with deep respect for the veterinarians, researchers and animal guardians whose work informs and strengthens this emerging field. My hope is that it ignites curiosity, encourages thoughtful practice and contributes to a future where functional fungi are recognised for their therapeutic potential across species.

> “Integrative medicine invites us to look beyond pathology and consider the animal's entire physiological landscape. *Dr Barbara Fougere, BVSc, MHSc, BHSc*”

A. TABLE OF CORE VETERINARY ACTIONS

IMPORTANT: The table below provides a concise overview of the core actions and evidence-informed veterinary applications of each functional mushroom. ***Section Two*** *offers a quick snapshot guide for rapid clinical reference.* ***Section Four*** *presents the extended evidence chapters, offering comprehensive species profiles that include taxonomy, bioactive chemistry, mechanisms of action and detailed clinical applications relevant to integrative veterinary practice.*

MUSHROOM	KEY VETERINARY ACTIONS
1 Reishi ***(Ganoderma lucidum)***	***The Calming Guardian / Mushroom of Immortality.*** Supports immune balance, stress resilience, liver detoxification and cardiovascular health. Excellent for aging, anxious, or medicated pets.
2. Turkey Tail ***(Trametes versicolor)***	***The Immune Defender.*** Enhances immune surveillance (PSK & PSP β-glucans), supports gut microbiota and complements oncology or chronic infection protocols.
3. Lion's Mane ***(Hericium erinaceus)***	***The Brain Booster*** **and Gut Warrior.** Promotes nerve growth, cognitive clarity and emotional balance. Useful for cognitive decline, anxiety and neurorehabilitation.
4. Cordyceps ***(Cordyceps militaris)***	***The Vitality Enhancer.*** Boosts energy, oxygen utilisation and recovery. Supports respiratory, adrenal and cardiovascular performance in active or senior animals.
5. Chaga ***(Inonotus obliquus)***	***The Antioxidant Shield.*** Rich in polyphenols and melanin compounds for antioxidant, liver and skin support. Ideal for detoxification and anti-inflammatory protocols.
6. Maitake ***(Grifola frondosa)***	***The Metabolic Harmoniser.*** D-fraction β-glucans promote immune balance, healthy glucose and lipid metabolism and recovery in chronic or metabolic conditions.

MUSHROOM	KEY VETERINARY ACTIONS
7. Shiitake *(Lentinula edodes)*	***The Immune Nourisher .*** Provides lentinan and eritadenine for immune, liver and cardiovascular support. Can be used as both an extract and cooked food addition for dogs.
8. Golden Oyster *(Pleurotus citrinopileatus)*	***The Longevity Mushroom.*** Natural source of ergothioneine for cellular protection, neuro-resilience and mitochondrial support. Complements Lion's Mane and Cordyceps in vitality blends

B. Functional Mushroom – Body Systems Map

Mushroom Species	Immune	Gut / Microbiome	Neurological	Metabolic / Endocrine	Oncology	Other Key Actions
Reishi (*Ganoderma lucidum*)	●	○	○	○	●	Calm / autonomic regulation
Turkey Tail (*Trametes versicolor*)	●	●	○	○	●	Microbiota–immune axis
Lion's Mane (*Hericium erinaceus*)	○	○	●	○	○	Neurotrophic / NGF pathways
Chaga (*Inonotus obliquus*)	●	○	○	○	●	Antioxidant & oxidative defence
Cordyceps (*Cordyceps militaris*)	○	○	○	●	○	Energy metabolism / oxygen utilisation

Mushroom Species	Immune	Gut / Microbiome	Neurological	Metabolic / Endocrine	Oncology	Other Key Actions
Maitake (*Grifola frondosa*)	○	○	○	●	○	Insulin signalling / metabolic stability
Shiitake (*Lentinula edodes*)	●	○	○	○	○	Cardiovascular / lipid metabolism
Golden Oyster (*Pleurotus citrinopileatus*)	○	●	○	○	○	Ergothioneine-rich antioxidant support

Notes

● **Strong evidence** - consistent preclinical + clinical + biochemical support.

○ **Supportive evidence** - moderate / adjunctive effects, species-dependent or mechanism-specific.

" **Other Key Actions"** - helps highlight clinically relevant traits without overcrowding columns.

Quality decoder:

Look for:

✓ 100 % fruiting body
✓ Full-spectrum extract
✓ Subcritical-water extraction
✓ Retained beta-glucans and prebiotic fibre

Question / avoid:

✗ Myceliated biomass / mycelium on grain
✗ Starch or fillers
✗ Isolated beta-glucans
✗ Proprietary blends (without details)

The mushroom quality pyramid

The path to potency: understanding mushroom product quality

OMG MUSHROOMS

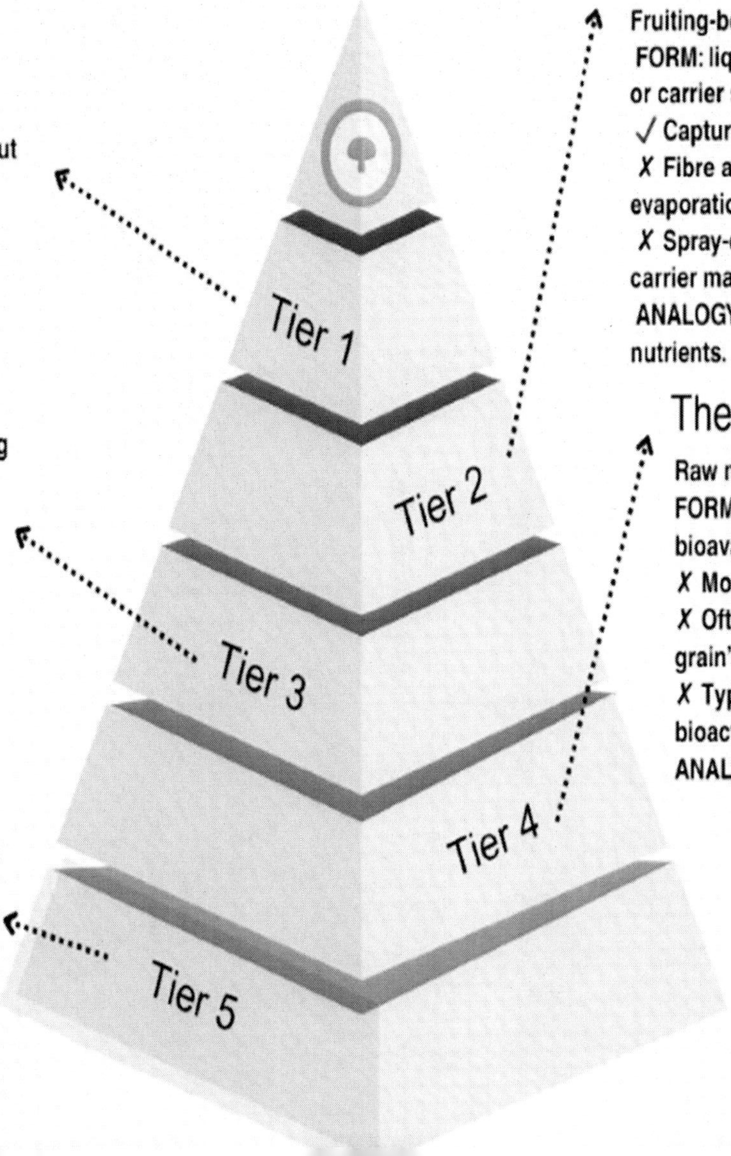

Scientifically superior (the full-spectrum gold standard)

Full-spectrum fruiting-body extraction (subcritical water – pressure and steam)

FORM: naturally concentrated extract – fine whole-food powder without carriers

✓ Employs pure water, controlled temperature and pressure for a solvent-free process that mirrors dual extraction without alcohol.

✓ Retains both water- and alcohol-soluble compounds, as well as natural prebiotic fibre and full nutritional synergy.

✓ A gentle, chemical-free technology recognised for comprehensive recovery of bioactive compounds and enhanced bioavailability.

ANALOGY: Whole-fruit smoothie v juice – everything retained, nothing wasted.

The basic extract (better, but limited)

Isolated hot-water extract (primarily beta-glucans)

FORM: liquid or spray-dried powder (often contains maltodextrin or carrier starch)

✓ Focuses mainly on immune-supporting beta-glucans.

✗ Misses the synergy of the whole mushroom and lacks alcohol-soluble compounds.

✗ Spray-dried powders typically include carriers or starch fillers.

ANALOGY: Vitamin C tablet v whole orange – one benefit, but missing the full spectrum.

The raw powder (fruiting body or mixed)

Unextracted mushroom powder (raw, ground form)

FORM: raw powder – not extracted, low bioavailability

✗ Minimal benefit as chitin blocks absorption of key compounds.

✗ Whether fruiting body or mycelium, potency remains low without extraction.

The dual extract (often marketed as 'premium')

Fruiting-body dual extraction (hot water and alcohol)

FORM: liquid extract or spray-dried powder (often contains maltodextrin or carrier starch)

✓ Captures both beta-glucans and triterpenes.

✗ Fibre and delicate compounds frequently lost during solvent evaporation or drying.

✗ Spray-dried powders often require maltodextrin, adding starch or carrier material.

ANALOGY: White bread v wholegrain bread – missing natural fibre and nutrients.

The foundation (commonly misunderstood)

Raw myceliated grain / biomass (usually unextracted)

FORM coarse powder – grain-rich biomass, not extracted, low bioavailability

✗ Mostly grain, not mushroom.

✗ Often labelled as 'myceliated biomass' or 'mycelium on grain'.

✗ Typically not extracted, so chitin remains indigestible and bioactives are poorly absorbed.

ANALOGY: Apple-flavoured porridge v real apple.

"OMG Mushrooms – pioneering Australia's subcritical-water, full-spectrum extraction."

1 Functional Mushrooms, Full-Spectrum Difference

1.1 A Scientific Foundation for a New Era in Animal Health

A new era in veterinary medicine is emerging, one that honours the irreplaceable value of conventional care, yet recognises that nutrition, microbiome health and immune modulation play far greater roles in animal wellbeing than previously understood. As companion animals live longer and their chronic health needs become more complex, veterinarians are increasingly integrating whole-food therapeutics to complement their clinical tools. Among these, functional mushrooms occupy a unique and rapidly expanding space.

These organisms are not simply culinary fungi; they are intricate biochemical systems containing molecules that interact with animal physiology on multiple levels. Their ability to influence immunity, metabolism, gut integrity, oxidative balance and neurological resilience has attracted growing international attention. Far from alternative, functional mushrooms represent a convergence of evolutionary biology, nutritional science and clinical insight–aligning closely with the terrain-based philosophy used in integrative veterinary medicine.

1.2 Nutritional and Biochemical Richness of Functional Mushrooms

Functional mushrooms are far more than therapeutic adjuncts–they are **nutrient-dense whole foods** with a biochemical profile unlike any other group of organisms. Their fruiting bodies contain a rich matrix of macronutrients, micronutrients and health-promoting bioactive compounds that act together to influence immunity, gut function, metabolism and oxidative balance. Understanding this foundation is essential for appreciating why whole-mushroom extracts, particularly SCWE preparations, are such powerful tools in veterinary Mycotherapy.

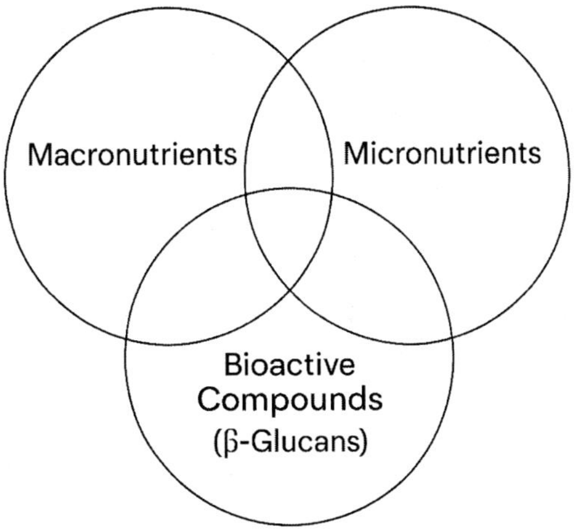

1.2.1 Macronutrients: functional carbohydrates, fibres and proteins

Whole mushrooms provide a diverse macronutrient profile that delivers far more than basic nutrition. Their carbohydrate fraction is composed of structurally complex polysaccharides, β-glucans, mannans, heteroglucans, and chitinous fibres, each contributing to gastrointestinal resilience and mucosal immunity. Unlike simple carbohydrates, these long-chain molecules reach the lower intestine intact, where they selectively nourish beneficial microbes and promote the production of short-chain fatty acids (SCFAs) such as butyrate, acetate and propionate. SCFAs are central to immune signalling, epithelial repair, metabolic homeostasis and neuro–immune communication, making the fungal fibre matrix uniquely valuable for animals with chronic inflammation, gut sensitivity or immune dysregulation.

The protein fraction of mushrooms, though modest in quantity, is rich in essential amino acids critical for cellular renewal. These amino acids support tissue repair, enzyme formation, neuromuscular balance and energy metabolism. Many species also contain bioactive peptides with antioxidant and antimicrobial functions, components that are lost or denatured when mushrooms are reduced to isolated fractions or high-heat dehydrated powders. This is one of the reasons full-spectrum SCWE extraction preserves a more physiologically active profile: it retains the natural peptide structures that contribute to immune defence and metabolic steadiness.

Collectively, these macronutrients form the structural backbone of the mushroom, creating the fibre–polysaccharide–peptide matrix responsible for many of the systemic benefits observed in veterinary practice, including improved stool quality, modulation of post-prandial inflammation, enhanced digestive resilience and stabilised energy utilisation.

1.2.2 Micronutrients: vitamins, minerals and antioxidants

The micronutrient density of mushrooms is often underestimated, yet it plays a substantial role in their therapeutic relevance. Mushrooms naturally supply B-group vitamins (B1, B2, B3, B5, B6, B7 and folate), which act as co-factors in cellular metabolism, neurotransmitter synthesis and mitochondrial energy production. These nutrients are essential for recovery, vitality and neuromuscular coordination in dogs and other companion animals. Their presence is central to metabolic steadiness and immune function .

Many species also contain ergosterol, a precursor to vitamin D2, supporting calcium balance, neuromuscular control and bone integrity, all particularly important in ageing animals, juveniles during growth, or patients with musculoskeletal stress. Mushrooms provide a spectrum of minerals including selenium, copper, phosphorus, iron, manganese and potassium. Selenium- and copper-dependent enzymes contribute to antioxidant defence, while iron and phosphorus support oxygen transport and skeletal development.

Importantly, the antioxidant capacity of whole mushrooms extends beyond vitamins and minerals. They contain a suite of phenolic compounds, glutathione, ergothioneine and other redox-modulating molecules that buffer oxidative stress, a recurring biological burden in chronic disease, immune dysfunction, metabolic syndrome and the ageing process. This natural antioxidant network acts synergistically; many of these compounds are sensitive to aggressive processing and therefore best preserved through low-temperature, solvent-free SCWE extraction.

1.2.3 Bioactive compounds: the therapeutic heart of functional mushrooms

Beyond nutrition, functional mushrooms contain a diverse array of bioactive molecules that influence physiology at multiple levels. Four principal groups are consistently recognised across Mycotherapy and veterinary research, each contributing distinct therapeutic actions. A fifth group of small-molecule antioxidants provides additional cellular protection.

i) βeta-glucans:

These well-studied polysaccharides bind to pattern-recognition receptors such as Dectin-1 and TLRs, helping regulate innate and adaptive immunity. β-glucans form the cornerstone of mushroom-mediated immune modulation across species.

Key physiological actions:

- enhance macrophage and Natural Killer cell (NK-cell) activity
- balance cytokine signalling
- support immune vigilance without overstimulation
- contribute to microbiome–immune crosstalk

ii) Terpenoids (including triterpenes and sterols):

Terpenoids are a large family of compounds with potent anti-inflammatory, hepatoprotective and antioxidant effects. Triterpenes dominate in species such as Reishi and Chaga, where they modulate inflammatory cascades and liver pathways. These properties are particularly relevant in animals with immune dysregulation, hepatic strain or chronic inflammatory conditions.

Key physiological actions:

- reduce inflammatory mediators e.g., *Nuclear factor kappa-light-chain-enhancer of activated B cells (*NF-κB*),* Cyclo-oxygenase-2 (COX-2)
- support hepatic function and detoxification
- provide antimicrobial and antioxidant effects
- help stabilise chronic inflammatory states

iii) Lectins:

Lectins are carbohydrate-binding proteins that influence cellular communication, viral recognition and immune coordination. Their ability to interface with the gastrointestinal and respiratory immune system is of growing interest in veterinary science.

Key physiological actions:

- modulate innate immune responses
- exert antiviral and antimicrobial effects
- influence gut–immune interaction
- support mucosal immunity

iv) Polysaccharides (non-β-glucan):

Beyond β-glucans, mushrooms contain heteropolysaccharides, mannans, chitin-like fibres and other structural carbohydrates that contribute to metabolic and gastrointestinal effects. These compounds underpin many of the gut-centred clinical uses of functional mushrooms in animals.

Key physiological actions:

- provide prebiotic substrate supporting beneficial microbiota
- reinforce epithelial integrity and mucosal resilience
- influence SCFA production and gut–immune signalling
- support metabolic steadiness and digestive function

v) Small-molecule antioxidants (polyphenols, ergosterol derivatives, ergothioneine):

Mushrooms contain a suite of low-molecular-weight antioxidants not captured in isolated hot-water or tincture extractions.

Key molecules include:

- polyphenols
- ergosterol derivatives
- ergothioneine, a unique, diet-derived antioxidant now recognised as a potential 'longevity vitamin'

Key physiological actions:

- protect mitochondria and cellular structures
- buffer oxidative stress
- support neurological and metabolic stability
- aid healthy ageing

Ergothioneine is naturally present in high amounts in Golden Oyster mushrooms – a notable advantage for species requiring cellular protection and metabolic resilience.

1.2.4 Why these nutrients matter more in a whole-food, full-spectrum SCWE extract

The therapeutic impact of mushrooms does not lie in isolated β-glucans or single compounds alone, but in the **entire biochemical orchestra** that includes macronutrients, micronutrients, peptides, prebiotic fibres, sterols, polyphenols and intracellular antioxidants. SCWE extraction retains this complete matrix without solvents, carriers or grain substrates, ensuring that the resulting powder behaves as a nutrient-dense whole food rather than a fractionated supplement.

This is especially important in veterinary practice, where gastrointestinal health, immune function and metabolic recovery are closely intertwined. By preserving the natural nutrient architecture, SCWE extracts support:

- **gut–immune axis stability** through the synergistic action of fibres, SCFAs and micronutrient cofactors
- **antioxidant defence** via ergothioneine, glutathione and mineral-dependent enzymes
- **metabolic steadiness** through intact B-vitamin complexes and amino acid availability
- **tissue repair and resilience** due to amino acids, peptides and bioavailable minerals
- **whole-system physiological balance**, mirroring how animals interact with fungi in nature

The addition of evidence-based micronutrient and macronutrient detail strengthens the case for whole-food mushroom extracts as functional nutritional agents – not merely carriers of β-glucans, but integrative biological systems delivering benefits through multiple pathways simultaneously.

> **Science Spotlight: Sub-critical Water Extraction (SCWE):** 'Sub-critical water' extraction uses **heat and pressure** to keep water in a liquid state above its normal boiling point (typically 120-180 °C). In this state, water's **polarity changes**, allowing it to dissolve **triterpenes, sterols, and other alcohol-soluble compounds** as effectively as ethanol - but **without losing polysaccharides or fibre.**
>
> This process produces a **full-spectrum, solvent-free extract** that mirrors dual extraction while maintaining the mushroom's natural prebiotic matrix and nutritional integrity. The Gold Standard.

1.3 Whole-Food Power for Pets and Practitioners

For pet owners, functional mushrooms provide a supplement that mirrors nature's design - powerful, pure and readily absorbed as a whole-food extract. For veterinarians, they offer a practical, evidence-aligned tool to support immune balance, recovery, healthy ageing and stress adaptation. Their value lies not in marketing language but in measurable biochemical and physiological effects.

As companion animals live longer and their health needs become more complex, preventive care has become an essential part of modern veterinary practice. Functional mushrooms bridge traditional wisdom with current scientific understanding, offering a safe, sustainable and biologically intelligent way to nurture wellbeing. Whether you are a clinician seeking reliable natural options or a devoted guardian wanting your animal to live their best life, these remarkable fungi have a meaningful role to play.

1.4 Multi System Mechanisms Relevant to Animal Health

Functional mushrooms exert their effects through a systems-biology model–multiple compounds acting across multiple pathways simultaneously. This is particularly relevant in veterinary care, where many chronic conditions do not arise from a single malfunction but from a network of metabolic, inflammatory and gastrointestinal interactions.

Modern research demonstrates that mushrooms can:

- modulate immune tone rather than simply stimulate it
- reduce oxidative and nitrosative stress
- support gastrointestinal integrity and microbiome balance
- influence glucose and lipid metabolism
- regulate inflammatory signalling at both mucosal and systemic levels
- provide neurotrophic and neuroprotective support

These cross-system effects make functional mushrooms valuable as **terrain-modulating agents,** supporting overall physiological resilience while complementing targeted veterinary interventions.

1.5 Why Whole-Food, Fruiting Body Only Extracts Matter

Not all mushroom products offer the same clinical potential. Preparations made from myceliated grain contain high levels of starch and minimal concentrations of the critical bioactive compounds found in fruiting bodies. Hot-water or alcohol extractions capture only fragments of the mushroom's full chemistry. (See also 2.1)

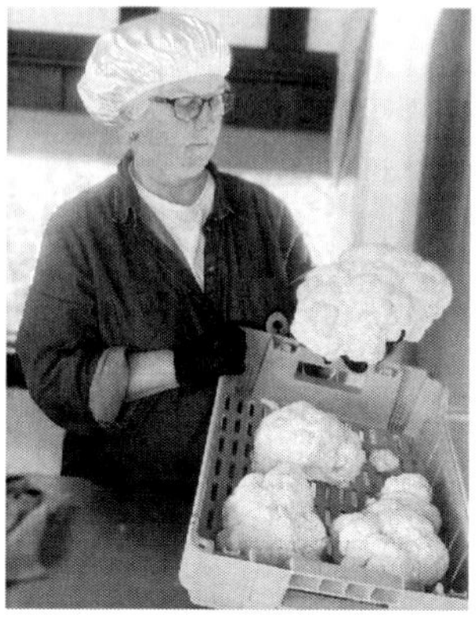

Whole-food, fruiting-body extracts preserve the complexity nature intended. When produced through SCWE, they retain:

- high-molecular-weight polysaccharides (β-glucans)
- triterpenes and sterols
- low-molecular-weight antioxidants
- peptides and nucleosides
- polyphenols
- the natural prebiotic fibre critical for gut and immune modulation

This fidelity is central to clinical reliability. Extracts that maintain the mushroom's *full-spectrum chemistry* align more closely with how these organisms have been used historically in traditional systems of medicine, while meeting the evidence expectations of modern veterinary practice.

1.6 Veterinary Aplications: An Emerging Evidence Base

Across global veterinary research, functional mushrooms are increasingly recognised for their capacity to influence multiple physiological systems relevant to animal health. Early studies in dogs, horses, livestock and laboratory species highlight effects on immune competence, gastrointestinal stability, metabolic steadiness, vaccination response, oxidative defence and recovery from physiological stress. These outcomes reflect the multi-modal nature of mushrooms, whose polysaccharides, phenolics, sterols, triterpenes and antioxidants act collectively rather than through a single mechanism.

Although the veterinary evidence base is still developing, several consistent patterns have emerged. Controlled studies, particularly those examining β-glucans, polysaccharopeptides and Pleurotus-derived compounds, demonstrate improved macrophage and dendritic-cell activity, enhanced natural-killer cell behaviour, better mucosal immunity, reduced markers of oxidative stress and favourable shifts in gut–microbiome composition. In working dogs and livestock, mushroom supplementation has been linked with improved exercise tolerance, reduced inflammatory load and steadier metabolic parameters under stress. These findings mirror decades of human and preclinical research, supporting the biological plausibility of mushrooms as adjuncts in veterinary medicine.

The growing interest in mycological therapeutics also reflects broader developments in integrative veterinary practice. As chronic, multifactorial conditions increasingly dominate companion-animal medicine, such as inflammatory disorders, metabolic dysregulation, cognitive decline, immune fragility and age-related comorbidity, there is heightened recognition of the value of interventions that modulate physiology gradually and systemically. Functional mushrooms sit naturally within this paradigm. Their actions are not rapid or symptomatic; instead, they support underlying biological networks that contribute to resilience, recovery and long-term stability.

Functional mushrooms do not inherently sit behind or beneath conventional medicine; their role depends entirely on clinical judgment, case presentation and the veterinarian's therapeutic philosophy. For some integrative practitioners, functional mushrooms are used as a first-line intervention in chronic, inflammatory or metabolic conditions where physiological modulation is preferred over symptomatic suppression. Others employ them alongside conventional treatments to support immune balance, moderate oxidative and inflammatory load, improve gastrointestinal integrity and reinforce metabolic and cellular resilience. Their flexibility across both primary and adjunctive roles reflects the breadth of mechanistic evidence underpinning Mycotherapy.

The emerging veterinary literature, supported by extensive human and translational research, establishes a credible scientific foundation for the clinical use of functional mushrooms across preventive, supportive and long-term integrative care. As quality standards, extraction methods and analytical transparency continue to advance, mushrooms are increasingly recognised as biologically coherent tools capable of influencing multiple physiological systems. Evidence continues to grow, and ongoing research suggests that functional mushrooms are poised to play an expanding role in veterinary practice, whether utilised as a foundational intervention or integrated alongside other therapeutic modalities.

> Research momentum is building, with multi-species studies confirming their value as non-pharmacological allies in long-term health strategies.

1.7 Safety, Species Considerations and Responsible Use

The functional species used in veterinary Mycotherapy - such as Reishi, Maitake, Lion's Mane, Shiitake, Turkey Tail, Chaga, Cordyceps and Golden Oyster -are well tolerated in animals when appropriately dosed. They are entirely distinct from toxic or hallucinogenic fungal species and have long histories of safe use.

Careful consideration is still warranted in:

- animals with severe hepatic or renal compromise
- individuals on anticoagulant or immunosuppressive therapy

- cases where dosing must be titrated slowly due to gastrointestinal sensitivity

This guide addresses such considerations in later chapters and provides veterinarians with dosing strategies and clinical adjustment frameworks to support safe integration.

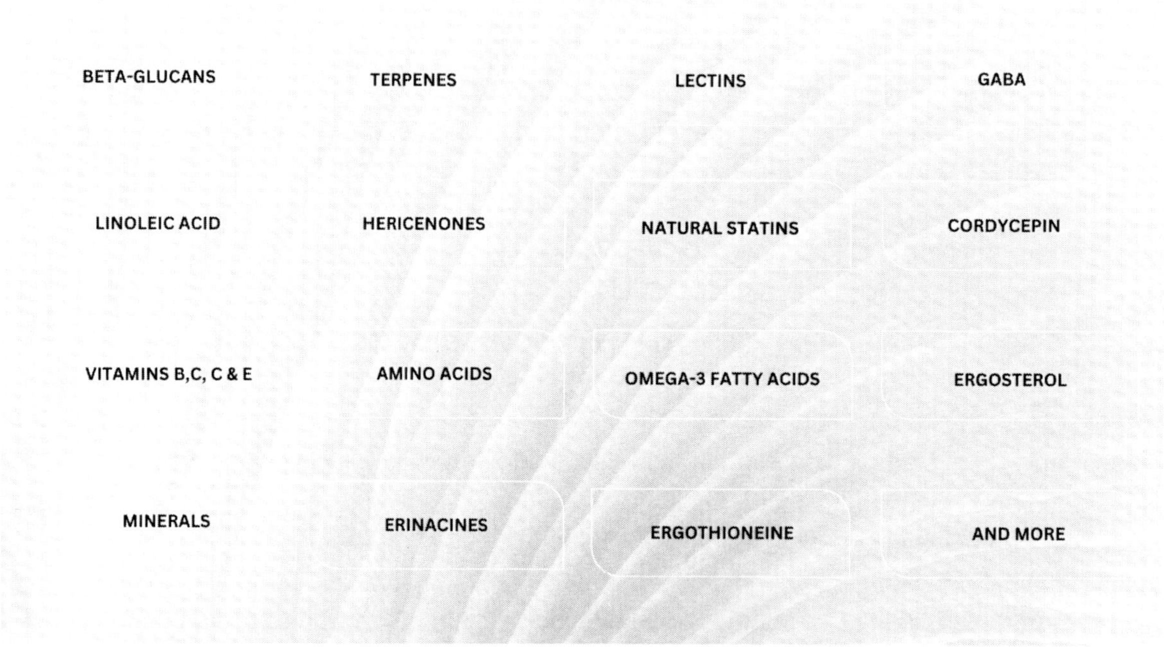

Each functional mushroom contains a naturally complex matrix of β-glucans, triterpenes, polyphenols, sterols, antioxidants, peptides and other small molecules that act on multiple physiological pathways.

1.8 Functional Mycotherapy: A Bridge Between Science, Nutrition and Integrative Care

Functional mushrooms offer a rare combination of nutritional value, biochemical complexity and therapeutic relevance. Their multi-pathway actions complement the goals of integrative veterinary medicine: supporting the whole animal, strengthening physiological resilience and promoting long-term wellbeing.

As this guide will demonstrate, each mushroom species contributes a unique profile of actions: calming, stabilising, nourishing, modulating or restoring, while maintaining a shared foundation of safety and whole-body support. Whether used for immune balance, metabolic steadiness, digestive harmony, cognitive ageing or recovery from chronic stress, functional mushrooms provide a clinically meaningful, evidence-aligned tool for modern animal care.

2 Selecting Functional Mushrooms

2.1 The Power of the Whole Mushroom

Each functional mushroom contains a naturally complex matrix of β-glucans, triterpenes, polyphenols, sterols, antioxidants, peptides and other small molecules that act on multiple physiological pathways. Increasing research demonstrates that these compounds do not work in isolation; instead, their interactions create broader and more balanced biological effects than any single constituent alone. This reflects a systems-biology model, where multiple bioactives influence immune, metabolic, neurological and antioxidant pathways simultaneously.

A key element of this synergy lies in the presence of **Biological Response Modifiers (BRMs)**. BRMs are multifunctional compounds - including β-glucans, proteoglucans, glycoproteins and triterpenes - that help modulate immune responsiveness rather than simply 'stimulating' it. Studies show that BRMs are most effective when preserved in their natural ratios, as found in full-spectrum fruiting-body preparations, where co-factors and supportive molecules enhance their stability, uptake and physiological impact. This is why reductions that focus only on isolated fractions (e.g., β-glucans alone) may not replicate the more comprehensive, regulated responses associated with the whole mushroom.

Scientific reviews consistently highlight that whole-mushroom or full-spectrum extracts demonstrate more reliable immunomodulatory, antioxidant and adaptogenic activity compared with isolated compounds. These effects are attributed to the structural complexity and natural synergy of the mushroom's biochemical network.

In Mycotherapy, this underscores a fundamental principle: the therapeutic value of medicinal mushrooms lies not in any single 'hero' molecule - and β-glucans are frequently promoted as the primary marker of quality - but in the integrity of the mushroom's full biochemical matrix. Research consistently shows that triterpenes, sterols, proteoglucans, peptides, polyphenols and other small molecules interact with β-glucans to form the Biological Response Modifiers that underpin the mushroom's broader functional effects.

2.2 Why Extraction Matters for Animal Physiology

From an integrative veterinary perspective, the extraction method used in medicinal mushroom preparations is central to their clinical usefulness. Dogs and cats have shorter gastrointestinal tracts, faster transit times and significantly lower hindgut fermentation capacity compared with humans. This means they are less able to break down the tough chitin-rich cell walls of fungi, and without proper extraction much of the mushroom's therapeutic potential simply passes through unutilised.

Animal studies consistently demonstrate that extraction increases the digestibility, bioavailability and physiological impact of mushroom compounds. Research in dogs has shown that processed or extracted mushroom materials improve digestibility and enhance the utilisation of β-glucans and other polysaccharides, supporting more efficient immune and metabolic responses *(de Godoy & Swanson, 2013; Bosch et al., 2015)*. In feline nutrition, studies confirm that extraction and processing increase the availability of fungal fibre and antioxidant compounds, promoting beneficial modulation of the gut environment and immune signalling (*Sparkes et al., 2015)*. Additional work in companion animals demonstrates that hot-water and Sub-critical-water extraction significantly improve the release of polysaccharide-protein complexes, triterpenes and other small bioactive molecules essential for biological response modification *(Vasanthi et al., 2020; Meng et al., 2016)*.

For these reasons, the role of extraction in ANIMAL MYCOTHERAPY cannot be overstated. Extraction is not simply a manufacturing step; it is a physiological necessity that allows dogs and cats to access the therapeutic potential locked within the mushroom's structural matrix.

> 'Water under pressure becomes a far more effective solvent. As temperature and pressure increase, water molecules are less tightly bound, allowing a much broader range of compounds to dissolve – including triterpenes and β-glucans. Sub-critical water extraction is therefore a clean, sustainable method for releasing the mushroom's full spectrum of active constituents.'
>
> 'After the extraction water is reduced and the solids re-dried, the resulting powder often behaves like a 2:1 whole-food concentrate, and in some cases may reach 5-10:1 equivalence depending on species.'
>
> *– Dr Christopher Hobbs Author of Medicinal Mushrooms – The Essential Guide*

At OMG Mushrooms, we use Sub-critical Water Extraction (SCWE), an advanced solvent-free technique that keeps water in a super-heated liquid phase to unlock both large and small bioactive molecules. SCWE releases β-glucans, proteoglucans, triterpenes, sterols, fibre-associated compounds and delicate antioxidants such as ergothioneine in their natural ratios. This creates a true full-spectrum extract that is significantly more accessible to the canine and feline digestive system and better aligned with the way animals absorb, utilise and respond to mushroom-based Biological Response Modifiers

2.3 Important Note on Alcohol or Solvent Extraction

Dual-extraction tinctures that rely on ethanol or other solvents are common in herbal medicine, but medicinal mushrooms have a fundamentally different biochemical profile and require a different approach. The primary immunologically active molecules in mushrooms – particularly β-glucans, proteoglucans, glycoproteins and many polysaccharide-protein complexes – are predominantly water-soluble. Alcohol alone does not efficiently extract these macromolecules and instead favours smaller, more lipophilic components such as certain terpenoids and phenolics. As a result, ethanol-based tinctures capture only a narrow fraction of the mushroom's chemistry and do not reliably deliver the full spectrum of Biological Response Modifiers that underpin mushroom-based immune modulation and adaptogenic support (Xia et al., 2022).

Modern extraction research on medicinal fungi confirms that water-based methods – including hot-water and sub-critical-water extraction – release a broader spectrum of immunologically active compounds than alcohol-dominant methods (Xia et al., 2022; Hattori et al., 2022; Meng et al., 2016). While in-vivo research in dogs and cats remains scarce, animal-model findings support the use of full-spectrum, solvent-free extraction methods in Mycotherapy.

From an animal-health perspective, solvent choice matters just as much as extract profile. Companion animals – particularly cats and small dogs – have limited capacity to metabolise ethanol and can experience mucosal irritation, gastrointestinal disturbance, dysbiosis and metabolic disruption from even modest residual alcohol. For this reason, solvent-based extracts intended for veterinary use should have any carrier solvents fully removed or, preferably, avoided altogether in favour of non-toxic, animal-appropriate extraction media.

> Sub-critical Water Extraction (SCWE) offers a clean and biologically appropriate solution for animals. By using elevated temperature and pressure to keep water in a liquid state above its normal boiling point, SCWE alters water's solvent properties and enhances its ability to solubilise both high-molecular-weight polysaccharides and smaller bioactive molecules. This allows SCWE to release β-glucans, proteoglucans, triterpenes, sterols and antioxidant compounds (including ergothioneine) without resorting to ethanol or other organic solvents and without grain-based carriers. For veterinary Mycotherapy, this results in a true full-spectrum extract that is solvent-free, physiologically appropriate for dogs and cats and aligned with the way animals absorb and respond to mushroom-derived Biological Response Modifiers.

Clinical Note for Veterinarians: Why alcohol tinctures are unsuitable for medicinal mushrooms in dogs and cats:

- Mushroom pharmacology differs from herbal pharmacology – key immune-active compounds are water-soluble and not efficiently extracted by alcohol.

- Alcohol-based tinctures do not deliver full-spectrum Biological Response Modifiers required for Mycotherapy.
- Companion animals, especially cats and small dogs, have reduced tolerance for ethanol – even trace residuals may cause mucosal irritation, gut disturbance or metabolic effects.
- Regulatory bodies including the National Animal Supplement Council (NASC), the European Medicines Agency (EMA) and the Australian Pesticides and Veterinary Medicines Authority (APVMA) all discourage the presence of solvent residues in animal supplements. As a result, best practice strongly favours solvent-free extraction methods such as sub-critical water extraction.
- Traditional and modern evidence supports water-based extraction of mushrooms – decoction, hot-water or sub-critical-water methods release the broadest compound spectrum.
- SCWE (Sub-critical Water Extraction) aligns with animal physiology – enabling release of both large polysaccharide complexes and small bioactives in a clean, solvent-free extract, appropriate for dogs and cats.

2.4 Fruiting Body vs Mycelium-On-Grain (MOG) Products

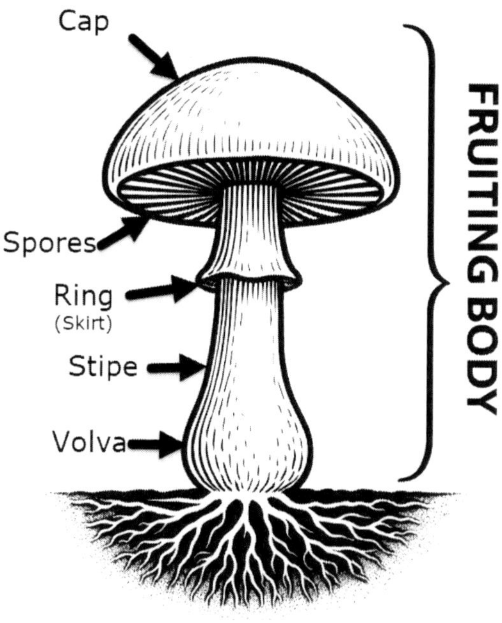

Mycelium network
(usually MOG – Mycelium on Grain)

In the veterinary nutraceutical market, particularly in Australia, there is increasing confusion about the difference between true fruiting-body extracts and mycelium on grain (MOG) products. This confusion is often exacerbated by marketing language that implies freeze-dried MOG powders are 'full spectrum' or equivalent to fruiting-body extracts (often these products have no extraction at all). Scientifically, these materials are not comparable. Mycelium grown on sterilised grain contains a high proportion of residual grain starch (alpha-glucans) and significantly lower levels of mushroom-specific beta-glucans, triterpenes, phenolic antioxidants and other bioactive compounds that underpin therapeutic value. Independent analyses consistently demonstrate that MOG can contain up to 50–70 per cent grain substrate, diluting potency - affecting the biological profile delivered to the animal.

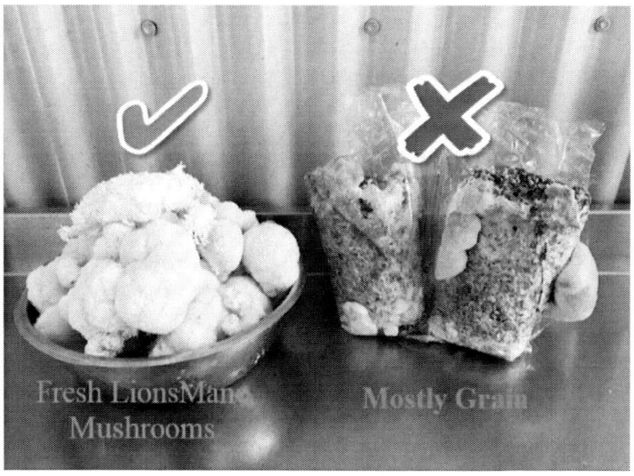

Fruiting bodies, by contrast, represent the fully developed reproductive structure of the mushroom and contain the highest concentration and diversity of bioactive compounds relevant to Mycotherapy (once extracted). Equally important is the presence of the mushroom's natural fibre matrix, which supports gut motility, microbial diversity and the production of beneficial metabolites such as short-chain fatty acids. When fruiting bodies are extracted using SCWE, this natural structure is preserved in a way that freeze-drying cannot replicate. SCWE retains heat-sensitive compounds, maintains polysaccharide complexity and protects the natural ratios present in nature.

Because many commercial products rely on mycelium grown on grain or non-extracted raw powders - approaches that are quick to produce and substantially cheaper - even correct species labelling does not ensure that an animal is receiving the full complement of functional bioactive compounds. Only whole-mushroom extraction methods, such as sub-critical water extraction (SCWE), preserve the complete biochemical profile of the fruiting body, including its natural fibre matrix. Without this integrity, the therapeutic profile becomes inconsistent and clinical outcomes far less predictable.

Given the rapid expansion of functional mushroom products in Australia, understanding this distinction is essential. The efficacy of any mushroom supplement is determined not only by species and dosage but by the integrity and traceability of the material itself. For this reason, OMG Mushrooms uses only certified organic fruiting bodies, never grain-grown mycelium, to ensure authenticity, bioactive density and reliable therapeutic outcomes. Golden Oyster is one of OMG Mushrooms' signature species, cultivated organically in Western Australia; its fruiting body is a naturally rich source of ergothioneine, a rare antioxidant now recognised as a potential longevity vitamin.

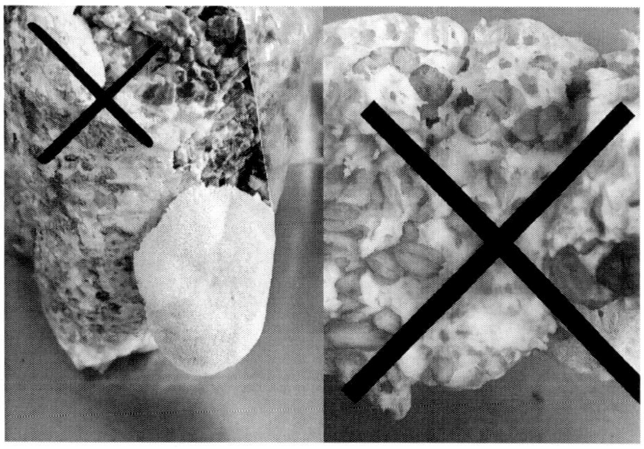

> Microscopic analysis consistently shows that mycelium-on-grain products may contain 50–70% grain starch and only modest amounts of fungal biomass, resulting in significantly reduced concentrations of β-glucans, proteoglucans and other clinically relevant compounds. *(Smith et al., 2018; Rogers, 2020)*

2.5 Why Product Authenticity Matters: Lessons from the Global Reishi Adulteration Study

Ensuring that a product truly contains the mushroom species stated on its label is essential for clinical reliability. A landmark analysis published in *Scientific Reports* (Nature Research) examined 19 commercially available supplements sold as *Ganoderma lucidum* (Reishi) in the United States *(Wu et al., 2017).* Using chromatographic and saccharide-mapping techniques, the researchers assessed whether each product contained the characteristic triterpenes and beta-glucans associated with authentic Reishi fruiting bodies.

The findings were alarming: only 5 of the 19 products (around 26 per cent) displayed chemical profiles consistent with genuine Reishi, while the majority contained starch-rich polysaccharides typical of grain substrates rather than mushroom tissue. In other words, most samples did not match the biochemical markers expected from the species advertised. The authors concluded that quality consistency within the retail mushroom supplement market is 'extremely poor', raising important questions about transparency and manufacturing practices.

Although this study analysed supplements purchased in the United States, it reflects a broader, well-documented issue highlighted by independent laboratories worldwide. Many products rely on mycelium on grain, grain fillers or misidentified species, resulting in inconsistent potency and unreliable therapeutic outcomes. For veterinarians and animal-health practitioners, this underscores the importance of selecting suppliers who can provide species authentication, substrate transparency, extraction data and full traceability from cultivation to final product. Without this, it becomes difficult to ensure that a supplement delivers the full range of compounds required for evidence-based Mycotherapy.

Quality Insight: what this means for animal practitioners

- Ingredient labels do not guarantee species authenticity or bioactive density.
- Many products marketed as mushroom supplements contain diluted MOG substrates rather than true fruiting bodies.
- The absence of mushroom-specific triterpenes and beta-glucans reduces therapeutic predictability.
- Reliable Mycotherapy requires traceable supply chains, validated extraction methods and third-party analytical testing.

- Because non-extracted powders and MOG products do not preserve the whole biochemical matrix of the mushroom, they provide incomplete and often inconsistent therapeutic profiles.
- Whole-mushroom extraction methods, such as Sub-critical water extraction, protect the natural ratios of polysaccharides, triterpenes, phenolics and fibre, ensuring a more predictable clinical outcome.

Clinical takeaway

For meaningful and reproducible outcomes in animals, choose mushroom extracts that provide:

- Genuine fruiting bodies
- Verified bioactive profiles
- Transparent cultivation and extraction data
- Absence of grain fillers or adulterants

> Quality is not a premium feature - it is the foundation of evidence-based Mycotherapy.

2.6 Understanding Extraction Integrity: Why Production Method Matters More Than Product Volume

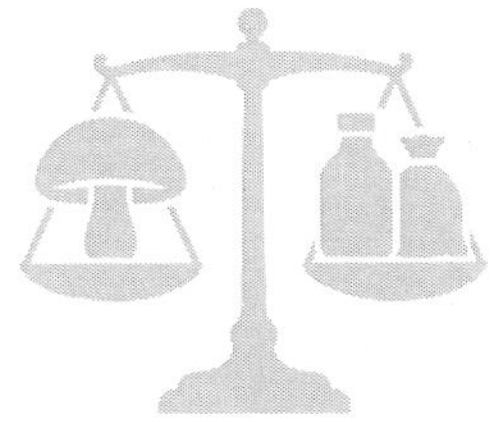

The commercial mushroom market offers a wide variety of powders, extracts and liquid formulations, yet the therapeutic value of these products differs substantially depending on the production method. While many products appear similar on the shelf, the amount of *true mushroom biomass* they contain, the integrity of their biochemical matrix and the labour required to produce them can vary dramatically. For practitioners seeking reliable, evidence-aligned functional support for animals, understanding these distinctions is essential.

Two dominant commercial forces influence the supplement landscape: **production cost** and **retail yield**. Products that generate a high number of saleable units per kilogram of starting material are often prioritised in mainstream marketing, even when they contain only small amounts of actual mushroom. In contrast, whole-food formats such as sub-critical water extracted (SCWE) powders are more labour-intensive, more resource-intensive and yield fewer retail units, yet retain the highest degree of structural and biochemical integrity. This section outlines how these differences arise and why they matter in clinical and wellness settings.

2.6.1 True mushroom content: The core determinant of quality

The most meaningful way to compare mushroom products is not by their marketing language but by their **actual mushroom content per unit**. When assessed this way, substantial differences emerge:

- **SCWE whole-food extracts** retain nearly the entire original mushroom matrix, providing the equivalent of ~100 g real mushroom material per 100 g jar. This includes β-glucans, prebiotic fibre, sterols, peptides, polyphenols and intracellular antioxidants such as ergothioneine.
- **Pure hot-water extract powders** offer concentrated fractions of water-soluble polysaccharides, but these extracts are rarely sold neat because they yield small volumes and are costly to produce.
- **Blended extract powders** often contain around 20 % extract and 80 % carrier, resulting in the equivalent of ~20 g mushroom material per 100 g jar.
- **Myceliated grain powders** consist largely of fermented grain substrate with minimal fruiting-body development. Despite often being marketed as 'mushroom powder', their true mushroom content is extremely low (often freeze dried and marketed as full spectrum).
- **Liquid tinctures** (water, glycerol or dual extracts) contain the least mushroom biomass per unit, often only 1–2 g mushroom-equivalent per 50 ml bottle.

Across all categories, SCWE whole-food extracts provide the most complete and concentrated representation of *real mushroom*. This distinction becomes particularly important in veterinary contexts where dosing accuracy and biochemical completeness are central to achieving physiological outcomes.

> The commercial mushroom market offers a wide variety of powders, extracts and liquid formulations, yet the therapeutic value of these products differs substantially depending on the production method.

2.6.2 Production integrity and labour intensity

Each extraction method carries a different level of technological complexity, resource demand and potential for modification or dilution. These differences influence the final product's integrity:

- **SCWE production** involves carefully controlled temperature–pressure environments, multi-stage extraction, re-drying and milling. It requires significant equipment, energy and hands-on oversight, but yields a 1:1 powder that preserves the mushroom's full biochemical orchestra.
- **Pure water and dual extracts** require managed decoction and solvent processing; once concentrated, they can be easily diluted into powders or liquids.
- **Extract blends** introduce opportunities to "stretch" yields using carriers such as maltodextrin, rice flour or fibre bases, increasing jar count without increasing mushroom biomass.

- **Myceliated grain** is comparatively simple and inexpensive to produce, with the majority of the biomass coming from the grain substrate rather than fungal tissue.
- **Liquid tinctures** are straightforward to produce in large volumes, with most of the final product consisting of solvents.

> The more a product can be diluted or blended, the greater its susceptibility to marketing-driven manipulation rather than integrity-driven formulation.

2.6.3 Accessing the internal bioactive compounds.

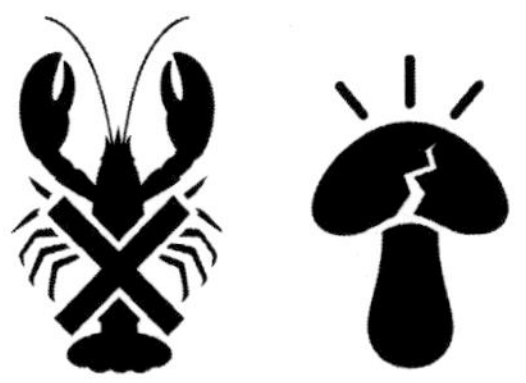

The therapeutic potential of mushrooms depends on accessing their internal bioactive compounds. Their cell walls are built from chitin – a rigid, indigestible polysaccharide similar to the exoskeleton of crustaceans. Without effective extraction, this barrier remains intact and many key constituents – β-glucans, proteoglucans, triterpenes, phenolics, peptides and intracellular antioxidants – are never fully released. Sub-critical Water Extraction (SCWE) breaks down the chitin matrix under controlled temperature and pressure, freeing the full spectrum of water- and heat-stable compounds while preserving the native fibre structure. The result is a whole-mushroom extract that more accurately reflects the natural biochemical profile and is markedly more bioavailable than unextracted powders, tinctures or myceliated-grain products.

> Chitin, the tough material that forms mushroom cell walls, is as hard to digest as a lobster shell. Without breaking it open, the bioactive compounds inside the mushroom cannot be fully accessed.

Summary

Although the supplement market often rewards high-yield, low-integrity formats, the functional and therapeutic value of a mushroom product is determined by its **true mushroom content, biochemical completeness and extraction honesty**, not by the number of jars or bottles produced per kilogram of material. SCWE whole-food extracts, while more labour-intensive and yielding fewer retail units, provide one of the highest-integrity formats available and align closely with traditional and evidence-based Mycotherapy principles.

By appreciating these distinctions, practitioners can make informed choices, optimise outcomes for animals and contribute to a more transparent and scientifically grounded use of medicinal mushrooms.

2.7 More than 'Beta-Glucans'

Functional mushrooms exert their benefits through a wide constellation of synergistic compounds, far beyond β-glucans. In veterinary Mycotherapy, retaining this full biochemical spectrum is essential, as different molecules contribute to immune modulation, metabolic steadiness, gut integrity and neurological resilience. Whole-food extraction, particularly sub-critical water extraction (SCWE), preserves this natural matrix of polysaccharides, triterpenes, phenolics, nucleosides and prebiotic fibre while avoiding the starch-heavy limitations of myceliated-grain powders. This whole-matrix integrity is fundamental to therapeutic consistency and underpins the clinical reliability of mushroom-based support across species.

Mushrooms are frequently discussed in terms of one or two dominant compounds - β-glucans, cordycepin, triterpenes, hericenones or PSK. Yet this focus captures only a fraction of the biochemical reality. Each fruiting body is a complex ecological matrix containing **hundreds of interacting molecules**: polysaccharides, triterpenes, sterols, glycoproteins, peptides, amino acids, phenolics, nucleosides, small-molecule antioxidants, vitamins and natural prebiotic fibres. These compounds evolved to work together, not in isolation.

Relying on a single marker compound to represent a functional mushroom is therefore reductive. Just as the nutritional value of an apple cannot be judged by its vitamin C content alone, the clinical potential of a mushroom cannot be inferred from β-glucan percentages or isolated actives. Whole-fruiting-body metabolomic surveys reveal extensive chemical diversity – including minor triterpenes, nucleosides, peptides and glycan structures - that collectively shape the immune, metabolic, hepatic, neurological and gut–microbiome effects observed in practice.

> Functional mushrooms are multi-compound wholefoods - not single-compound extracts.

2.7.1 Why whole-food extraction matters

Traditional hot-water or alcohol extraction can favour specific compound classes while losing others. Ethanol extracts capture triterpenes but exclude water-soluble polysaccharides; hot-water methods extract β-glucans but may degrade heat-sensitive antioxidants, nucleosides and phenolics. Myceliated-grain powders, meanwhile, introduce predominantly starch-based α-glucans with minimal secondary metabolites.

In contrast, **full-spectrum whole-food extracts** preserve the full breadth of the mushroom's chemical fingerprint:

- high-molecular-weight polysaccharides
- small, delicate antioxidants
- prebiotic fibres
- nucleosides and glycoproteins
- sterols, aromatic compounds and metabolites only present in fruiting bodies

Preserving this diversity allows the extract to behave like whole food in the body – supporting nutrient utilisation, immune patterning, gut–brain physiology and microbial balance.

2.7.2 Why Sub-critical Water Extraction (SCWE) is superior

Sub-critical Water Extraction (SCWE) is a solvent-free method that uses pressurised hot water to broaden solubility and release a much wider range of compounds than traditional extraction. Metabolomic comparisons show that SCWE:

- increases phenolic and antioxidant yield
- preserves nucleosides and other labile small molecules
- recovers polysaccharides of varied molecular weights
- retains natural prebiotic fibre
- delivers extracts closer to the mushroom's native chemical ecosystem

These outcomes have been demonstrated across multiple medicinal mushroom species, including:

- **Reishi** – co-extraction of polysaccharides and diverse ganoderic acids
- **Lion's Mane** – preservation of hericenones alongside polysaccharides and soluble fibre
- **Turkey Tail** – improved recovery of PSP/PSK complexes and phenolics
- **Cordyceps** – enhanced extraction of cordycepin and nucleoside partners
- **Maitake, Shiitake, Chaga, Golden Oyster** – recovery of sterols, phenolics, triterpenes, antioxidants and species-specific compounds such as ergothioneine in Golden Oyster

2.7.3 Why Sub-critical Water Extraction (SCWE) Matters

SCWE whole-food extracts offer advantages essential to clinical practice:

- preserve both large (β-glucans, triterpenes) and small (ergothioneine, phenolics, nucleosides) molecules
- retain natural prebiotic fibre for gut and microbiome support
- maintain synergistic compound networks rather than isolated fractions
- mimic whole-food behaviour within the body
- avoid grain-derived α-glucans and starch found in myceliated-grain powders

This full-matrix integrity is the foundation of terrain-based Mycotherapy – supporting immunity, metabolic steadiness, neurological function and gut–brain signalling in a way that single-compound extracts cannot achieve.

2.7.4 Sub-critical Water Extraction vs Conventional Extraction

Extraction Type	Compounds Captured	Nutrient Diversity	Retains Prebiotic Fibre	Biological Synergy
OMG SCWE Whole-Food Extract	50 - 400 + bioactives	✓ Broad	✓ YES	✓ FULL Matrix
Alcohol / hot-water extract	1 - 5 key actives	**X** Limited	**X** No	**X** Partial
Myceliated grain powder	Mostly α-glucans & starch	**X** Low	**X** No	**X** Minimal

> *Extracts standardised only to β-glucans or a single marker completely miss the broader chemical orchestra, which is what drives clinical effects.*

Mushroom	Minimal-extraction compounds	Approx. total known compounds
Reishi	2–3	400–500+
Chaga	2–3	200–300+
Lion's Mane	2–4	200–300+
Maitake	2–3	100–200+
Cordyceps	2–3	100–200+
Turkey Tail	2–3	100–200+
Shiitake	2–3	100–150+
Golden Oyster	3–4	150–250+

Mushrooms contain far more than the handful of compounds commonly referenced on supplement labels. While minimal extraction may highlight two or three marker compounds, modern metabolomic studies show that most medicinal species contain **200–500+ distinct bioactive molecules**, including β-glucans, polysaccharide–protein complexes, triterpenes, sterols, phenolics, glycoproteins, nucleosides, peptides and intracellular antioxidants such as ergothioneine. These compounds do not act in isolation; they exert their effects synergistically, creating the complex biochemical interactions that underpin Mycotherapy.

Because these constituents are embedded within a chitin–glucan matrix, **only whole-mushroom extraction methods that fully open the cell wall - such as Sub-critical Water Extraction - can access the full biochemical spectrum.** This complexity helps explain why fruiting-body, SCWE-based extracts consistently outperform simplified or fractionated preparations in practice.

3. A Note on Chinese-Sourced Fruiting Bodies: What Veterinarians Should Know

3.1 Sourcing fruiting bodies – Evidence, provenance and common misconceptions

As functional mushrooms become more widely used in veterinary practice, questions often arise regarding the origin of medicinal mushroom raw materials—particularly those sourced from China. These concerns are understandable, yet they often stem from misunderstandings about modern cultivation standards, global supply-chain realities and the biological requirements necessary to grow authentic, fruiting-body mushrooms at scale.

3.2 China as the global centre of mushroom expertise

China is the birthplace of mushroom cultivation, with documented practice extending back nearly a thousand years. More than **90 % of the world's mushrooms** - including almost all functional species used in research - are grown there under **di dao** principles, which emphasise growing mushrooms in their **correct ecological origin** using native trees, substrates and microbiomes. This ecological authenticity directly influences the mushroom's biochemical profile, including β-glucan structure, phenolics, triterpenes and ergothioneine.

This is why globally recognised professional brands, including **Real Mushrooms in Canada**, whose veterinary advisory board includes **Dr Rob Silver** - source their raw fruiting-body materials from China before applying their own extraction and standardisation processes.

3.3 Irradiation myths and Australian import realities

A persistent misconception is that *all* mushroom material imported into Australia is gamma-irradiated. <u>This is incorrect.</u>

- Certified organic mushroom material **cannot be irradiated under Australian organic standards.**
- Companies importing for **human or veterinary use** are able to use **non-irradiation pathways** provided they follow strict biosecurity protocols and supply documentation verifying cultivation, processing and pest-free status.
- OMG Mushrooms uses **no irradiation** at any stage.

- All extraction is performed in Australia using **sub-critical water extraction (SCWE)** under controlled conditions, preserving native fibre and full-spectrum bioactive compounds.

3.4 Fruiting body vs. myceliated grain – the real quality divide

From a biochemical and therapeutic standpoint, the far more important distinction is not geographic origin, but **fruiting body vs mycelium-on-grain (MOG)**.

Some Australian-grown 'medicinal mushrooms' are in fact **myceliated-grain products**, where the majority of biomass is non-fungal starch. Independent analyses show myceliated grain may contain:

- **50–70 % grain starch**,
- **very low β-glucans**,
- **minimal triterpenes, phenolics or secondary metabolites**,
- and no true fruiting-body architecture.

When vets compare Australian-grown MOG to Chinese-grown fruiting bodies, they are comparing two entirely different categories of material - not two versions of the same thing.

4. Quality assurance, verification and traceability

Because veterinarians require transparency, OMG Mushrooms undertook an **18-month verification process** before partnering with its producer, including:

- multi-stage certification checks (USDA Organic, EU Organic, JAS, China Organic)
- FSSC 22000 and HACCP audit reviews
- independent pesticide, heavy-metal and microbial testing
- documentation of cultivation substrates (native timbers, organic grains)
- confirmation of non-irradiation pathways
- regular batch-level Certificates of Analysis
- Australian re-testing upon arrival

Every batch is tested **twice**—once before export and again on arrival in Australia—for fungal purity, β-glucans, ergosterol, alpha-glucans (to detect adulteration), microbial safety and secondary metabolites relevant to veterinary use.

This dual testing at source and destination provides traceability unmatched by most domestic producers.

4.1 Why this matters to veterinary practice

For clinicians selecting functional mushrooms, origin is less important than:

- Was the product grown from **whole fruiting bodies**?
- Does the material contain the **full biochemical matrix** relevant to Mycotherapy?
- Is the extract **non-irradiated and solvent-free**?
- Are **β-glucan, ergosterol and secondary metabolites** verified?
- Is extraction performed using a **method that preserves fibre and intracellular antioxidants** (e.g., SCWE)?
- Is documentation **transparent, batch-specific and accessible**?

When these criteria are met, Chinese-sourced fruiting bodies represent some of the **highest-quality medicinal mushrooms available worldwide** - which is why many of the world's leading functional-mushroom companies, research groups, and integrative veterinary practitioners rely upon them

5. Comparison of Common Mushroom Material Types in Veterinary Mycotherapy

Criteria	Australian Myceliated Grain (MOG)	Australian Small-Scale Fruiting Body Cultivation	Chinese Di Dao Fruiting Body Cultivation (Native-Origin)
Primary biomass	Mycelium + grain substrate (often 50–70 % grain starch)	True fruiting body	True fruiting body grown on native timbers / forest substrates
β-glucan content	Low (diluted by grain-derived α-glucans)	Moderate–high depending on species	High; aligns with global research-standard fruiting-body levels
Secondary metabolites (triterpenes, phenolics, ERGO, etc.)	Minimal; not expressed without fruiting	Present but variable due to scale, substrate and strain access	Robust and species-typical; reflects centuries of strain development and di dao practices
Alignment with published research	Weak – most studies use fruiting bodies, not MOG	Strong when fruiting bodies are used	Strongest match to global pharmacological and veterinary research literature

Criteria	Australian Myceliated Grain (MOG)	Australian Small-Scale Fruiting Body Cultivation	Chinese Di Dao Fruiting Body Cultivation (Native-Origin)
Typical cultivation substrates	Grain (rice, oats, sorghum)	Sawdust, straw, supplemented mixes	Native logs, hardwoods, forest substrates, species-specific media
Expression of full metabolomic profile	Very limited	Partial to full depending on strain and substrate	Full-spectrum biochemical expression characteristic of research-grade mushrooms
Extraction suitability	Poor – high starch load, low fungal density	Suitable	Excellent; optimised for high-yield SCWE and hot-water extraction
Testing & standardisation	Variable; often limited beyond microbial checks	Good but inconsistent between growers	Extensive: organic certification, heavy metals, pesticides, β-glucans, ERGO, speciation confirmation (HPTLC/DNA/NMR)
Irradiation risk	Low but varies by producer	Low	Zero when imported through non-irradiation biosecurity pathways (required for organic certification)
Scalability for supplement-grade material	High volume, low potency	Limited, inconsistent	High volume, high potency; aligns with global nutraceutical supply
Clinical relevance in Mycotherapy	Low	Moderate–high	High; matches research-validated profiles used in human and veterinary studies
Representative products	MOG powders marketed as "extracts" or "mushroom powders"	Gourmet + some medicinal	Research-grade fruiting-body extracts used by leading global brands

Veterinarians evaluating functional mushroom products should prioritise biological authenticity and biochemical density, not geographic origin alone. Fruiting bodies - whether grown in Australia or in their native Chinese mountain regions - offer the metabolic completeness, β-glucan structure and secondary metabolite profile that align with the Mycotherapy evidence base. In contrast, myceliated-grain material represents a biologically different product, with significantly reduced relevance to published research and markedly lower concentrations of key therapeutic compounds.

SECTION TWO

1

Mycotherapy Full Spectrum Extract Products

1.1 Why Choose 'Full Spectrum' Extracts?

The therapeutic value of a functional mushroom extract is determined not simply by the species selected but by the integrity of its chemistry, the extraction method and the absence of unnecessary carriers. OMG Mushrooms employs sub-critical water extraction (SCWE) to produce whole-food fruiting-body extracts that retain the mushroom's full biochemical matrix with exceptional fidelity. SCWE uses heat and pressure to expand the solvent capacity of water, enabling the release of both high - and low-molecular weight compounds including: β-glucans, triterpenes, sterols, polyphenols, peptides, nucleosides and ergothioneine, without reliance on alcohol, chemical solvents or grain-based substrates. This approach mirrors the principles of Mycotherapy by preserving the synergy, balance and complexity of the natural organism rather than reducing it to isolated fractions.

Only certified organic fruiting bodies are used, ensuring that no starch, grain, myceliated filler or undeclared excipients appear in the final product. The extracts behave as true whole-food concentrates: rich in polysaccharides, triterpenoids and small-molecule antioxidants, but also retaining the prebiotic fibres and structural components that support gastrointestinal modulation, immune steadiness and metabolic resilience in animals. Rigorous batch-level testing, transparent sourcing and quality assurance support clinical confidence in dosing, tolerance and reproducibility.

OMG Mushrooms' formulations are developed in consultation with integrative veterinarians and informed by global research trends in immunology, neurobiology, metabolism and gut–immune interactions. This results in practitioner-ready extracts and blends that are tailored for real-world challenges in veterinary practice, while maintaining the highest standards of purity, potency and ethical production. For clinicians seeking a full-spectrum extract that aligns with both scientific evidence and the foundational principles of Mycotherapy, OMG Mushrooms provides a clinically robust and trustworthy solution.

* * *

1.1.1 Key attributes at a glance

• Sub-critical water extraction (SCWE).

A solvent-free, grain-free method using heat and pressure to release both large and small molecules. SCWE preserves thermolabile antioxidants such as ergothioneine and yields a high-potency whole-food extract without alcohol or chemical solvents.

• Certified organic fruiting bodies only.

No mycelium, no grain, no starch and no fillers. This avoids alpha-glucan dilution, protects phytochemical diversity and prevents metabolic destabilisation in sensitive or insulin-dysregulated animals.

• Full-spectrum chemistry preserved.

SCWE extracts retain the mushroom's complete profile – polysaccharides, triterpenes, sterols, polyphenols, peptides, nucleosides, cordycepin, ergothioneine and natural prebiotic fibre – supporting multi-system modulation.

• Clinically informed formulations.

Created in collaboration with integrative veterinarians and aligned with evidence paths relevant to oncology, immune modulation, gut–brain axis dynamics, metabolic stability and healthy ageing.

• Practitioner-ready blends.

Synergistic combinations designed for real-world clinical presentations, allowing veterinarians to pair species with complementary actions and avoid under-dosed or incomplete products.

• Transparent, ethical and rigorously tested.

Certified organic supply chains, independent third-party testing, and Australian-owned production ensure purity, potency, safety and reproducibility – core requirements for reliable veterinary Mycotherapy.

* * *

2. Mycotherapy Options for Integrative Veterinary Practice

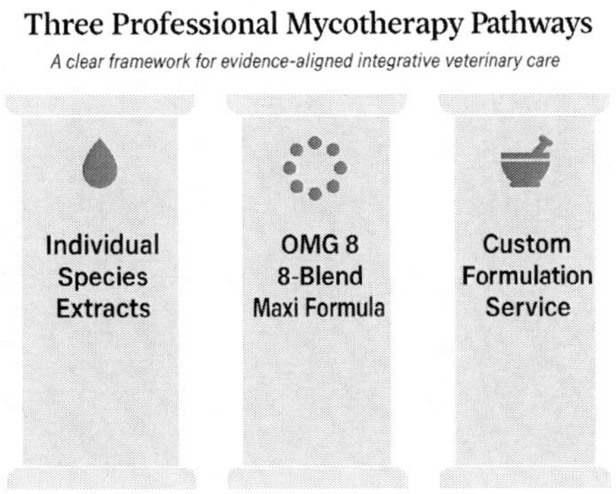

Modern integrative veterinary care benefits greatly from evidence-aligned full-spectrum mushroom extracts that can be tailored to both species and clinical presentation. OMG Mushrooms partners with veterinarians to provide high-quality formulations that respect the principles of Mycotherapy, maintain the integrity of the whole mushroom, and deliver consistent therapeutic outcomes in practice. To support different therapeutic goals, dosing preferences and case complexities, three professional pathways are offered:

1• Individual mushroom species

Single full-spectrum extracts (Reishi, Lion's Mane, Turkey Tail, Chaga, Maitake, Shiitake, Cordyceps and Golden Oyster) for targeted protocols or for integrating into existing care plans.

2• The OMG 8-blend maxi formula

A broad-spectrum professional formula combining the eight functional species most widely used in clinical practice. Golden Oyster provides an ergothioneine-rich cornerstone for cellular protection, antioxidation and healthy ageing.

3• Custom formulation service

Collaborative development of bespoke blends tailored to the patient's presentation: immune modulation, neurological support, stress resilience, recovery following chronic disease, hepatic support, gastrointestinal regulation or metabolic balance.

This tiered flexibility enables veterinarians to design protocols that are both species-appropriate and therapeutically precise.

2.1 Clinical value and efficacy

While high-quality full-spectrum extracts may appear more costly than raw powders or mycelium-on-grain products, practitioners consistently find that their **concentration, purity and bioavailability** yield superior clinical reliability.

Fruiting-body extracts contain significantly higher levels of β-glucans, triterpenes and other small bioactive molecules compared with myceliated grain substrates, which may contain 50–70 per cent non-fungal starch *(Smith et al., 2018; Rogers, 2020).* The natural structural fibre of fruiting bodies also supports slower gastric transit, improved tolerability and prebiotic activity influencing the gut–immune axis.

Extraction further elevates efficacy. Sub-critical Water Extraction (SCWE) enhances the availability of polysaccharides, proteoglucans, phenolics and antioxidants, allowing therapeutic response at lower dosing volumes than raw or freeze-dried powders. For veterinarians, this translates to:

- greater predictability
- improved patient compliance
- lower required doses
- more consistent response patterns
- reduced formulation variability

Full-spectrum extracts therefore offer superior overall value and higher clinical confidence, especially in complex cases.

Why settle for a fraction when nature offers the whole?

2.2 Custom blends for clinical practice

Because every animal presents uniquely, OMG Mushrooms offers a professional formulation service designed to help integrative veterinarians optimise outcomes.

We provide:

A • Bespoke formulations

Targeted combinations of functional mushrooms chosen to support specific therapeutic outcomes such as immune modulation, cognitive support, gastrointestinal balance, stress resilience, hepatic detoxification or metabolic stability.

B • Collaborative case design

Veterinarians can liaise directly with the OMG Mushrooms team to align mushroom profiles with clinical goals, creating reliable adjuncts to multimodal treatment plans.

C • Full-spectrum quality assurance

All extracts are produced using SCWE to ensure purity, potency, structural integrity and consistency across batches. For broad-spectrum support, many practitioners choose the **OMG 8-Blend Maxi Formula**, featuring Reishi, Lion's Mane, Cordyceps, Turkey Tail, Maitake, Shiitake, Chaga and Golden Oyster – the latter providing naturally occurring ergothioneine for cellular protection and healthy ageing.

> “Nutrition is not an adjunct to veterinary care; it is its foundation. *Dr Susan Wynn, DVM, DACVIM (Nutrition)*”

2

Unified Dosing Guidance

2. Unified Dosing Guidance for Veterinary Mycotherapy

Functional mushrooms exert their therapeutic influence through a broad constellation of synergistic compounds – β-glucans, triterpenes, phenolics, flavonoids, nucleosides, peptides, sterols and natural prebiotic fibres. Sub-critical water extraction (SCWE) captures this full biochemical matrix by using heat and pressure to expand water's solvating capacity and release both large and small molecules. The extract is then concentrated through water reduction and re-drying, yielding a whole-food concentrate free from carriers or grain-derived starches.

Because SCWE extracts retain the mushroom's natural complexity and are often equivalent to **2:1** and, in some species, up to **5–10:1** concentration, dosing is expressed as **mg/kg of finished SCWE extract powder** using a standardised tier model across all species.

2.1. Tier-Based Dosing Model (SCWE Full-Spectrum Extracts)

These dosing tiers apply universally to all mushroom species within this guide.

Tier 1 – Wellness / Maintenance (10–30 mg/kg/day)

- general wellness, mild immune support
- early inflammatory changes
- senior animals
- preventative support across life stages

Tier 2 – Moderate / Supportive (30–60 mg/kg/day)

- chronic inflammatory conditions
- microbiome or gastrointestinal modulation
- recovery from illness
- metabolic or stress-related dysregulation
- early cognitive decline

Tier 3 – Intensive / Adjunctive (60–100 mg/kg/day)

- oncology support
- chronic immune dysregulation
- refractory inflammatory conditions
- neurodegeneration

(Tier 3 ideally under integrative veterinary supervision.)

Titration guidance: Begin at the lower end of the chosen tier and increase gradually over 5–7 days. Sensitive or medically compromised animals may require slower dose titration.

2.2 How to calculate mg/kg → grams → teaspoon dosing

Mushroom dosing in this guide is expressed as milligrams of extract per kilogram of bodyweight per day (mg/kg/day). This ensures accurate, weight-adjusted dosing across all breeds and species.

To calculate the correct dose *(and convert to teaspoons if required)*:

- **Step 1** - Identify the animal's weight (in kilograms).
- **Step 2** - Select the dosing tier (e.g., Tier 1 = 10–30 mg/kg/day).
- **Step 3** - Multiply weight × mg/kg to obtain the total daily mg.
- **Step 4** - Convert mg → grams → teaspoons using the OMG Mushrooms standard:
    - **¼ teaspoon = 0.5 g (500 mg)**
    - **½ teaspoon = 1 g (1,000 mg)**
    - **1 teaspoon = 2 g (2,000 mg)**

This unified dosing system ensures clinical precision for veterinarians and practical simplicity for owners.

The final calculation provides the **total daily amount of extract**, which may be divided into one or two doses depending on the clinical goal.

> *To calculate the correct dose, multiply bodyweight (kg) by the target mg/kg range. For example, a typical 21 kg dog receiving Tier 1 support would require 210–630 mg per day. Begin at the lower end and titrate gradually over 5–7 days.*

Example – Tier 1 Dosing Using an Average 21 kg Dog

Low end:
21 kg × 10 mg/kg = 210 mg/day
≈ 0.21 g/day
≈ ⅛–¼ teaspoon
Mid-range:
21 kg × 20 mg/kg = 420 mg/day
≈ 0.42 g/day
≈ just under ½ teaspoon
Upper end:
21 kg × 30 mg/kg = 630 mg/day
≈ 0.63 g/day
≈ ½ teaspoon

Summary: A typical 21 kg dog in Tier 1 requires 210–630 mg per day, which equates to approximately ¼–½ teaspoon per day of SCWE full-spectrum extract.

2.3. Dogs – Unified Weight-Based Table (SCWE Extracts)

For SCWE full-spectrum fruiting-body extracts only

Standard OMG Mushroom Conversion:

- **¼ tsp = 0.5 g**
- **½ tsp = 1 g**
- **1 tsp = 2 g**

Tier-to-Teaspoon Approximation (per 10 kg bodyweight):

- Tier 1 (10–30 mg/kg) → 0.10–0.30 g → ⅛–¼ tsp per 10 kg
- Tier 2 (30–60 mg/kg) → 0.30–0.60 g → ¼–½ tsp per 10 kg
- Tier 3 (60–100 mg/kg) → 0.60–1.00 g → ½–1 tsp per 10 kg

These approximations scale smoothly across all dog sizes.

* * *

Size category	Approx. weight	Tier 1 (mg/kg → g → tsp)	Tier 2 (mg/kg → g → tsp)	Tier 3 (mg/kg → g → tsp)
Toy	1–5 kg	10–30 mg/kg 0.01–0.15 g *pinch–⅛ tsp*	30–60 mg/kg 0.03–0.30 g *pinch–¼ tsp*	60–100 mg/kg 0.06–0.50 g *⅛–½ tsp*
Small	5–10 kg	10–30 mg/kg 0.05–0.30 g *⅛–¼ tsp*	30–60 mg/kg 0.15–0.60 g *¼–½ tsp*	60–100 mg/kg 0.30–1.00 g *½–1 tsp*
Medium	10–25 kg	10–30 mg/kg 0.10–0.75 g *⅛–½ tsp*	30–60 mg/kg 0.30–1.50 g *¼–1 tsp*	60–100 mg/kg 0.60–2.50 g *½–1¼ tsp*
Large	25–40 kg	10–30 mg/kg 0.25–1.20 g *¼–¾ tsp*	30–60 mg/kg 0.75–2.40 g *¾–1¼ tsp*	60–100 mg/kg 1.50–4.00 g *¾–2 tsp*
Giant	>40 kg	10–30 mg/kg 0.40–1.50 g *½–1 tsp*	30–60 mg/kg 1.20–3.00 g *1–1½ tsp*	60–100 mg/kg 2.40–5.00 g *1¼–2½ tsp*

Larger dogs may require proportionally lower mg/kg at higher body weights, yet unified tiers maintain clinical clarity and remain safe.

2.4. Cats – Adjusted Tier Ranges (SCWE Extracts)

Cats metabolise mushroom polysaccharides effectively but have heightened taste sensitivity, shorter gastrointestinal transit, and lower tolerance for alcohol-based extracts – making SCWE an ideal solvent-free method.

Species	Tier 1 (mg/kg → g → tsp)	Tier 2 (mg/kg → g → tsp)	Tier 3* (mg/kg → g → tsp)
Adult cat (4–5 kg)	**8–25 mg/kg** **0.03–0.12 g** ***pinch–⅛ tsp***	**25–50 mg/kg** **0.10–0.25 g** ***⅛ tsp***	**60–80 mg/kg** **0.25–0.35 g** ***⅛–¼ tsp***
Senior cat (4–5 kg)	**5–20 mg/kg** **0.02–0.10 g** ***pinch–⅛ tsp***	**20–40 mg/kg** **0.08–0.20 g** ***pinch–⅛ tsp***	**50–70 mg/kg** **0.20–0.30 g** ***⅛–¼ tsp***

*Keep cats in the lower half of Tier 3 unless oncology-directed and supervised.

Practical guidance:

- Introduce over 5–7 days
- Divide Tier 3 doses into two daily feeds
- Mix with wet food for improved acceptance

2.5 Equine Dosing Framework (SCWE Extracts)

Horses metabolise polysaccharides well, but their hindgut fermentation, metabolic variability (EMS/PPID), and laminitis sensitivity require a separate dosing model.

Daily SCWE Extract Dosing – 500 kg Standard Horse

Tier	Clinical context	Total daily dose (SCWE)
Tier 1	Wellness, maintenance, early inflammatory support	**2–4 g/day**
Tier 2	Metabolic regulation, immune modulation, recovery	**4–7 g/day**
Tier 3*	Intensive, oncology, chronic immune dysregulation*	**7–10 g/day**

**Tier 3 ideally under veterinary supervision.*

Equine dosing notes:

- Divide into 1–2 feeds
- Titrate over 5–7 days
- Prioritise fruiting-body-only extracts
- Avoid myceliated grain in all EMS, PPID or laminitic horses (*For laminitis-specific guidance, refer to the dedicated laminitis chapter and use this dosing table for quantities.)*

2.6. Clinical Workflow for Integrative Veterinarians

Step 1 – Determine the therapeutic objective

1. Immune support – Turkey Tail, Reishi, Maitake
2. Oncology adjunct – Turkey Tail, Reishi, Chaga, Maitake

3. Neurological support – Lion's Mane, Reishi
4. Stress/adrenal regulation – Reishi, Chaga
5. Gastrointestinal and microbiome modulation – Turkey Tail, Shiitake, Lion's Mane
6. Metabolic/energy support – Cordyceps, Maitake
7. Healthy ageing and vitality – Golden Oyster, Reishi, Chaga

Step 2 – Select the appropriate dosing tier

Use Tier 1, 2 or 3 according to clinical presentation.

Step 3 – Start low, titrate gradually

- Begin at 10–20 % of the intended dose
- Increase over 5–7 days
- Observe stool, appetite, sleep, behaviour

Step 4 – Combine mushrooms strategically (see section 4 for assistance)

- Immune + oncology: Turkey Tail + Reishi (+ Chaga)
- Gut + immune: Turkey Tail + Lion's Mane
- Neurological: Lion's Mane + Reishi
- Stress/adrenal: Reishi + Chaga
- Vitality/ageing: Golden Oyster + Cordyceps + Reishi

Limit to 2–3 mushrooms concurrently unless under veterinary oversight.

Step 5 – Assess clinical response (4–6 weeks)

Universal indicators:

- inflammation patterns
- stool quality
- appetite and energy
- sleep/behaviour
- coat/skin condition

Case-specific markers include:

- oncology: comfort, appetite, treatment tolerance

- cognitive: orientation, engagement, sleep–wake cycles
- hepatic: ALT/ALP trends
- gastrointestinal: stool consistency, vomiting, dysbiosis
- stress/anxiety: reactivity, settling behaviours
- senior care: mobility, stamina, interaction

Adjust dose, tier or pairing accordingly.

2.7. Clinical Adjustment Matrix

Functional mushrooms are broadly well tolerated across species, yet certain clinical presentations require thoughtful adjustment of dose, titration speed and species selection. The following guidance is not a comprehensive disease manual but a practical framework highlighting situations in which Mycotherapy may need to be moderated, tailored or introduced more gradually than standard recommendations. These principles support safe and effective integration alongside conventional veterinary care. Functional mushrooms should be viewed as adjunctive tools within a multimodal plan - not as replacements for established medical management - and dosing should always reflect the individual animal's physiology, history and ongoing clinical assessment.

Gastrointestinal sensitivity

- Start at ½ of the low end of Tier 1
- Titrate over 7–10 days
- Prioritise Lion's Mane, Turkey Tail, Shiitake
- Use Chaga cautiously at high tiers

Hepatic disease

- Favour Reishi, Chaga, Shiitake
- Avoid high Chaga in oxalate-sensitive animals
- Begin in low Tier 1
- Monitor ALT/ALP values

Renal disease

- Avoid high-tier Chaga
- Prefer Lion's Mane, Turkey Tail, Reishi
- Remain within Tier 1

Anxiety / behavioural stress

- Reishi primary agent
- Add Chaga if needed
- Tier 1–2
- Evening dosing may optimise calmness

Geriatric animals

- Begin at 5–10 mg/kg
- Titrate slowly
- Prioritise Lion's Mane, Golden Oyster, Reishi
- Maintain hydration and nutritional stability

Oncology (adjunctive)

- Core pairing: Turkey Tail + Reishi
- Add Chaga or Maitake if indicated
- Use Tier 2–3
- Monitor appetite, stool quality and vitality

> To heal the animal, we must consider the whole of its life, not merely the condition before us. *Dr Richard Pitcairn, DVM, PhD*

3. Functional Mushroom Prescribing Checklist

Clinical Workflow for Integrative Veterinarians (SCWE Full-Spectrum Extracts)

1. Patient Overview

Checklist Item	*Tick*	*Notes*
Medically stable for adjunctive support	*[ ]*	
Primary diagnosis confirmed	*[ ]*	
Medications documented	*[ ]*	
Baseline bloods / imaging available	*[ ]*	
Other____________________	*[ ]*	

2. Terrain Assessment (tick all that apply)

Physiological Domain	*Tick*	*Notes*
Chronic inflammation	*[ ]*	
Immune dysregulation / depletion	*[ ]*	
GI sensitivity / dysbiosis	*[ ]*	
Oxidative load / ageing	*[ ]*	
Neurological or behavioural strain	*[ ]*	
Hepatic or metabolic burden	*[ ]*	
Cardiovascular / respiratory stress	*[ ]*	
Post-surgical or post-illness recovery	*[ ]*	
Other ____________________	*[ ]*	

3. Contraindications & Caution Flags

Item	*Tick*	*Notes*
Autoimmune disease	*[ ]*	
Immunosuppressive medication	*[ ]*	
Chemotherapy underway	*[ ]*	
Bleeding disorders / peri-surgical	*[ ]*	
Severe hepatic compromise	*[ ]*	
Renal compromise	*[ ]*	
Known mushroom allergy	*[ ]*	
Other ____________________	*[ ]*	

4. Primary Therapeutic Targets (tick to guide selection)

Target Domain	*Tick*
Immune support	*[ ]*
Neurotrophic / cognitive	*[ ]*
Oxidative resilience	*[ ]*
Gut–immune axis	*[ ]*
Metabolic modulation	*[ ]*
Stress adaptation	*[ ]*
Performance / vitality	*[ ]*
Other ____________	*[ ]*

5. Mushroom Strategy

Strategy Type	*Tick*	*Selection Options*
Single Species	*[ ]*	*Reishi [ ] Turkey Tail [ ] Lion's Mane [ ] Chaga [ ]* *Maitake [ ] Shiitake [ ] Cordyceps [ ] Golden Oyster [ ]*
Synergistic Blend	*[ ]*	*Reishi [ ] Turkey Tail [ ] Lion's Mane [ ] Chaga [ ]* *Maitake [ ] Shiitake [ ] Cordyceps [ ] Golden Oyster [ ]*
Broad-Spectrum	*[ ]*	*OMG 8-Blend Maxi Formula*

6. Dose Selection (SCWE Extract Only – tick tier)

Tier	*Dose Range*	*Indication*	*Tick*
Tier 1	*10–30 mg/kg/day*	*Wellness / general support*	*[ ]*
Tier 2	*30–60 mg/kg/day*	*Moderate or chronic conditions*	*[ ]*
Tier 3	*60–100 mg/kg/day*	*Intensive support / oncology (supervision)*	*[ ]*

7. Prescribing Summary

Item	*Notes*
Selected mushroom(s)	
Rationale (based on domains)	
Dose and Tier	
Administration instructions	
Monitoring plan	
Other ________________	

8. Review & Follow-Up

Follow-Up Item	*Notes*
Reassess in 7–14 days	
Adjust dose or combination	
Review bloods / markers if applicable	
Document clinical response	
Schedule next review	
Other ______________	

SECTION THREE

Condensed guide to Functional Mushrooms

FUNCTIONAL MUSHROOMS IN INTEGRATIVE VETERINARY PRACTICE

Functional mushrooms represent one of the most promising frontiers in integrative veterinary care – bridging traditional Mycotherapy with modern clinical insight. Each species offers a distinct matrix of bioactive compounds that can influence immune balance, digestive integrity, neurological function and systemic resilience. For practitioners seeking to broaden their therapeutic toolkit beyond conventional pharmacology, these evidence-supported fungi provide opportunities for targeted nutritional and physiological support in both acute and chronic presentations.

The following profiles summarise eight well-researched medicinal mushrooms used in veterinary Mycotherapy, highlighting their fruiting-body constituents, key mechanisms of action and practical considerations for clinical use. This section offers a concise, accessible overview intended to support quick decision-making in practice and to serve as a reliable starting point for clinicians new to functional mushrooms.

* * *

> These snapshots also act as a gateway to deeper learning. Readers who wish to explore the **scientific foundations** – including taxonomy, bioactive chemistry, mechanistic pathways and detailed clinical applications – are encouraged to continue to **SECTION FOUR**, where the extended evidence chapters provide comprehensive species-specific monographs for integrative veterinary practice.

1

REISHI - Clinical Brief

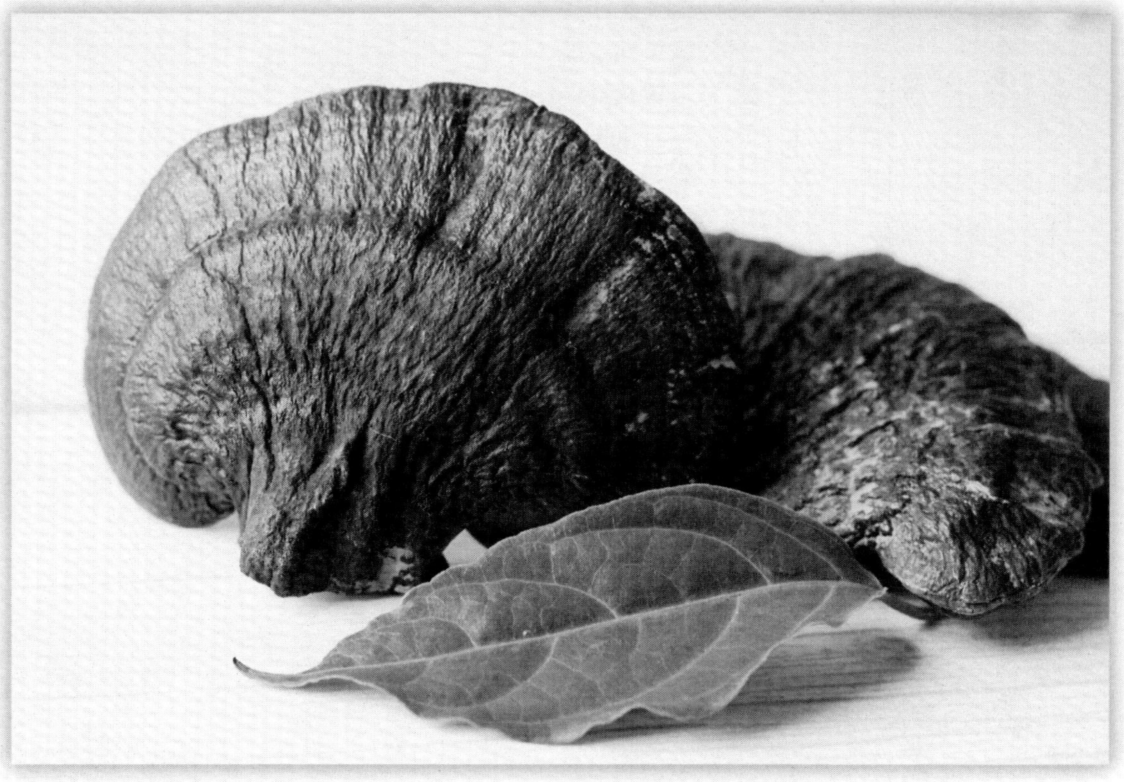

REISHI *(Ganoderma lucidum) - The Calming Guardian & Mushroom of Immortality*

1.1 General Information:

Reishi, traditionally known as the 'mushroom of immortality or the calming mushroom', has a long history of use in Asian medicine for supporting longevity, immune balance and emotional resilience. In veterinary Mycotherapy, Reishi acts as a gentle adaptogen – modulating stress responses, promoting calm without sedation, and supporting restorative sleep patterns. Its broad immunomodulatory and antioxidant effects make it valuable for animals experiencing chronic inflammation, immune dysregulation or age-associated decline.

Reishi also offers hepatoprotective, cardiovascular and respiratory support, which is particularly relevant for older animals or those receiving long-term medication. As a daily tonic, it helps build resilience, supports emotional wellbeing and contributes to healthier ageing across species.

KEY POWER: THE CALMING GUARDIAN – ADAPTOGEN / IMMUNE MODULATOR / STRESS BALANCER

Top Effects

- Supports balanced immune defence by enhancing innate surveillance (macrophages, NK cells) while reducing excessive inflammatory signalling.
- Helps regulate chronic inflammation and oxidative stress through triterpenes, polysaccharides and antioxidant compounds.
- Contributes to hepatic, cardiovascular and nervous-system steadiness, supporting ageing animals or those on long-term medication.
- Assists vitality, appetite and resilience in chronic disease, and is commonly used within integrative oncology protocols.
- Promotes calmer behaviour and autonomic balance, supporting animals experiencing anxiety, environmental stressors, convalescence or trauma recovery.

Immune and stress support

- Reishi polysaccharides (notably β-glucans), proteoglucans and triterpenes modulate T-cell and macrophage activity, improving immune balance. Triterpenes also reduce mast-cell degranulation and histamine release, supporting animals with atopic or allergic tendencies. Reishi aids HPA *(Hypothalamic-Pituitary-Adrenal)* axis. axis regulation, enhances stress recovery and promotes restorative sleep.

Neurologic and cognitive support

- Reishi's antioxidant and anti-inflammatory compounds protect neuronal structure in preclinical models, reducing oxidative load on the central nervous system. While controlled veterinary evidence is limited, Reishi is frequently paired with Lion's Mane for cognitive ageing, neuroinflammation and gentle behavioural support in senior pets.

Liver and detoxification

- Protects liver cells from toxin-induced damage and may assist in stabilising liver enzymes in medicated animals.

- Triterpenoids and antioxidant compounds support hepatic detoxification pathways and reduce lipid peroxidation.
- Combines effectively with Chaga or Shiitake in hepatic support protocols, particularly in older animals or those with chronic inflammatory or metabolic burden.
- Use cautiously in animals with advanced hepatic disease; consult the prescribing veterinarian.

Cardiovascular and respiratory support

- Reishi terpenes contribute to improved circulation and smooth-muscle relaxation, useful for cardiovascular support in senior or performance animals. Preclinical evidence suggests improved oxygen utilisation and respiratory comfort.

Microbiome and digestive support

- Reishi's fibre and polysaccharides have prebiotic activity, helping maintain favourable gut microbial balance. SCWE maintains the natural fibre matrix, enhancing its gastrointestinal and immune-associated benefits.

1.2 Pairings with other mushrooms

- **With Turkey Tail** – synergistic immune modulation and oncology support.
- **With Lion's Mane** – combined neuroprotective, adaptogenic and gut–brain axis support.
- **With Cordyceps** – enhanced energy regulation, recovery and metabolic resilience.
- **With Chaga** – strengthened hepatic and metabolic balance, antioxidant defence and allergy-modulating potential.
- **With Golden Oyster** – cellular resilience, healthy-ageing support and ERGO-enhanced antioxidant protection.

> Synergistic pairings or triads of mushrooms can act across multiple physiological pathways, broadening the supportive effect and contributing to a full-spectrum, terrain-based Mycotherapy strategy.

1.3 Vet Use Note

Clinical application

- Reishi is traditionally prepared as a decoction (hot-water extraction) for polysaccharides or as a dual extract for triterpenes. For veterinary practice, full-spectrum SCWE extracts are preferred because they retain the complete biochemical matrix – polysaccharides, triterpenes, polyphenols, sterols, peptides and the natural prebiotic fibre – without solvents or grain-based carriers.

Safety considerations

Reishi is generally well tolerated, but caution is warranted in:

- animals on **antihypertensives**, due to potential mild blood-pressure-lowering effects
- animals receiving **immunosuppressive therapy**
- animals with **advanced hepatic or renal compromise**
- peri-surgical patients due to potential platelet-aggregation effects
- individuals with known mushroom hypersensitivity
- Monitor for mild gastrointestinal upset when first introduced.

OMG Mushrooms SCWE advantage

OMG Mushrooms SCWE full-spectrum extracts preserve the complete profile of beneficial compounds – polysaccharides, triterpenes, polyphenols, peptides and ergothioneine – in their natural ratios. This solvent-free method enhances bioavailability and ensures a whole-mushroom extract that is physiologically appropriate, safe and effective for companion animals.

Custom blends

When broader immune, inflammatory or neuroendocrine support is needed beyond single-mushroom therapy, OMG Mushrooms collaborates with integrative veterinarians to design personalised SCWE full-spectrum blends centred around Reishi. These may incorporate synergistic species such as Turkey Tail (immune modulation), Lion's Mane (neurocognitive stability), Chaga (antioxidant and hepatic support) or Cordyceps (stress physiology and metabolic reinforcement). These tailored formulations allow Reishi to function within a wider therapeutic matrix suited to complex clinical presentations.

* * *

Unified Dosing Guidance (SCWE Full-Spectrum Extracts)

Tier 1 – Wellness / Maintenance: 10–30 mg/kg/day

Tier 2 – Moderate / Supportive Conditions: 30–60 mg/kg/day

Tier 3 – Intensive / Adjunctive Protocols (e.g., oncology): 60–100 mg/kg/day - *Use under veterinary supervision.*

Unified dosing guidance

Dosing for this mushroom follows the standard SCWE full-spectrum extract ranges used across all species in this guide. These mg/kg tiers apply specifically to whole-mushroom SCWE extracts and should not be compared with myceliated-grain powders or non-extracted mushroom products. Begin at the lower end of the tier and titrate gradually over 5–7 days, with additional caution in sensitive or medically compromised animals.

> *For extended dosing considerations – including species notes, titration strategies and clinical modifiers – practitioners can refer to **Section 2, point 3** of this guide.*

1.4 Interesting Research - Reishi and animals

Within veterinary contexts, *Ganoderma lucidum* (Reishi) is recognised for its potent immunomodulatory and anti-inflammatory properties, largely attributed to its β-glucans and triterpenes. Studies in dogs demonstrate enhanced immune responsiveness, improved vaccine antibody titres, and favourable gut-health outcomes without adverse effects. Reishi's bioactive compounds support immune homeostasis, stress resilience, and cellular protection, making it a valuable adjunct in integrative veterinary practice for chronic inflammatory or neoplastic conditions.

1. The Role of Medicinal Mushrooms in Cancer Treatment: Bioactive Compounds and Therapeutic Potential, 2025

Comprehensive review outlining the anticancer and immunomodulatory properties of medicinal mushrooms including Ganoderma lucidum. Key mechanisms identified include β-glucan-driven immune activation, triterpenoid-induced apoptosis, and suppression of metastasis and angiogenesis. Findings are largely preclinical but indicate promising adjunctive roles in oncology and potential cross-applicability to veterinary oncology models.

2. Functional Properties of Ganoderma lucidum Supplementation in Canine Nutrition, 2024

A controlled trial in adult beagles assessed dietary Ganoderma lucidum inclusion at varying doses (5-15 mg/kg BW). Supplementation showed no negative effects on nutrient digestibility or general health. Dogs receiving 15 mg/kg exhibited enhanced phagocytic activity, increased MHC-II expression on B cells, and higher post-vaccination IgG titres, suggesting dose-dependent immunostimulatory benefits relevant to veterinary practice.

3. Effect of Ganoderma lucidum on Serum Lipid Profiles: A Systematic Review and Meta-Analysis on Animal Studies, 2023

This meta-analysis evaluated animal studies exploring Ganoderma lucidum's lipid-lowering potential. The mushroom demonstrated consistent reductions in total cholesterol and triglycerides across species, with minimal reported adverse effects. These findings suggest possible roles in managing dyslipidaemia and supporting metabolic health in companion animals, warranting targeted veterinary trials.

4. Modulation of Immune Response through Nutraceutical Interventions: Implications for Canine and Feline Health, 2024

Reviewed article discussing nutritional modulation of immunity in small animals, highlighting Ganoderma lucidum as a key immunonutrient. Reishi's polysaccharides and triterpenes are noted for enhancing cellular immunity and reducing inflammatory load, aligning with emerging nutraceutical strategies for immune support in dogs and cats.

1.5 Summary:

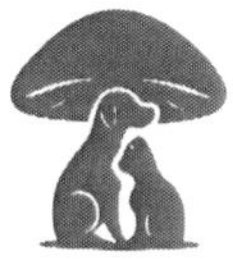

Reishi is widely recognised as one of the most comprehensive functional mushrooms in veterinary Mycotherapy, valued for its triterpenes, β-glucans and polysaccharides that collectively support immune modulation, balanced inflammatory activity and systemic resilience. Traditionally regarded as the 'mushroom of calm', Reishi has long been used to support stress adaptation and emotional balance. Emerging evidence suggests it may help promote autonomic stability, stress resilience and restorative sleep patterns in animals affected by anxiety, ageing or chronic illness, though veterinary-specific studies remain limited. These adaptogenic qualities make Reishi particularly relevant for animals experiencing chronic stress, environmental pressures or behavioural tension.

Beyond its calming profile, Reishi contributes meaningfully to immune balance through modulation of cytokine activity, enhancement of innate immune surveillance and support during chronic inflammatory states. Its triterpenes also exhibit hepatoprotective, cardiovascular-supportive activity in preclinical models, offering further value for senior animals, those with metabolic strain or those undergoing long-term medication. Although most data come from translational and preclinical research, the convergence of traditional use, modern pharmacology and practitioner experience positions Reishi as a reliable, whole-system support mushroom within integrative veterinary care.

> Reishi is widely recognised as one of the most comprehensive functional mushrooms in veterinary Mycotherapy,

Key Sources (Summary)

- Gao et al., 2003
- Lin, Biochemical Pharmacology, 2005
- Chu et al., 2017
- Wasser, 2014
- Memorial Sloan Kettering Cancer Center, 2024
- European Mycotherapy School (MykoTroph), 2023

> “Medicinal mushrooms have tremendous potential in veterinary medicine, particularly for supporting immune function and improving quality of life in chronic disease.”
> *Source: Silver, Veterinary Herbal Medicine (Elsevier, 2006)*

2

TURKEY TAIL - Clinical Brief

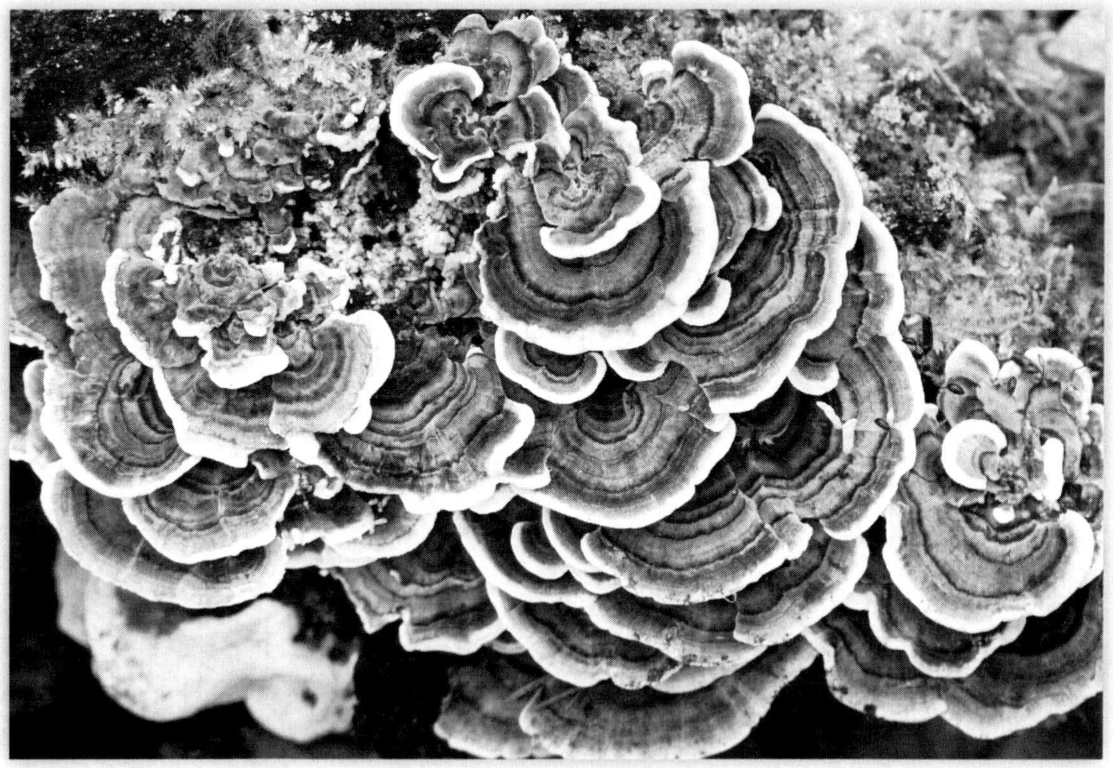

TURKEY TAIL *(Trametes versicolor) - The Immune Defender*

2.1 General Information:

Turkey Tail, the immune defender, is one of the most extensively researched functional mushrooms in both human and veterinary Mycotherapy. Celebrated for its robust immune-modulating properties, it supports resilience, recovery and balanced host defence. Rich in β-glucans and unique polysaccharopeptides (PSK: polysaccharide-Krestin; PSP: polysaccharide-peptide), Turkey Tail promotes the activity of macrophages, NK cells and dendritic cells – the key cellular components of immune surveillance.

In dogs, early veterinary research has shown promising improvements in immune resilience and quality of life, particularly in animals receiving integrative support alongside cancer care. Beyond oncology, Turkey Tail contributes to everyday wellness by supporting the gut microbiome, reducing oxidative stress and strengthening natural defence pathways in ageing, convalescent or immune-compromised animals.

KEY POWER: *THE IMMUNE DEFENDER - CELLULAR DEFENCE AND RECOVERY*

Top Effects:

- Strengthens immune defence through β-glucans and polysaccharopeptides (PSK and PSP).
- Supports animals experiencing chronic immune stress or undergoing chemotherapy.
- Promotes microbiome balance and intestinal integrity through prebiotic activity.
- Reduces oxidative stress and inflammatory load.
- Enhances vitality and recovery in ageing or convalescent animals.
- Helps support immune-associated skin health through balanced inflammatory signalling.
- Valuable adjunct under veterinary supervision for immune, inflammatory and oncology protocols.

Immune System Support

- Polysaccharopeptides (PSK and PSP) activate macrophages, NK cells and dendritic cells, improving immune surveillance and supporting balanced Th1/Th2 responses.
- Early research in other species suggests that polysaccharopeptides may influence antibody responses, though veterinary-specific evidence is still emerging.
- May help enhance resilience during periods of immune challenge, convalescence or chronic inflammatory stress.
- Demonstrated synergistic immune benefits when combined with Reishi or Chaga.

Gut and Microbiome Support

- PSP exhibits prebiotic activity that promotes beneficial gut flora such as Bifidobacterium and Lactobacillus.
- Supports microbial balance in animals recovering from antibiotic use or chronic gastrointestinal inflammation.
- Helps maintain digestive regularity and contributes to improved nutrient assimilation in senior pets.

- Gut–immune axis support may assist immune-associated skin conditions.
- By supporting balanced immunity and improving microbial diversity, Turkey Tail may assist animals with recurrent yeast-related skin or ear concerns where dysbiosis or immune imbalance play a role.'

Liver and Metabolic Support

- Supports detoxification pathways and reduces oxidative load on hepatic tissue.
- May contribute to improved glucose and lipid metabolism, supporting metabolic balance in ageing animals.
- Useful in multi-mushroom hepatic support protocols (e.g. with Reishi or Chaga).

Antioxidant and Anti-Inflammatory Benefits

- Polyphenols and polysaccharopeptides help counter oxidative stress and reduce inflammatory mediators.
- Assists recovery from chronic inflammatory or degenerative conditions.
- Provides systemic antioxidant defence, supporting cellular resilience.

2.2 Pairings with Other Mushrooms:

- **With Reishi** – antiviral synergy and balanced immune modulation.
- **With Chaga or Maitake** – oncology support, immune priming, antioxidant defence and metabolic stability.
- **With Lion's Mane** – gut–brain axis reinforcement and cognitive support.
- **With Golden Oyster** – complementary neuroprotective and mitochondrial support for long-term resilience and cellular vitality.

> Synergistic pairings or triads of mushrooms can act across multiple physiological pathways, broadening the supportive effect and contributing to a full-spectrum, terrain-based Mycotherapy strategy.

2.3 Vet Use Note: (SCWE Full-Spectrum Extracts)

Clinical application

Turkey Tail is an excellent adjunct in integrative oncology, chronic immune dysregulation, convalescence and age-related immune decline. It is well suited to multi-modal protocols where immune alignment and cellular support are key goals.

Safety considerations

Turkey Tail is generally well tolerated. Monitor for:

- mild gastrointestinal changes in sensitive animals
- interactions with immunosuppressive medications
- theoretical additive effects in animals receiving antihypertensives
- signs of hypersensitivity in mushroom-reactive individuals

Avoid raw mushrooms; use only fruiting-body extracts.

OMG Mushrooms SCWE advantage

OMG Mushrooms SCWE full-spectrum extracts preserve the complete matrix of beneficial compounds – β-glucans, polysaccharopeptides, polyphenols, triterpenes and natural fibre – without solvents or grain carriers. This enhances bioavailability and provides a reliable, clinically appropriate whole-mushroom extract for veterinary use.

Custom blends

For cases requiring integrated immune regulation, gastrointestinal steadiness or adjunctive oncology support, OMG Mushrooms can work with clinicians to develop personalised SCWE full-spectrum blends incorporating Turkey Tail. Synergistic partners may include Reishi (immune and inflammatory balance), Maitake (metabolic and immune synergy), Lion's Mane (gut–brain axis modulation) or Golden Oyster (ergothioneine-rich cellular protection). These blends support individualised, multi-system Mycotherapy strategies.

* * *

Unified Dosing Guidance (SCWE Full-Spectrum Extracts)

Tier 1 – Wellness / Maintenance: 10–30 mg/kg/day

Tier 2 – Moderate / Supportive Conditions: 30–60 mg/kg/day

Tier 3 – Intensive / Adjunctive Protocols (e.g., oncology): 60–100 mg/kg/day - *Use under veterinary supervision.*

Unified dosing guidance

Dosing for this mushroom follows the standard SCWE full-spectrum extract ranges used across all species in this guide. These mg/kg tiers apply specifically to whole-mushroom SCWE extracts and should not be compared with myceliated-grain powders or non-extracted mushroom products. Begin at the lower end of the tier and titrate gradually over 5–7 days, with additional caution in sensitive or medically compromised animals.

> *For extended dosing considerations – including species notes, titration strategies and clinical modifiers – practitioners can refer to* Section 2, point 3 *of this guide.*

2.4 Interesting Research - Turkey Tail and animals

Trametes versicolor (Turkey Tail) is best known for its polysaccharopeptide (PSP) and polysaccharide-K (PSK) complexes, which exhibit strong immunostimulatory and antitumour activity. Veterinary studies in dogs with haemangiosarcoma have shown extended survival times and delayed metastasis with PSP supplementation, marking one of the few controlled clinical trials in companion animals. Turkey Tail is increasingly applied in veterinary oncology protocols as an evidence-supported adjunct to conventional therapies for immune and quality-of-life support.

1. Integrative Veterinary Oncology: Part I-Diet, Herbs, Essential Oils, and Supplements, 2025

Comprehensive review of integrative oncology strategies noting *Trametes versicolor* (Turkey Tail) among key medicinal mushrooms used as adjunctive support in canine cancer care. The article reports that Turkey Tail supplementation significantly delayed metastatic progression and improved survival in dogs, underscoring its potential as a supportive immune-oncologic nutraceutical within evidence-based veterinary practice.

2. Current State of Scientific Research and Prospects for Using Basidiomycetes in Veterinary Medicine, 2023

Extensive literature review evaluating numerous medicinal mushrooms, including *Trametes versicolor*. The authors conclude that basidiomycetes provide promising natural resources for developing veterinary feed additives and therapeutic agents. Their β-glucans, triterpenes, and phenolic compounds contribute to immunomodulatory, antioxidant, antimicrobial, and anti-inflammatory actions with applications across livestock, aquaculture, poultry, and companion-animal health.

3. Single Agent Polysaccharopeptide Delays Metastases and Improves Survival in Naturally Occurring Hemangiosarcoma, 2012

A pivotal double-blind canine clinical trial assessing polysaccharopeptide (PSP) from *Coriolus versicolor*. High-dose PSP markedly delayed metastatic progression and produced the longest survival times reported in canine hemangiosarcoma. The study demonstrated safety, dose-response benefit, and translational relevance for oncology patients when advanced treatments are limited.

4. Coriolus versicolor Mycotherapy in Veterinary Oncology, 2011

Professional summary by Dr Franck Floch (DVM, Oncovet France) describing veterinary applications of PSP-rich *Coriolus versicolor* in managing cancer. The discussion highlights increasing clinician and client interest in adjunctive mushroom-based therapies, improved owner awareness, and integration of Turkey Tail within multimodal oncology protocols to enhance immune competence and quality of life in pets with cancer.

5. Medicinal Mushrooms: Their Therapeutic Properties and Current Medical Usage with Special Emphasis on Cancer Treatments, 2011

Scholarly compendium reviewing the biochemical and clinical foundations of medicinal mushrooms, with emphasis on anticancer activity. The authors document scientific validation for products such as *Coriolus versicolor* extracts used in veterinary formulations (e.g., K9 Immunity). The report reinforces that mushroom-derived polysaccharides are credible immunonutrients supported by mechanistic and applied research.

6. Turkey Tail Mushrooms for Canine Hemangiosarcoma, 2012 (Expanded Clinical Detail)

This seminal canine trial investigated whether an oral *Coriolus versicolor* PSP product could slow metastasis and extend survival in naturally occurring hemangiosarcoma. Fifteen client-owned dogs were randomised to daily doses of 25, 50, or 100 mg/kg. Monthly imaging and necropsy confirmation revealed that higher PSP doses significantly prolonged survival, with no adverse biochemical effects. This represents one of the earliest well-documented veterinary oncology studies demonstrating Turkey Tail's clinical efficacy.

2.3 Summary:

Turkey Tail is one of the best-documented medicinal mushrooms for immune modulation,recognised for its polysaccharopeptides PSK and PSP, which activate macrophages, natural killer cells and dendritic cells. Evidence from oncology, immunology and translational medicine demonstrates its ability to support immune surveillance, balance Th1/Th2 responses and assist recovery during immune suppression, chronic inflammation or convalescence. Early veterinary reports and preclinical work support its potential as a safe adjunct in animals with reduced immune resilience or those receiving chemotherapy and radiation.

Beyond its immunological actions, Turkey Tail supports gastrointestinal integrity through prebiotic polysaccharides that promote microbial diversity and short-chain fatty-acid production. These effects, combined with its broad defence-enhancing profile, make Turkey Tail suitable for animals with chronic immune conditions, recurrent infections, gut–immune dysregulation or age-related immune decline. Its excellent safety record and evidence-based immune mechanisms position it as a cornerstone mushroom in integrative veterinary practice. Turkey Tail remains a key component of modern Mycotherapy.

> Turkey Tail is one of the best-documented medicinal mushrooms for immune modulation.

Key Sources (Summary)

- Torkelson et al., 2017
- Ooi & Liu, 2000
- Standish et al., 2008
- Kidd, Alternative Medicine Review, 2000
- Japanese Cancer Research Association (PSK data), 1970–present
- Memorial Sloan Kettering Cancer Center, 2024

> “Animals thrive when we support the systems nature designed, not just suppress the symptoms we see. *Dr Barbara Royal, DVM*”

3

LION'S MANE Clinical Brief

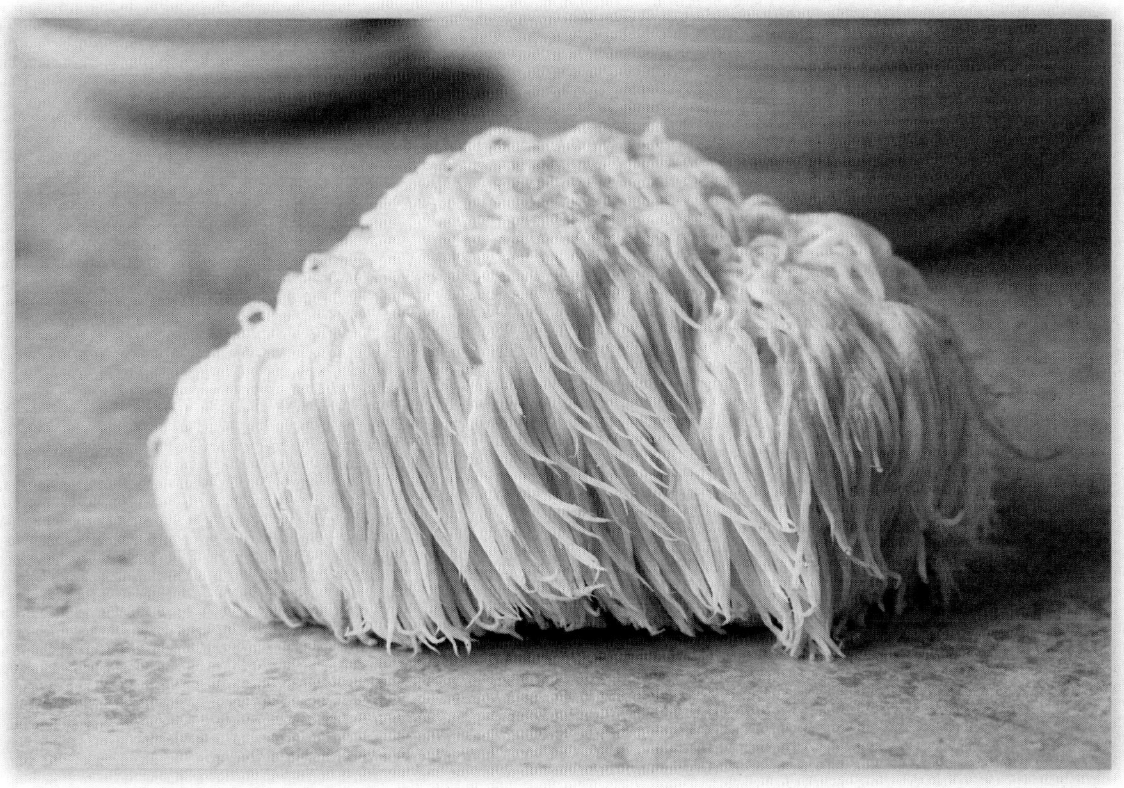

LION'S MANE *(Hericium erinaceus) - The Brain Booster and Gut Warrior*

3.1 General Information:

Often called the 'brain mushroom,' Lion's Mane is known for supporting memory, focus, and overall nervous system function. Its natural compounds – hericenones and erinacines – are thought to stimulate nerve growth and enhance communication within the brain. Many pet owners report their older animals becoming more alert, interactive, and emotionally balanced after consistent use.

Lion's Mane also supports calm behavior and a healthy stress response, making it potentially beneficial for both aging and anxious pets.

KEY POWER: NERVE GROWTH & COGNITIVE SUPPORT – *THE 'NOOTROPIC' MUSHROOM FOR NEURO AND GUT HEALTH*

Top Effects:

- Enhances nerve regeneration and cognitive clarity by stimulating Nerve Growth Factor (NGF) and Brain-Derived Neurotrophic Factor (BDNF).
- Supports healthy aging and mental sharpness in senior pets.
- May improve adaptation to stress, ease anxiety and slow mild behavioural decline.
- Protects neurons against oxidative and inflammatory injury.
- May help improve memory, focus and coordination in working and performance animals.
- Supports liver, cardiovascular and digestive balance through anti-inflammatory pathways (based on preliminary research).

Neurological and Cognitive Support

- Bioactive erinacines and hericenones stimulate neurogenesis and myelin repair showing protective effects in lab models of spinal cord injury, epilepsy and neurodegeneration.
- May assist with canine cognitive dysfunction (doggy dementia) and senior-onset anxiety when used long-term.
- Complements Reishi for calming effects and enhanced stress adaption support.

Liver and Metabolic Support

- Antioxidant compounds in Lion's Mane may help protect liver cells (hepatocytes) from toxin-induced stress. In non-veterinary studies, it has been associated with reduced cholesterol levels and support of normal lipid metabolism – promising findings that warrant further research in pets.
- Preliminary evidence suggests Lion's Mane could enhance liver detoxification enzymes and help reduce inflammatory load, although more veterinary-specific studies are needed.

Immune and Inflammatory Balance

- Polysaccharides (like β-glucans) in Lion's Mane can modulate macrophage and lymphocyte activity, promoting a balanced immune response.
- In studies, Lion's Mane reduced neuroinflammation associated with aging or traumatic brain injury.

- Serves as a potential adjunct for managing chronic inflammation, easing joint stiffness, and combating fatigue.

Digestive and Microbiome Support

- Traditionally used in Chinese medicine for stomach ailments, Lion's Mane has shown mucosal protective effects in gastritis models (helping shield the stomach lining).
- Acts as a prebiotic for beneficial gut flora, which can enhance nutrient absorption and support serotonin production along the gut-brain axis.
- May help reduce the frequency of inflammatory bowel flare ups when used alongside veterinary diets.

Cardiovascular and Longevity Support

- In research outside of veterinary trials, Lion's Mane has demonstrated potential to lower 'bad' LDL *(Low-Density Lipoprotein)* cholesterol and triglycerides, suggesting possible heart-health benefits for animals.
- Its antioxidant activity may protect blood vessel linings (vascular endothelium) from oxidative damage, potentially supporting longevity and sustained energy in active pets.

3.2 Pairings with Other Functional Mushrooms:

- **With Reishi** – stress modulation, autonomic balance and complementary neurological support.
- **With Turkey Tail** – broad immune support and adjunctive oncology care that also benefits the nervous system.
- **With Chaga** – enhanced digestive resilience and antioxidant synergy.
- **With Cordyceps** – stamina, energy metabolism and neural recovery.
- **With Golden Oyster** – dual neuroprotection and mitochondrial support for long-term brain vitality.

> Synergistic pairings or triads of mushrooms can act across multiple physiological pathways, broadening the supportive effect and contributing to a full-spectrum, terrain-based Mycotherapy strategy.

3.3 Vet Use Note:

Clinical application

Lion's Mane is highly valued in integrative veterinary practice for neurological and cognitive support. It is particularly useful in senior animals experiencing cognitive decline, age-related anxiety, behavioural slowing or reduced engagement. Lion's Mane also contributes to gut–brain axis balance and may support recovery following neurological injury or chronic neuroinflammation. It pairs effectively with Reishi for stress-adaptation and with Turkey Tail or Golden Oyster in longevity and neuroprotective protocols.

Safety considerations

Lion's Mane is generally well tolerated. Monitor for:

- mild soft stools at higher doses
- changes in appetite or stool when initiating in sensitive animals
- theoretical interactions with CNS-active medications (e.g. anti-seizure or anxiolytic drugs)
- signs of hypersensitivity in mushroom-reactive individuals

Use only fruiting-body extracts. Avoid unprocessed raw mushrooms.

OMG Mushrooms SCWE advantage

OMG Mushrooms SCWE full-spectrum extracts preserve the complete matrix of bioactive compounds – β-glucans, hericenones, erinacines, polyphenols and natural fibre – without solvents or grain carriers. This whole-food extraction enhances bioavailability and provides a reliable, physiologically appropriate extract for neurological, gastrointestinal and immune support in animals.

Custom blends

For extended neurological, cognitive or gut–brain support, OMG Mushrooms collaborates with integrative veterinarians to create personalised SCWE full-spectrum blends in which Lion's Mane forms the neurotrophic core. Synergistic additions may include Reishi (neuroendocrine calming), Turkey Tail (immune–gut interaction), Cordyceps (neuro-metabolic resilience) or Golden Oyster (mitochondrial and redox stability). These bespoke blends provide nuanced support for animals with multi-factorial neurological or behavioural presentations.

* * *

Unified Dosing Guidance (SCWE Full-Spectrum Extracts)

Tier 1 – Wellness / Maintenance: 10–30 mg/kg/day

Tier 2 – Moderate / Supportive Conditions: 30–60 mg/kg/day

Tier 3 – Intensive / Adjunctive Protocols (e.g., oncology): 60–100 mg/kg/day - *Use under veterinary supervision.*

Unified dosing guidance

Dosing for this mushroom follows the standard SCWE full-spectrum extract ranges used across all species in this guide. These mg/kg tiers apply specifically to whole-mushroom SCWE extracts and should not be compared with myceliated-grain powders or non-extracted mushroom products. Begin at the lower end of the tier and titrate gradually over 5–7 days, with additional caution in sensitive or medically compromised animals.

> *For extended dosing considerations – including species notes, titration strategies and clinical modifiers – practitioners can refer to* Section 2, point 3 *of this guide.*

3.4 Interesting Research - Lion's Mane and animals

Hericium erinaceus (Lion's Mane) has gained strong interest in veterinary medicine for its neuroprotective, metabolic, and gut–brain axis benefits. In aged dogs, controlled feeding trials demonstrate two parallel effects:

1. **enhanced systemic antioxidant and repair-related metabolites**, and
2. **favourable restructuring of the gut microbiota**, including reduced pro-inflammatory taxa and a lower Firmicutes/Bacteroidetes ratio.

These changes occur alongside the mushroom's well-established neurotrophic actions - hericenones and erinacines stimulate nerve growth factor (NGF) - providing therapeutic potential for cognitive ageing, anxiety modulation, and peripheral nerve recovery in companion animals.

1. Gut Microbiota Modulation in Aged Dogs, 2022

A 16-week controlled study in eighteen aged dogs assessed how two inclusion levels of *Hericium erinaceus* (0.4 g/kg and 0.8 g/kg BW) altered gut microbial composition. High-dose supplementation significantly reduced the Firmicutes/Bacteroidetes ratio – a pattern associated with improved metabolic balance and reduced obesity risk in dogs. Beneficial fibre associated taxa such as Bacteroidetes and Prevotella increased, while pro-inflammatory or dysbiosis-linked genera (Campylobacter, Streptococcus, Tyzzerella) decreased. Microbial richness and evenness were maintained, indicating that Lion's Mane reshaped the microbiome without disturbing ecological stability. These findings support its role in enhancing immune tone, mucosal health, and metabolic resilience in senior dogs.

2. Hericium erinaceus Extract Exerts Beneficial Effects on Gut-Neuroinflammaging-Cognitive Axis in Elderly Mice, 2023

Study demonstrating that oral *Hericium erinaceus* extract remodels the gut microbiome by increasing beneficial bacteria and reducing pathogens, producing a measurable prebiotic effect. Supplementation decreased hippocampal inflammation and improved cognitive performance in aged mice, suggesting modulation of the gut-brain axis as a potential nutritional strategy to delay neuroinflammaging-mechanistically relevant to geriatric veterinary neurology.

3. PSXI-7 Effects of Hericium erinaceus on Health of Aged Dogs, 2022

Controlled 16-week feeding trial in adult and aged dogs evaluating two dietary inclusion levels (0.4 g and 0.8 g per kg BW). No adverse effects on body weight or blood chemistry were observed, confirming safety. Higher doses increased serum choline, ascorbate, acetone, and formate, compounds associated with antioxidant defence, membrane synthesis, and tissue repair-indicating *H. erinaceus* supports metabolic resilience and cellular renewal in senior dogs.

4. Lion's Mane (*Hericium erinaceus*): A Potential Treatment for Neurologic Disorders in Veterinary Medicine, 2023

Review authored by veterinary clinicians proposing *H. erinaceus* as a neuro-trophic and anti-inflammatory adjunct for animals. Potential applications include radial and spinal nerve injuries, degenerative myelopathy, intervertebral disc disease, seizures, cognitive decline, and anxiety-related disorders. The authors emphasise *H. erinaceus*' role in promoting nerve regeneration, supporting proprioception, and enhancing quality of life in geriatric and neurologically impaired pets.

5. Gut Microbiota Profiling in Aged Dogs after Feeding Pet Food Containing Hericium erinaceus, 2023

Metagenomic assessment of 18 senior dogs fed 0.4 g or 0.8 g *H. erinaceus* per kg BW for 16 weeks. High-dose intake (HE-H) significantly shifted microbial diversity-raising *Bacteroidetes* and reducing *Firmicutes* and *Campylobacteraceae* populations. These microbiome improvements suggest enhanced immune regulation and potential anti-obesity effects, supporting the inclusion of Lion's Mane in functional geriatric pet diets.

6. Multimodal Assessment of Hericium erinaceus and Valeriana officinalis for Canine Anxiety, 2025

Open-label canine study integrating EEG, neurochemical assays, and behavioural scoring. *H. erinaceus* and *Valeriana officinalis* both reduced anxiety-related behaviours without adverse events. *H. erinaceus* specifically modulated serotonin and dopamine pathways and decreased theta-band activity in frontal/temporal EEG regions. These results indicate potential for *H. erinaceus* as a natural anxiolytic complement, though controlled trials are warranted.

Scientific Rationale to include GOLDEN OYSTER

Recent studies (2022-2024) have identified **ergothioneine (ERGO)** as a naturally occurring thiol compound that accumulates in tissues with high oxidative and metabolic activity - especially the brain, liver, kidneys and eyes.

It's actively transported into cells via the **OCTN1 transporter**, protecting neurons from oxidative stress, inflammation and mitochondrial dysfunction - the same pathways Lion's Mane influences via NGF and BDNF signalling.

> Thus, while Lion's Mane supports *neuroregeneration and growth*, Golden Oyster supports *neuroprotection and longevity*.

Together, they form a complementary dual pathway:

- **Lion's Mane (Hericium erinaceus)** → *Nerve Growth & Regeneration* (via NGF/BDNF)
- **Golden Oyster (Pleurotus citrinopileatus)** → *Oxidative Protection & Mitochondrial Defense* (via ERGO + β-glucans)

This combination can be particularly powerful for:

- **Senior animals** with age-related cognitive decline.
- **Working and performance animals** exposed to metabolic and oxidative stress.
- **Neuroinflammatory conditions** where both regeneration and protection are required.

3.5 Summary:

Lion's Mane is emerging as one of the most important neurotrophic mushrooms in integrative veterinary care. Its unique compounds – including hericenones, erinacines and β-glucans – demonstrate the ability to promote nerve growth factor activity, support neuronal regeneration and enhance neuroplasticity. Translational and preclinical evidence suggests potential benefits for cognitive function, myelination and neurological resilience, making Lion's Mane particularly valuable for ageing animals, those recovering from neurological stress or injury, and individuals with gut–brain axis imbalance.

Beyond its neurotrophic actions, Lion's Mane also provides gastrointestinal support through its prebiotic fibres and polysaccharides, which help strengthen mucosal integrity and contribute to microbiome diversity. These effects may support animals experiencing digestive sensitivity, stress-related gastrointestinal signs or immune-mediated gut issues. Its gentle adaptogenic properties may further assist behavioural calm and autonomic balance in anxious or reactive animals.

When paired with Golden Oyster Mushroom – a naturally ergothioneine-rich species, Lion's Mane forms a complementary neuroprotective–neuroregenerative pairing. The combination supports mitochondrial health, cellular defence and long-term brain vitality, delivering a wider spectrum of neurological and metabolic resilience for companion and performance animals. Although veterinary-specific studies remain limited, the convergence of traditional applications, preclinical research and emerging practitioner experience strongly supports Lion's Mane as a versatile, evidence-aligned mushroom for neurological, gastrointestinal and behavioural wellness.

> Lion's Mane is emerging as one of the most important neurotrophic mushrooms in integrative veterinary care.

Key Sources (Summary)

- Cho et al 2022
- Mori et al., 2009
- Wong et al., 2020
- Friedman, 2015
- Zhang et al., International Journal of Medicinal Mushrooms, 2016
- Memorial Sloan Kettering Cancer Center, 2024
- Japanese pharmacognosy data on erinacines (1994–present)

> "Lion's Mane supports neurological and digestive resilience at the same time, highlighting the importance of the gut–brain axis in whole-body vitality. *Dr Christopher Hobbs, PhD*"

4

CHAGA Clinical Brief

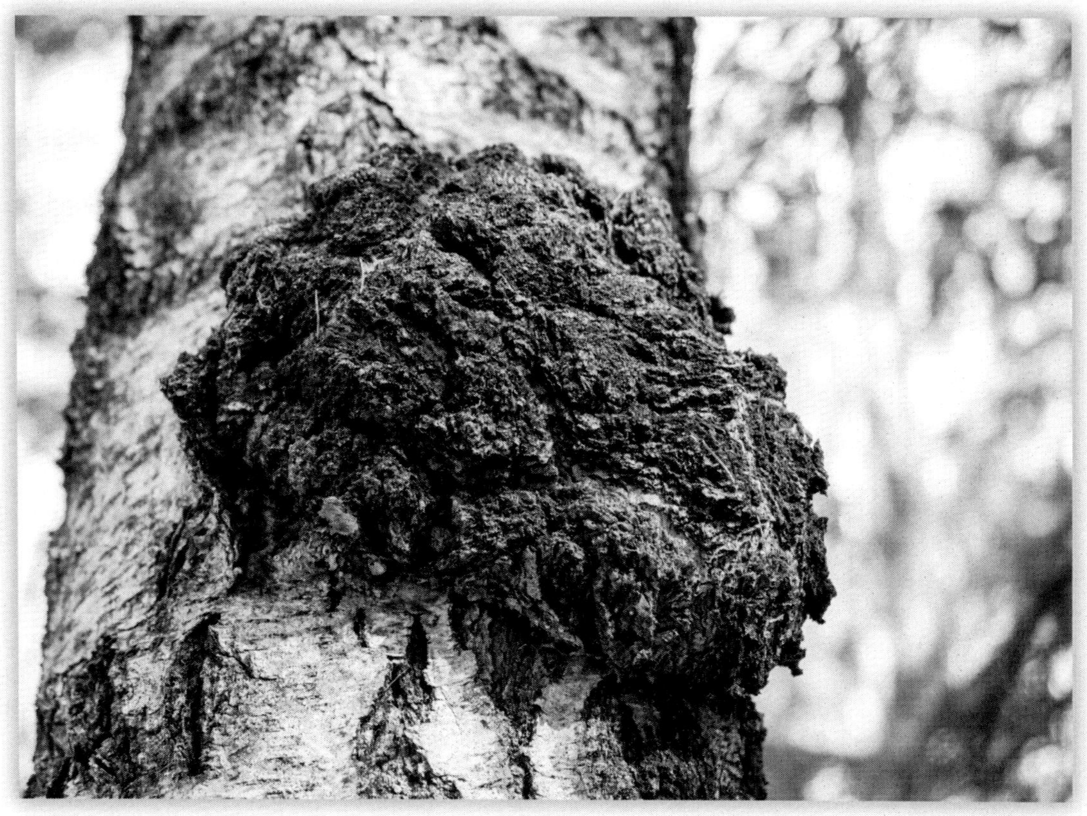

CHAGA (*Inonotus obliquus*) - *The Antioxidant Shield*

4.1 General Information

Chaga is widely regarded as one of nature's most concentrated antioxidant sources. Traditionally used across Russia, Siberia and Northern Europe, its medicinal reputation has been documented since the 16th century. In veterinary wellness, interest in Chaga has grown due to its exceptionally high levels of polyphenols, melanins, triterpenes (including betulinic acid), and polysaccharides that collectively help buffer oxidative stress and support immune, gastrointestinal and metabolic resilience.

Although robust veterinary clinical trials remain limited, translational evidence from human studies, rodent models and in vitro work suggests that Chaga may help regulate inflammation, promote cellular repair, support hepatic detoxification pathways and improve skin and mucosal health. Early practitioner reports also highlight potential benefits for animals experiencing environmental toxicity, chronic inflammatory conditions or age-related oxidative burden.

KEY POWER: *THE ANTIOXIDANT SHIELD - POTENT ANTIOXIDANT /CELLULAR RESTORATION SUPPORT*

Top Effects

- Exceptional free-radical scavenging capacity from melanin, polyphenols and betulinic acid.
- Helps regulate oxidative stress and fatigue in in aging or environmentally stressed animals.
- Supports balanced immune responses and tissue repair during chronic inflammatory processes.
- Protects the gastrointestinal mucosa and liver from chemical or environmental toxins.
- May aid glucose and lipid metabolism, contribution to healthy weight and energy balance (extrapolated from preclinical studies).
- Enhances vitality, recovery and coat condition in senior or convalescent animals.

Immune System Support

- β-glucans and melanins enhance macrophage and NK-cell activity, supporting broad innate defence.
- Modulates cytokine patterns, promoting balanced Th1/Th2 responses (preclinical).
- Demonstrates anti-allergic potential by reducing IgE-mediated inflammatory signalling (emerging evidence).
- Useful adjunct for immune-compromised or allergy-prone animals.
- Shows synergistic immune support when paired with Reishi or Turkey Tail.

Digestive and Gut Support

- Traditionally used for gastritis and gastric discomfort; polysaccharides soothe GI mucosa.
- Prebiotic fibre supports beneficial gut microflora and contributes to gut–immune balance.
- May reduce loose stools associated with stress or dietary changes.
- Useful for animals with sensitive digestion or low-grade inflammatory bowel tendencies.

Liver and Detoxification Support

- Triterpenes and polyphenols protect hepatocytes against oxidative damage (preclinical evidence).
- May support detoxification enzyme pathways during increased toxin or medication load.
- Frequently paired with Reishi for comprehensive liver and allergy-support protocols.

Antioxidant and Cellular Defence

- One of nature's richest antioxidant sources – polyphenols, melanins and SOD-like activity *(SOD -superoxide dismutase – a key antioxidant enzyme).*
- Helps reduce oxidative DNA damage and supports mitochondrial health.
- Supports tissue repair and recovery after illness or environmental toxin exposure.

Metabolic and Endocrine Support

- May support healthy glucose regulation and insulin sensitivity (rodent models).
- Possible benefit in metabolic syndromes associated with inflammation and oxidative stress.
- Adaptogenic profile may aid overall vitality and stress resilience.

Skin & Coat Health

- Antioxidant and anti-inflammatory compounds may assist itchy, inflamed or sensitive skin.
- Traditional use for irritated skin conditions; emerging evidence for cellular protection in keratinocytes.
- Supports coat gloss and overall dermal integrity during ageing or chronic inflammation.

Cardiovascular Support (light evidence)

- Preclinical studies suggest improvements in lipid metabolism and systemic inflammatory load.
- Antioxidant activity contributes to vascular resilience and overall cardiovascular wellness.

4.2 Pairings with Other Functional Mushrooms:

- **With Reishi** – immune modulation, allergy support and hepatic balance.
- **With Turkey Tail** – oncology adjunct and immune resilience.

- **With Lion's Mane** – gut–brain axis support and digestive comfort.
- **With Cordyceps** – endurance, recovery and metabolic support.
- **With Golden Oyster** – enhanced antioxidant and tissue-protective synergy for animals exposed to oxidative or environmental stress.

> Synergistic pairings or triads of mushrooms can act across multiple physiological pathways, broadening the supportive effect and contributing to a full-spectrum, terrain-based Mycotherapy strategy.

4.3 Vet Use Note (SCWE full spectrum extract)

Clinical application

Supports animals experiencing oxidative stress, chronic inflammation, immune imbalance, environmental toxin exposure, skin irritation, digestive sensitivity or age-related decline. May serve as a supportive adjunct in oncology, detoxification and senior vitality programmes.

Safety considerations

- High natural oxalate content – avoid in animals with a history of calcium-oxalate stones.
- Use caution with hypoglycaemic, anticoagulant or antihypertensive medications.
- Introduce gradually to minimise gastrointestinal sensitivity.
- Avoid raw or unextracted Chaga; use fruiting-body SCWE extracts only.

OMG Mushrooms SCWE advantage

SCWE full-spectrum extraction preserves Chaga's complete matrix of polysaccharides, triterpenes, polyphenols, melanins and natural fibre. Solvent-free and grain-free, ensuring veterinary-appropriate bioavailability and clinical reliability.

Custom blends

When enhanced antioxidant, hepatic, dermatological or chronic-inflammatory support is required, OMG Mushrooms works with veterinarians to design SCWE full-spectrum Chaga-centred blends. Synergistic species may include Reishi (inflammatory modulation), Turkey Tail (immune balance and gastrointestinal support), Cordyceps (mitochondrial and metabolic steadiness) or Golden Oyster (ergothioneine-mediated cellular protection). These tailored combinations allow Chaga to function as part of a comprehensive redox-modulating strategy.

* * *

Unified Dosing Guidance (SCWE Full-Spectrum Extracts)

Tier 1 – Wellness / Maintenance: 10–30 mg/kg/day

Tier 2 – Moderate / Supportive Conditions: 30–60 mg/kg/day

Tier 3 – Intensive / Adjunctive Protocols (e.g., oncology): 60–100 mg/kg/day - *Use under veterinary supervision.*

Unified dosing guidance

Dosing for this mushroom follows the standard SCWE full-spectrum extract ranges used across all species in this guide. These mg/kg tiers apply specifically to whole-mushroom SCWE extracts and should not be compared with myceliated-grain powders or non-extracted mushroom products. Begin at the lower end of the tier and titrate gradually over 5–7 days, with additional caution in sensitive or medically compromised animals.

> *For extended dosing considerations – including species notes, titration strategies and clinical modifiers – practitioners can refer to Section 2, point 3 of this guide.*

4.5 Interesting Research - Chaga and animals

Inonotus obliquus (Chaga) offers broad antioxidant, antiviral, and anticancer potential through its melanin, polyphenol, and betulinic acid content. Veterinary-oriented studies highlight its ability to inhibit canine bladder-cancer organoid growth and enhance chemotherapeutic response while maintaining cellular integrity. Additional evidence shows antiviral activity against multi-feline respiratory and gastrointestinal viruses, supporting Chaga's inclusion in veterinary formulations targeting oxidative stress, immune dysfunction, and tumour control.

1. Anti-Cancer Activity of Chaga Mushroom (*Inonotus obliquus*) Against Dog Bladder Cancer Organoids, 2024

Ground-breaking in vitro and in vivo study using canine bladder-cancer organoids demonstrated potent antitumour effects of Chaga extract. Treatment arrested the cell cycle, induced apoptosis, and suppressed expression of cancer-stem-cell markers (CD44, C-MYC, SOX2, YAP1). ERK-pathway inhibition and reduced cyclin expression were observed. In xenograft mice, Chaga reduced tumour mass and necrosis was evident. Combined use with chemotherapeutic agents enhanced efficacy, highlighting Chaga's potential as an adjunct to veterinary oncology protocols targeting drug-resistant tumours.

2. Identification of *Inonotus obliquus* Polysaccharide with Broad-Spectrum Antiviral Activity Against Multi-Feline Viruses, 2016

Laboratory evaluation identified Chaga-derived polysaccharides (IOPs) with low cytotoxicity and direct virucidal action against multiple feline pathogens-including calicivirus, herpesvirus-1, influenza H3N2/H5N6, panleukopenia, and feline infectious peritonitis virus. IOPs block viral binding and absorption, demonstrating strong promise as natural, broad-spectrum antiviral agents for feline respiratory and gastrointestinal infections.

3. Current State of Scientific Research and Prospects for Using Basidiomycetes in Veterinary Medicine: A Literature Review, 2023

Comprehensive review of pharmacological data on higher fungi, including *Inonotus obliquus*. The authors describe Chaga's documented hypoglycaemic, antioxidant, immunostimulant, and antimicrobial properties, citing applications in gastrointestinal disorders, infections, cancer, and metabolic disease. The paper concludes that basidiomycete-based Mycotherapy represents a scientifically validated and expanding field within veterinary medicine, with *I. obliquus* a leading candidate for future therapeutic formulations.

4.6 Summary

Chaga stands out as the antioxidant powerhouse of functional mushrooms. Chaga mushroom is a versatile medicinal fungus offering a range of potential health benefits for animals. Its robust antioxidant, immune-modulating, anti-inflammatory, and adaptogenic properties make it a valuable tool in integrative veterinary medicine. Chaga can help protect cells from oxidative damage, support the immune system (enhancing defence while taming excessive reactions), and complement therapy for conditions like chronic inflammation, cancer, metabolic disorders, and skin issues. Emerging research and centuries of traditional use both underscore Chaga's multi-system benefits – from supporting liver and gut function to contributing to metabolic and cardiovascular wellness. Importantly, these benefits come with a relatively low risk profile, as long as sensible precautions (regarding oxalates, interactions, and quality control) are observed. In summary, Chaga is a potent natural adjunct that can promote balance and resilience in the canine and feline body. Used judiciously, it may improve outcomes and well-being in a variety of clinical scenarios, though it should always be integrated as part of a comprehensive treatment plan. The growing interest in veterinary mycotherapy is backed by increasing evidence, and Chaga stands out as a promising medicinal mushroom ally for our animal companions. All interventions should be personalized, and ongoing research will continue to clarify Chaga's role – but current knowledge suggests it can be a safe, effective, and holistic supplement in the hands of informed veterinary professionals.

Chaga stands out as the antioxidant powerhouse of functional mushrooms.

Key Sources (Summary)

- Pepin, 2025
- Alhallaf et al., 2024
- Memorial Sloan Kettering Cancer Center, 2025
- Heliyon Journal Review, 2024
- Additional peer-reviewed studies referenced within the monograph

> “Healing happens when we restore connection – within the body, within the environment, and within the bond between human and animal. *Dr Edward Bassingthwaighte, BVSc (Hons)*”

5

CORDYCEPS Clinical Brief

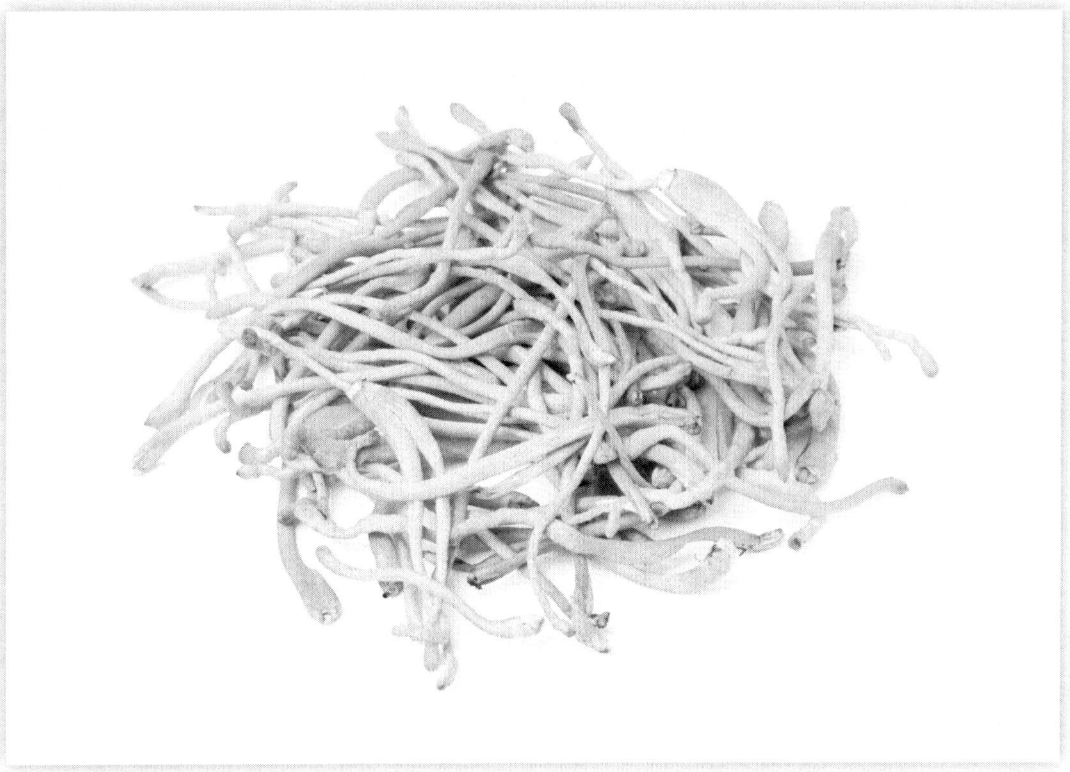

CORDYCEPS *(Cordyceps militaris)* - *The Vitality–Endurance Enhancer*

5.1 General Information

Cordyceps is a natural vitality enhancer long valued in traditional medicine for supporting stamina, respiratory function and healthy ageing. Modern research highlights its role in improving cellular energy through enhanced ATP production, supporting oxygen utilisation and promoting recovery after exertion. For animals, Cordyceps is particularly suited to active, working or senior pets needing metabolic, respiratory or endurance support, as well as those recovering from illness or chronic stress.

KEY POWER: THE VITALITY–ENDURANCE ENHANCER - *SUPPORTS ENERGY METABOLISM AND ADAPTOGENIC RESILIENCE IN ACTIVE AND AGEING ANIMALS.*

Top Effects

- Enhances stamina, oxygen use and recovery in active or performance animals.
- Supports healthy adrenal response and resilience to physical or emotional stress.
- Improves mitochondrial ATP production and cellular energy metabolism.
- Helps maintain healthy immune balance during training or chronic illness.
- Promotes cardiovascular and respiratory efficiency.
- Supports liver and kidney detoxification and recovery after exertion or medication.
- Contributes to longevity through antioxidant and anti-fatigue mechanisms.

Energy and Performance Support

- Cordycepin and adenosine derivatives support cellular ATP synthesis and cellular utilisation, improving endurance, post-training recovery.
- Helps reduce lactic-acid accumulation, enhancing muscular efficiency and exercise tolerance.

Adrenal and Stress Support

- Acts as a natural adaptogen, helping normalise cortisol and adrenal output.
- Beneficial for stress-sensitive, aging, or high-performance animals.
- Complements Reishi for adrenal and allergy modulation.

Immune System Support

- Polysaccharides support macrophage activity, T-cell and NK-cell activity while moderating excessive cytokine responses.
- Supports immune competence in older animals or those recovering from infection or chemotherapy.
- Cordycepin exhibits antimicrobial and antiviral potential in pre-clinical studies.

Cardiovascular and Respiratory Support

- Vasodilatory and mild hypotensive effects help improve blood flow and oxygen delivery.
- May help regulate lipid profiles in preclinical studies.

- Supports respiratory function and airway comfort in mild bronchial inflammation.

Liver - Kidney - Detoxification

- Demonstrates protective effects against toxin- or medication-induced hepatic and renal stress.
- Aids clearance of metabolic by-products following exertion.
- May improve renal blood flow and filtration efficiency.

Anti-Aging and Longevity Support

- Supports antioxidant enzyme activity (superoxide dismutase, catalase, glutathione peroxidase).
- Helps maintain mitochondrial integrity and reduce fatigue-related oxidative stress.
- Complements Lion's Mane and Golden Oyster (ergothioneine) for cognitive and metabolic clarity in senior animals.

5.2 Pairings with Other Mushrooms:

- **with Reishi** - liver, adrenal and allergy support.
- **with Turkey Tail or Chaga or Maitake** - immune and oncology adjunct.
- **with Lion's Mane** - neuro-metabolic support and fatigue recovery synergy.
- **with Golden Oyster** - mitochondrial and metabolic reinforcement for endurance, recovery and healthy ageing.

> Synergistic pairings or triads of mushrooms can act across multiple physiological pathways, broadening the supportive effect and contributing to a full-spectrum, terrain-based Mycotherapy strategy

5.3 Vet Use Note

Clinical Application

Cordyceps is suited to active, working and senior animals; recovery after illness; respiratory weakness; chronic fatigue; metabolic instability; and as a supportive adjunct in oncology protocols.

Safety Considerations

- Generally well tolerated; introduce gradually to minimise gastrointestinal sensitivity.
- Use caution in animals with suspected autoimmune disease.
- Avoid or monitor closely in suspected hormone-sensitive cancers.
- Potential mild interaction with anticoagulants; monitor when combined with blood-thinning medications.
- Avoid unextracted or myceliated-grain powders; use fruiting-body extracts only.

OMG Mushrooms SCWE Advantage

OMG Mushrooms SCWE full-spectrum extracts preserve the complete matrix of Cordyceps' key bioactive compounds - including cordycepin, adenosine and related nucleosides, β-glucans, fungal sterols, polyphenols and trace antioxidants - without solvents or grain carriers.

This whole-food profile supports superior bioavailability, consistent clinical outcomes and improved tolerability compared with conventional hot-water extracts or myceliated-grain powders.

Custom Blends

OMG Mushrooms collaborates with integrative veterinarians to develop personalised SCWE full-spectrum formulations incorporating Cordyceps for endurance support, respiratory capacity, metabolic stability, senior vitality or oncology-adjunct protocols. Complementary species may include Reishi (stress and immune regulation), Lion's Mane (neuro-metabolic synergy), Turkey Tail (immune tone), Maitake (endocrine and metabolic alignment) or Golden Oyster (mitochondrial resilience). These custom blends allow precision support for patients requiring sustained energy and recovery optimisation.

* * *

Unified Dosing Guidance (SCWE Full-Spectrum Extracts)

Tier 1 – Wellness / Maintenance: 10–30 mg/kg/day

Tier 2 – Moderate / Supportive Conditions: 30–60 mg/kg/day

Tier 3 – Intensive / Adjunctive Protocols (e.g., oncology): 60–100 mg/kg/day - *Use under veterinary supervision.*

Unified dosing guidance

Dosing for this mushroom follows the standard SCWE full-spectrum extract ranges used across all species in this guide. These mg/kg tiers apply specifically to whole-mushroom SCWE extracts and should

not be compared with myceliated-grain powders or non-extracted mushroom products. Begin at the lower end of the tier and titrate gradually over 5–7 days, with additional caution in sensitive or medically compromised animals.

> *For extended dosing considerations – including species notes, titration strategies and clinical modifiers – practitioners can refer to **Section 2, point 3** of this guide.*

5.4 Interesting Research RESEARCH - Cordyceps and animals

Cordyceps militaris is valued in veterinary integrative care for its adaptogenic, immunomodulatory, and performance-enhancing properties. Research indicates that Cordyceps β-glucans and cordycepin improve vaccine responsiveness, antioxidant status, and immune function in animals. Emerging clinical applications in dogs include support for vitality, respiratory performance, and endocrine balance, positioning Cordyceps as a multifaceted mushroom for both preventive and therapeutic use

1. Elucidation of Physicochemical Properties of Polysaccharides Extracted from Cordyceps militaris Fruiting Bodies with Different Drying Treatments and Their Effects on Ulcerative Colitis in Zebrafish, 2022

Study using a zebrafish colitis model demonstrated that polysaccharides from differently dried *C. militaris* fruiting bodies modulated inflammatory and immune responses, reduced intestinal ulceration, and promoted tissue recovery. Results indicate that fruiting-body compounds possess anti-inflammatory and immunoregulatory potential applicable to gastrointestinal disorders in veterinary species.

2. A Study of the Aphrodisiac Properties of Cordyceps militaris in Streptozotocin-Induced Diabetic Male Rats, 2021

Experimental findings revealed that *C. militaris* improved reproductive function in diabetic male rats by increasing testosterone, reducing oxidative stress, and normalising sexual behaviour indices. While based on a rodent model, the data suggest endocrine-supportive properties relevant to metabolic and reproductive disorders in companion animals.

3. Adjuvant Activity of Cordycepin, a Natural Derivative of Adenosine from Cordyceps militaris, to Boost Immune Responses Against a Commercial Rabies Vaccine, 2024

Animal-model evaluation showed that cordycepin enhanced humoral and cellular immune responses to a commercial rabies vaccine without adverse effects. Findings highlight the potential of *C. militaris* compounds as natural immunopotentiators to improve vaccine efficacy in veterinary applications.

4. Cordyceps for Dogs with Cancer - Clinical Insights and Veterinary Applications, 2023

Veterinary-oriented overview discussing the integration of *Cordyceps* supplements into canine cancer care. Summarises emerging evidence that bioactive cordycepin and polysaccharides may support mitochondrial energy production, reduce treatment-related fatigue, enhance immunity, and complement chemotherapy or radiation. Advocates cautious use under veterinary supervision.

5. Cordyceps - An Adaptogenic Mushroom for Dogs and Cats' Adrenal Health, 2022

Educational review detailing adaptogenic and anti-inflammatory effects of *Cordyceps* for dogs and cats. Discusses its use for improving stamina, supporting adrenal and respiratory function, and assisting recovery from chronic illness or stress. Highlights its suitability for inclusion in holistic veterinary wellness programs.

5.5 Summary

Cordyceps is a key functional mushroom in veterinary Mycotherapy for supporting energy metabolism, recovery and respiratory resilience. Its signature nucleoside analogues – including cordycepin and adenosine – together with polysaccharides and peptides, are associated with improved mitochondrial function, oxygen utilisation and ATP production in preclinical studies. Translational evidence suggests Cordyceps may support stamina, exercise tolerance and post-exertional recovery in performance animals, as well as assist senior or convalescent animals experiencing fatigue or reduced vitality.

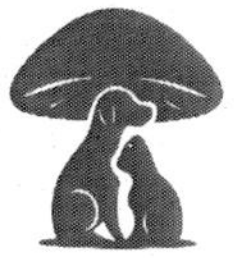

Beyond its effects on energy pathways, Cordyceps exhibits immunomodulatory and anti-inflammatory properties, helping to balance cytokine activity and support host defence without excessive immune stimulation. Preclinical data indicate potential benefits for respiratory function, including bronchodilatory and anti-inflammatory actions in lung tissue, which may translate into support for animals with chronic respiratory stress or environmental irritant exposure. Cordyceps may also aid glucose and lipid metabolism and support renal function, making it a useful adjunct in metabolic or age-related decline when integrated thoughtfully within a broader veterinary treatment plan.

When paired with Lion's Mane and Golden Oyster (ergothioneine-rich), Cordyceps contributes to a complementary neuro-metabolic foundation that supports vitality, resilience and healthy ageing in both companion and performance animals.

Key Sources (Summary)

- Tuli et al., *Life Sciences*, 2013
- Das et al., *Journal of Ayurveda and Integrative Medicine*, 2010
- Zhou et al., *Phytotherapy Research*, 2009
- Tzeng et al., *Journal of Agricultural and Food Chemistry*, 2006
- Wasser, functional mushroom reviews, 2011–2023
- Traditional Tibetan and Chinese materia medica on Cordyceps species

> “Fungi are a reminder that the familiar can also be strange, and that life’s complexity is far beyond what we see.”
> *Source:* Sheldrake, *Entangled Life* (2020)

6

MAITAKE Clinical Brief

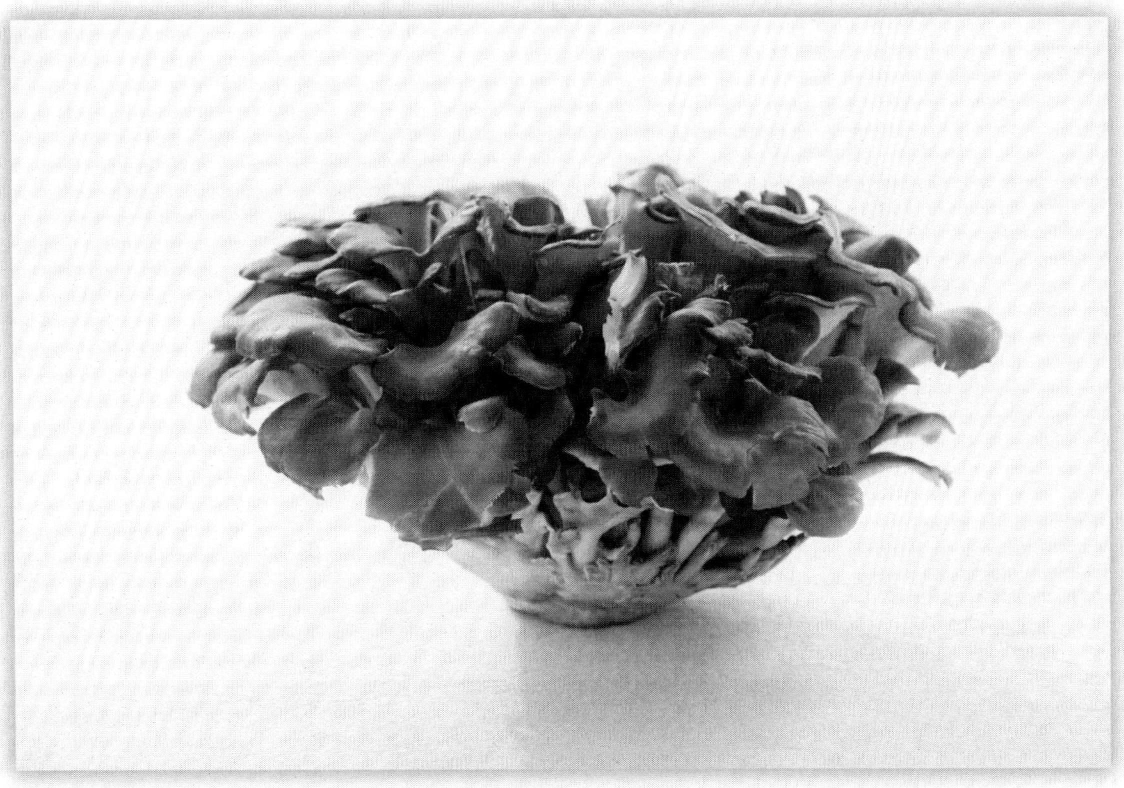

MAITAKE *(Grifola frondosa) - The Metabolic Harmoniser*

6.1 General Information

Maitake, also known as the 'Dancing Mushroom,' is prized for its rich D-fraction β-glucans, which modulate immunity and support balanced glucose and lipid metabolism. In both human and veterinary contexts, it is recognised for enhancing immune vigilance, supporting insulin sensitivity and improving vitality in aging or overweight animals. Maitake can also complement oncology care by strengthening the body's natural immune defences.

Although less commonly featured in pet formulations, Maitake deserves renewed attention for its broad metabolic and immune benefits. Its under representation stems largely from fewer direct veterinary studies, despite extensive laboratory and human research confirming its safety and efficacy.

KEY POWER - *THE METABOLIC HARMONISER*. THE 'DANCING MUSHROOM' IS REGARDED AS A SUPPORTER OF IMMUNOMETABOLIC HARMONY AND OVERALL VITALITY.

Top Effects

- Supports immune function and white blood cell activity.
- Helps balance blood glucose and lipid levels in overweight or insulin-resistant pets.
- Aids liver detoxification and antioxidant status.
- May assist recovery and appetite in chronically ill animals.
- Enhances resilience during chemotherapy or stress.

Immune and Oncology Support

- D-fraction β-glucans activate macrophages and NK cells to strengthen tumour surveillance and modulating cytokine balance.
- Demonstrated in animal and in-vitro studies to enhance immune responsiveness.
- Supports overall vitality in animals receiving integrative oncology protocols.

Metabolic and Endocrine Support

- Helps regulate insulin activity and lipid metabolism.
- May reduce markers of oxidative stress and improve liver enzyme profiles.
- Useful adjunct for metabolic syndrome, obesity, or aging pets with low energy.

Digestive and Gut Health

- Promotes beneficial gut bacteria and assists nutrient assimilation.
- Gentle on digestion and synergistic with Turkey Tail and Chaga for microbiome balance.

Why Maitake is often left out

Maitake has a strong research foundation in human and laboratory models but comparatively fewer veterinary-specific studies. As a result, some supplement ranges overlook it in favour of species with more direct animal data. However, its **β-glucan profile, metabolic benefits and safety record** make it a valuable inclusion for both preventive care and targeted veterinary support.

6.2 Pairings with Other Mushrooms:

- **with Reishi** – metabolic–inflammatory balance with additional hepatic steadiness and immune regulation in ageing or inflamed animals.
- **with Turkey Tail** – enhanced immune nourishment and gut–immune axis reinforcement, particularly in animals with recurrent infections or chronic immune fragility.
- **with Lion's Mane** – gut–brain and metabolic–cognitive synergy for animals with stress-linked digestive issues or early cognitive changes.
- **with Cordyceps** – metabolic endurance and improved energy utilisation for overweight, lethargic or senior animals with reduced vitality.
- **with Golden Oyster** – endocrine, lipid and glucose modulation supported by ERGO-driven mitochondrial and antioxidant protection in metabolic or ageing cases.

> Synergistic pairings or triads of mushrooms can act across multiple physiological pathways, broadening the supportive effect and contributing to a full-spectrum, terrain-based Mycotherapy strategy

6.3 Vet Use Note

Maitake is traditionally prepared using hot-water extraction to release its β-glucans and polysaccharide–protein complexes. In modern veterinary Mycotherapy, full-spectrum SCWE extracts are preferred because they maintain the complete metabolic matrix: β-glucans, glycoproteins, sterols, phenolics and pre-biotic fibre. This ensures predictable immune, metabolic and endocrine-modulating effects in companion animals, without alcohol residues or grain-derived carriers.

Clinical application

- Maitake is particularly relevant in metabolic dysregulation, early endocrine imbalance, overweight animals and age-related metabolic slowdown.
- Its β-glucans modulate insulin sensitivity and support healthier lipid metabolism, making it suitable for animals with weight gain, early insulin resistance or inflammatory–metabolic interplay.
- Maitake offers immune nourishment in chronic, recurrent or age-related immune fragility, without overstimulation.
- It supports hepatic clarity, gastrointestinal steadiness and healthier inflammatory tone in multi-systemic presentations.

- Maitake integrates effectively into metabolic, endocrine, immune and geriatric protocols.

Safety considerations

Maitake is generally well tolerated, but clinical caution is warranted in:

- animals with unstable diabetes or those receiving insulin or hypoglycaemic agents
- animals on immunosuppressive therapy
- advanced hepatic or renal compromise where metabolic turnover may be unpredictable
- peri-surgical patients due to very mild platelet-influencing potential in sensitive individuals
- gastrointestinally sensitive animals, where gradual titration is recommended

Monitor for mild soft stools when first introduced, particularly in small dogs or cats.

OMG Mushrooms SCWE advantage

OMG Mushrooms SCWE full-spectrum extracts preserve the complete profile of beneficial compounds – polysaccharides, triterpenes, polyphenols, peptides and ergothioneine – in their natural ratios. This solvent-free method enhances bioavailability and ensures a whole-mushroom extract that is physiologically appropriate, safe and effective for companion animals.

Custom blends

When broader metabolic, endocrine or immune support is needed, OMG Mushrooms can produce tailored SCWE full-spectrum formulations centred on Maitake. Synergistic partners may include Reishi (inflammatory balance), Golden Oyster (mitochondrial protection and antioxidant stability), Lion's Mane (gut–brain axis support) or Turkey Tail (immune resilience). These personalised blends allow veterinarians to address complex multi-systemic cases in which Maitake plays a central metabolic-regulatory role.

***

Unified Dosing Guidance (SCWE Full-Spectrum Extracts)

Tier 1 – Wellness / Maintenance: 10–30 mg/kg/day

Tier 2 – Moderate / Supportive Conditions: 30–60 mg/kg/day

Tier 3 – Intensive / Adjunctive Protocols (e.g., oncology): 60–100 mg/kg/day - *Use under veterinary supervision.*

Dosing for this mushroom follows the standard SCWE full-spectrum extract ranges used across all species in this guide. These mg/kg tiers apply specifically to whole-mushroom SCWE extracts and should

not be compared with myceliated-grain powders or non-extracted mushroom products. Begin at the lower end of the tier and titrate gradually over 5–7 days, with additional caution in sensitive or medically compromised animals.

> *For extended dosing considerations – including species notes, titration strategies and clinical modifiers – practitioners can refer to **Section 2, point 3** of this guide.*

6.4 Interesting Research - Maitake and animals

Within veterinary contexts, Maitake is emerging as a supportive agent in oncology, metabolic balance, and immune health. Early *in vitro* and clinical studies indicate potential to enhance immune competence, assist glycaemic regulation, and provide adjunctive benefits in canine cancer care. Although most data remain preclinical, the safety and tolerability observed in dogs reinforce its relevance for integrative Mycotherapy in companion animals.

1. Potential Growth Inhibitory Effect of Maitake D-Fraction on Canine Cancer Cells, 2004

In vitro investigation on three canine cancer cell lines (CF33, CF21, CL-1) demonstrated that Maitake D-fraction, a purified β-glucan extract, potently inhibited cell proliferation and induced cell death. Other β-glucan products tested showed no such cytotoxicity, confirming the unique bioactivity of D-fraction. The findings suggest Maitake D-fraction may serve as a valuable adjunct for veterinary oncology, offering selective antiproliferative activity with potential immune-enhancing effects.

2. Antihypertensive and Metabolic Effects of Whole Maitake Mushroom Powder and Its Fractions in Two Rat Strains, 2002

Although performed in rats, this seminal study provides foundational metabolic insights relevant to veterinary nutrition. Maitake fractions significantly lowered blood pressure, enhanced insulin sensitivity, and improved lipid metabolism in hypertensive and diabetic models. These physiological outcomes highlight Maitake's adaptogenic potential to support cardiovascular and metabolic balance, mechanisms that may extend to companion animals under clinical supervision.

3. Maitake PETfraction - Single Agent in Dogs with Lymphoma (Clinical Trial), 2007

A prospective clinical trial in 15 dogs with intermediate-to-high-grade lymphoma evaluated oral Maitake PETfraction as monotherapy. The extract was well tolerated, with no hematologic or biochemical toxicity observed. Although no complete tumour regressions occurred, partial responses and stable disease were documented in several dogs. The study confirmed safety and indicated immunologic activity, establishing Maitake PETfraction as a viable supportive option in integrative cancer care for canines.

4. Supplements for Small Animal Cancer Patients - Including Maitake PETfraction, 2021

Comprehensive veterinary review summarising evidence for nutraceuticals in oncology, including Maitake PETfraction. The paper notes that mushroom β-glucans may aid immune modulation, reduce inflammation, and improve tolerance to conventional therapy. Maitake's inclusion is based on its clinical safety record and experimental antitumour findings, reinforcing its role as an adjunct supplement within integrative treatment protocols for dogs with cancer.

6.5 Summary

Maitake (Grifola frondosa) is the metabolic and immune harmoniser of the functional mushroom world. Maitake is particularly valued for its β-glucan fractions, notably the D-fraction and related polysaccharides, which demonstrate strong immunomodulatory and metabolic effects. Preclinical and clinical research in humans shows that Maitake can enhance innate and adaptive immune responses, supporting macrophage, natural killer cell and T-cell activity while helping to regulate cytokine balance. In veterinary contexts, this translates into potential support for animals with chronic immune challenges, oncology protocols or recurrent infections, where Maitake may act as a gentle but effective immunological ally.

Maitake is also notable for its impact on metabolic health. Studies indicate that Maitake extracts can support healthy blood glucose regulation, improve insulin sensitivity and positively influence lipid profiles. These properties make it especially relevant for animals with metabolic syndrome, overweight or obesity, and endocrine conditions such as insulin resistance. In addition, Maitake is often regarded as a 'women's mushroom' in traditional and integrative practice due to its supportive role in hormonal and metabolic balance, which may have translational relevance in female animals experiencing hormonal or peri-menopausal-like changes (e.g. desexed bitches with weight or coat changes). Used as part of a comprehensive nutritional and lifestyle programme, Maitake offers a well-rounded profile for immune, metabolic and endocrine support.

> Maitake (Grifola frondosa) is the metabolic and immune harmoniser of the functional mushroom world.

* * *

Key Sources (Summary)

- Kodama et al., *Journal of Medicinal Food*, 2003–2005 (D-fraction data)
- Konno, *International Journal of Medicinal Mushrooms*, 2010
- Kubo & Nanba, 1997–1999 (immunomodulation and metabolic effects)
- Talpur et al., *Molecular and Cellular Biochemistry*, 2002
- Wasser, Grifola frondosa reviews, 2011–2023
- Traditional Japanese and Chinese records on Maitake use

> “Mushroom polysaccharides have been used for their immune stimulating activity for centuries. Medicinal mushrooms exert their antineoplastic effects by activating immune responses. Hot water extracts of mushroom polysaccharides have been shown to act through T-cell, natural killer (NK) cell, B-cell and macrophage-dependent immune responses. Of relevance to aggressively metastatic neoplasms like HSA are studies that show the potential to prevent metastasis. A blend of mushroom polysaccharides was shown to inhibit lung metastasis through immune regulation involving cytokine signaling and immune response in the tumor microenvironment. *Erin Bannink, DVM, Diplomate ACVIM (oncology) / Steve Marsden, DVM, ND, MSOM, Lac, Dipl.Ch*”

7

SHIITAKE Clinical Brief

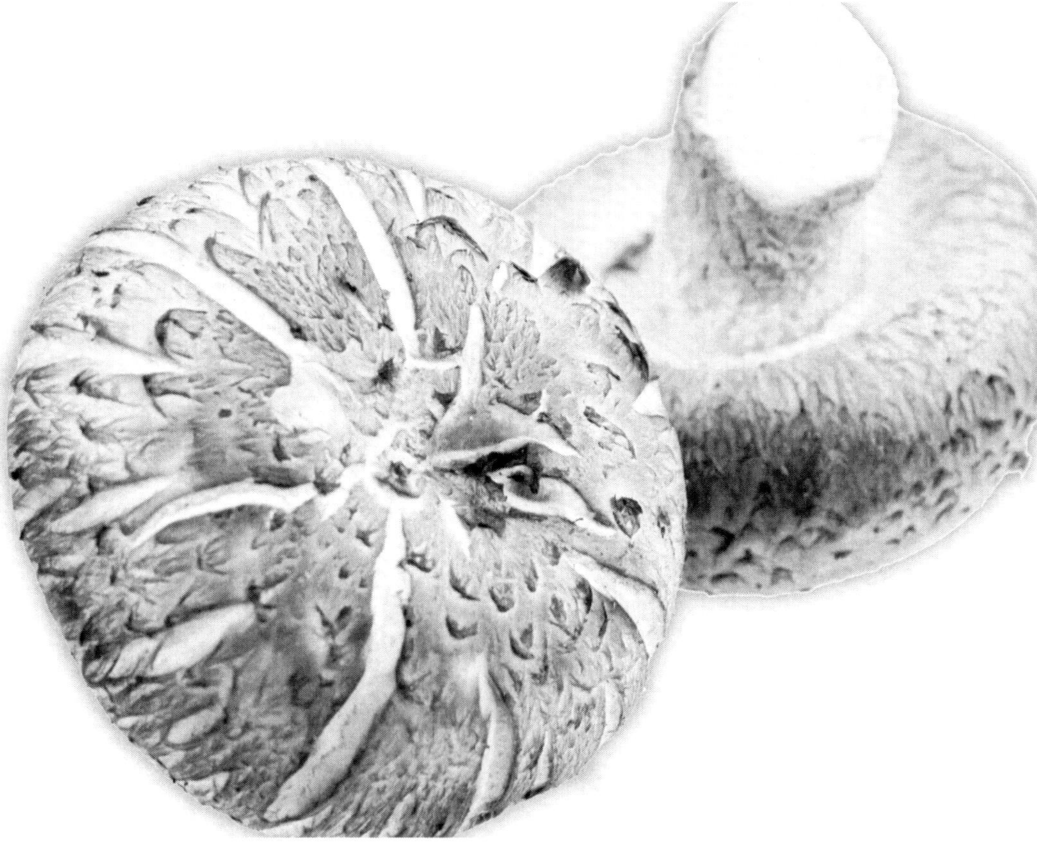

SHIITAKE *(Lentinula edodes) - The Immune Nourisher*

7.1 General Information

Shiitake is one of the world's most recognised medicinal and culinary mushrooms, offering a distinctive combination of lentinan beta-glucans, eritadenine and diverse polysaccharides that support immune function, hepatic detoxification and cardiovascular balance. In veterinary practice, Shiitake is valued for its role in integrative oncology, recovery from chronic infections and support of compromised liver function.

Although widely studied in human medicine and used extensively in traditional healing systems, Shiitake is often overshadowed in veterinary settings by Turkey Tail or Reishi. Nonetheless, it remains one of the safest and most accessible mushrooms for companion animals and can also be introduced as a cooked functional food to support immune and digestive wellness in dogs.

KEY POWER: THE IMMUNE NOURISHER - CELLULAR DEFENCE AND DETOXIFICATION SUPPORT

Top Effects:

- Promotes immune balance and cellular defence.
- Supports healthy liver function and detoxification pathways.
- Provides antimicrobial and antiviral benefits in chronic conditions.
- Helps regulate cholesterol and supports cardiovascular health.
- Contributes to skin and coat health through antioxidant effects.

Immune and Oncology Support

- Lentinan βeta-glucans support macrophage and natural killer (NK) cell activation.
- Pre-clinical models show improved survival markers and quality of life benefits in oncology contexts.
- Complements Turkey Tail and Maitake in integrative cancer support protocols.

Liver and Cardiovascular Support

- Eritadenine may help regulate cholesterol and improve lipid metabolism.
- Supports hepatic detoxification pathways and healthy bile flow.
- Useful for animals recovering from medication - related hepatic stress or toxin exposure.

Digestive and Culinary Use

- Cooked Shiitake mushrooms can safely be added to dog diets as a nutrient-rich functional food.
- Cooking breaks down tough chitin cell walls, improving digestibility and nutrient bioavailability.
- Small, well-cooked portions can support immune resilience and gastrointestinal health.

Why Shiitake is often left out

Despite its excellent safety profile and long-standing medicinal history, Shiitake is sometimes under-represented in pet supplements. The reason lies not in a lack of efficacy, but in the limited number of controlled veterinary studies. Most evidence comes from human and preclinical models - all showing consistent, positive outcomes for immune and hepatic health that translate well to companion animal care.

7.2 Pairings with Other Functional Mushrooms

- **with Reishi** – immune modulation and hepatic balance.
- **with Maitake** – metabolic support and antioxidant synergy.
- **with Turkey Tail** – immune resilience and oncology support.
- **with Lion's Mane** – gut–brain axis and digestive reinforcement.
- **with Golden Oyster** – cardiometabolic and immune-support synergy with longevity-focused antioxidant protection.

> Synergistic pairings or triads of mushrooms can act across multiple physiological pathways, broadening the supportive effect and contributing to a full-spectrum, terrain-based Mycotherapy strategy

7.3 Vet Use Note

Clinical Application

Shiitake is suitable for animals needing immune enhancement, hepatic support, recovery after chronic infections, cardiovascular balance or adjunctive oncology care. It is also useful for senior animals with declining vitality or digestive resilience.

Safety Considerations

- Generally well tolerated; introduce gradually for gastrointestinal-sensitive animals.
- Avoid raw Shiitake; always use cooked or extracted forms.
- Use caution in animals with active autoimmune conditions.
- Monitor lipid and hepatic parameters in metabolic or hepatic disease protocols.
- Avoid myceliated grain powders; use fruiting-body extracts only.

OMG Mushrooms SCWE Advantage

OMG Mushrooms SCWE full-spectrum extracts preserve the complete profile of Shiitake's bioactive compounds – including beta-glucans, eritadenine, polysaccharides, polyphenols and trace antioxidants – in their natural ratios. This solvent-free method provides excellent bioavailability and ensures a whole-mushroom extract appropriate for veterinary use.

Custom Blends

For wider immune, hepatic or metabolic programmes, OMG Mushrooms works with clinicians to create personalised SCWE full-spectrum blends incorporating Shiitake alongside complementary species such as Reishi (inflammatory and hepatic modulation), Turkey Tail (gut-immune support), Maitake (metabolic balance) or Golden Oyster (oxidative-stress protection). These formulations strengthen Shiitake's role within integrated, whole-system Mycotherapy plans.

***

Unified Dosing Guidance (SCWE Full-Spectrum Extracts)

Tier 1 – Wellness / Maintenance: 10–30 mg/kg/day

Tier 2 – Moderate / Supportive Conditions: 30–60 mg/kg/day

Tier 3 – Intensive / Adjunctive Protocols (e.g., oncology): 60–100 mg/kg/day - *Use under veterinary supervision.*

Unified dosing guidance

Dosing for this mushroom follows the standard SCWE full-spectrum extract ranges used across all species in this guide. These mg/kg tiers apply specifically to whole-mushroom SCWE extracts and should not be compared with myceliated-grain powders or non-extracted mushroom products. Begin at the lower end of the tier and titrate gradually over 5–7 days, with additional caution in sensitive or medically compromised animals.

> *For extended dosing considerations – including species notes, titration strategies and clinical modifiers – practitioners can refer to Section 2, point 3 of this guide.*

***

7.4 Interesting Research - Shiitake and animals

Shiitake (*Lentinula edodes*) is valued for its rich β-glucan (lentinan) content and array of bioactive nutrients that support immune modulation, antioxidant defence, and metabolic balance. In veterinary nutrition, shiitake has shown promise for enhancing antioxidant capacity, improving lipid metabolism, and supporting gastrointestinal health in dogs. Its demonstrated safety and multi-system benefits make it a valuable adjunct in integrative companion-animal care.

1. Shiitake Mushroom Powder Supplementation Increases Antioxidative Activity in Dogs, 2024

A controlled dietary study demonstrated that shiitake mushroom powder enhanced antioxidant defences and improved lipid metabolism in healthy dogs. After four weeks of supplementation, plasma total cholesterol levels decreased significantly, while superoxide dismutase (SOD) activity and leukocyte sirtuin-1 (SIRT1) expression increased. No adverse effects were observed on appetite, body weight, or general health. These findings highlight shiitake's potential as a functional dietary adjunct for oxidative-stress management and cardiovascular support in companion animals.

2. Effects of Supplementation with Shiitake Powder (*Lentinula edodes*) on Anti-Oxidative Activities and Energy/Lipid Metabolism in Healthy Dogs, 2022

Complementary research confirmed shiitake's metabolic and antioxidant benefits in canines. In this controlled trial, daily supplementation with varying doses of shiitake powder elevated SOD activity, improved energy utilisation, and lowered plasma cholesterol. Enhanced SIRT1 expression suggested a role in mitochondrial regulation and metabolic efficiency. The data reinforce shiitake's safety and functional value as a nutraceutical in veterinary nutrition.

3. A Supplement with *Lentinula edodes*, Bromelain & Quercetin: Antioxidant & Gut-Health Effects in Kennel Dogs, 2023

In a randomised controlled study on American Staffordshire Terriers, a daily feed supplement containing shiitake mushroom powder, bromelain, and quercetin improved gut health and stress biomarkers over 28 days. Treated dogs showed reduced fecal calprotectin, cortisol, and markers of intestinal fermentation, alongside increased short-chain fatty acids-indicating enhanced microbiota balance and anti-inflammatory effects. No adverse events were recorded, supporting the inclusion of shiitake as a safe, multifunctional ingredient for gastrointestinal and immune support in dogs.

7.5 Summary

Shiitake (*Lentinula edodes*) bridges nutrition and therapy, offering both culinary nourishment and clinically relevant bioactive compounds that support immune, metabolic and cardiovascular wellness. Its key functional constituents include lentinan (a beta-glucan with documented immunomodulatory and adjunctive oncology applications), eritadenine (associated with cholesterol regulation) and a diverse matrix of polysaccharides and polyphenols that contribute to balanced immune function.

In translational and early veterinary contexts, Shiitake may help improve immune surveillance, support recovery following infection and provide adjunctive benefit in chronic inflammatory or neoplastic conditions, particularly when used alongside other immunomodulatory mushrooms. Its combination of nutritional value, safety profile and therapeutic potential makes Shiitake a versatile option within integrative veterinary Mycotherapy.

Beyond its immune actions, Shiitake plays a role in cardiometabolic health, with eritadenine and Shiitake-derived sterols demonstrating lipid-modulating effects that may support cardiovascular wellness in senior or overweight animals. Its natural prebiotic fibres also help maintain gastrointestinal integrity and microbiome diversity, complementing whole-diet interventions aimed at gut-immune balance. While most research originates from human and rodent models, the convergence of culinary safety, long traditional use and modern mechanistic insights positions Shiitake as a highly relevant 'food-as-medicine' option for companion animals.

> Shiitake bridges nutrition and therapy, offering both culinary nourishment and therapeutic potential.

Key Sources (Summary)

- Chihara et al., early lentinan studies, 1970s–1990s
- Wasser, *International Journal of Medicinal Mushrooms*, 2002–2023
- Hibasami et al., *Oncology Reports*, 2000
- Fukushima et al., *Journal of Nutrition*, 2001 (cholesterol and eritadenine)
- Hobbs, C., *Medicinal Mushrooms: The Essential Guide*, 2017
- Traditional East Asian dietary and medicinal records on Shiitake

> "Mushrooms are miniature pharmaceutical factories, producing hundreds of compounds for the benefit of not only the mushrooms themselves but also the animals that ingest them. *Source: Stamets, Mycelium Running (2005)*"

8

GOLDEN OYSTER Clinical Brief

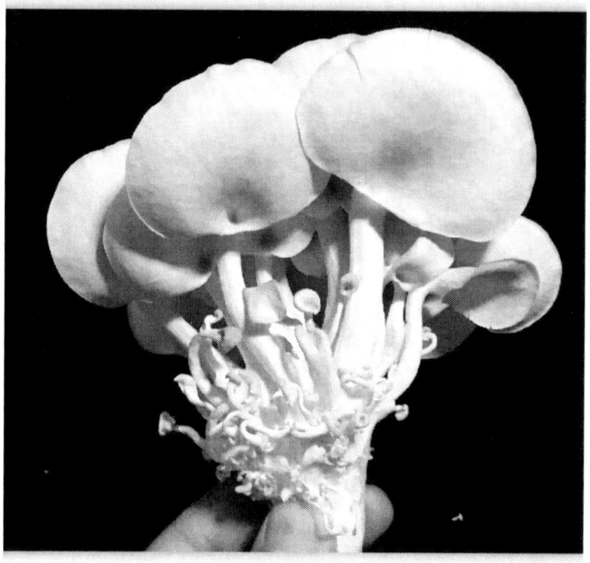

GOLDEN OYSTER *(Pleurotus citrinopileatus) - The Longevity Mushroom*

8.1 General Information

Golden Oyster is one of OMG Mushrooms' signature species, celebrated for its naturally high levels of **ergothioneine (ERGO)** – a unique thiol antioxidant increasingly recognised as a potential 'longevity vitamin'. Ergothioneine accumulates in key animal tissues including the brain, liver, kidneys and muscles, where it protects mitochondria, reduces oxidative damage and supports long-term cellular vitality.

In companion animals, Golden Oyster contributes to healthy ageing, neuroprotection, liver balance and metabolic resilience. When paired with Lion's Mane, the combination offers complementary neuro-support: **Lion's Mane encourages neuronal regeneration, while Golden Oyster protects those neurons from oxidative injury**, forming a powerful longevity-focused synergy.

Although direct canine and feline trials are still emerging, the expanding body of animal-model ERGO research provides a strong mechanistic basis for translational veterinary use. Its whole-food profile, broad safety and antioxidant potency position Golden Oyster as a valuable addition to modern Mycotherapy. These findings support the veterinary positioning of Golden Oyster as a neurometabolic and longevity-supportive mushroom.

KEY POWER: *THE LONGEVITY VITAMIN – ERGOTHIONEINE-DRIVEN CELLULAR VITALITY AND ANTIOXIDANT DEFENCE.*

Top Effects

- Cellular protection through naturally concentrated ergothioneine – a unique thiol antioxidant that accumulates in key organs such as the liver, kidneys and brain.
- Supports healthy aging and mitochondrial efficiency.
- Helps maintain muscle recovery and energy metabolism in working dogs and performance horses.
- Provides anti-fatigue and stress modulation support via polysaccharides and beta-glucans.
- Enhances immune resilience against oxidative load and environmental stress.
- Supports liver balance and digestive comfort through prebiotic fibres and natural enzymes.
- Demonstrates anti-inflammatory potential relevant to joint health and stability in aging pets.

Immune System Support

- Helps normalise immune response and reduce oxidative inflammation.
- May enhance vaccine-titre responses and post-infection recovery.
- Supportive addition to oncology protocols under integrative supervision.

Neurologic and Cognitive Support

- Ergothioneine crosses the blood-brain barrier via the Ergothioneine Transporter (ETT; formerly OCTN1).
- Protects neurons against oxidative stress and inflammatory damage.
- May assist ageing pets with cognitive decline (canine cognitive dysfunction) or stress sensitivity.
- Synergist with Lion's Mane for dual neuroprotective and neurodegenerative support – particularly in senior pets or stress-sensitive animals.

Liver and Metabolic Support

- Supports detoxification pathways and reduces lipid peroxidation.

- May aid lipid metabolism and healthy weight management.
- Useful in senior animals or those receiving long-term medication.
- Synergistic with Reishi for hepatic balance and allergy support.

Microbiome and Digestive Support

- Contains natural enzymes (lipase and amylase) that support digestion.
- Fibre-rich matrix offers gentle prebiotic effects for microbiome diversity.
- May improve nutrient absorption and gut–immune balance.

Cardiovascular Support

- May help normalise cholesterol and triglyceride levels via lovastatin-like metabolites.
- Supports endothelial function and circulatory health in active and senior animals.

Antioxidant and Longevity Benefits

- Ergothioneine acts as a direct cytoprotectant against oxidative and environmental stressors.
- Supports glutathione-related pathways and cellular repair.
- May influence longevity pathways, including Nrf2 activation, contributes to healthier ageing.

8.2 Pairings with Other Mushrooms:

- **with Lion's Mane** – neuroprotection and neuroregeneration with added mitochondrial and redox stability for cognitive and stress-related concerns.
- **with Reishi** – inflammatory modulation, hepatic steadiness and stress-physiology support with enhanced cellular resilience in ageing or inflamed animals.
- **with Cordyceps** – endurance, respiratory efficiency and mitochondrial reinforcement for active and performance breeds.
- **with Turkey Tail** – immune surveillance and oncology resilience strengthened by Golden Oyster's antioxidant and cytoprotective buffering.
- **with Maitake** – metabolic balance, endocrine steadiness and oxidative-stress reduction in overweight, ageing or metabolically vulnerable animals.

> Synergistic pairings or triads of mushrooms can act across multiple physiological pathways, broadening the supportive effect and contributing to a full-spectrum, terrain-based Mycotherapy strategy

8.3 Vet Use Note

Clinical application

Golden Oyster is appropriate for animals requiring antioxidant support, cognitive and neurological maintenance, liver balance, metabolic resilience, immune modulation or senior vitality programmes. Ideal for ageing pets, performance animals, those under chronic oxidative stress or those requiring gentle adjunctive care during illness.

Safety considerations

- Generally well tolerated; introduce gradually for gastrointestinal-sensitive animals.
- Use caution in severe hepatic insufficiency; monitor energy levels and appetite.
- Safe for long-term use as part of antioxidant and longevity-support protocols.
- Not recommended to replace primary therapy in neurological or metabolic disease.
- Avoid myceliated grain powders; use fruiting-body extracts only.

OMG Mushrooms SCWE advantage

OMG Mushrooms SCWE full-spectrum extracts preserve the complete beneficial matrix of Golden Oyster – including polysaccharides, beta-glucans, polyphenols, peptides and naturally occurring ergothioneine – in their original ratios. This solvent-free method ensures high bioavailability and delivers a whole-food extract appropriate for companion-animal physiology.

Custom blends

When additional longevity, antioxidant or neuroprotective synergy is indicated, OMG Mushrooms formulates personalised SCWE full-spectrum blends using Golden Oyster's ergothioneine-rich profile as a therapeutic foundation. Synergistic additions may include Lion's Mane (neurotrophic support), Reishi (calming and immune modulation) or Cordyceps (metabolic and mitochondrial reinforcement). These custom blends enable precision Mycotherapy tailored to individual animals requiring advanced cellular resilience and healthy-ageing support.

> Golden Oyster is emerging as the longevity and neuroprotective mushroom in veterinary wellness.

* * *

Unified Dosing Guidance (SCWE Full-Spectrum Extracts)

Tier 1 – Wellness / Maintenance: 10–30 mg/kg/day

Tier 2 – Moderate / Supportive Conditions: 30–60 mg/kg/day

Tier 3 – Intensive / Adjunctive Protocols (e.g., oncology): 60–100 mg/kg/day - *Use under veterinary supervision.*

Unified dosing guidance

Dosing for this mushroom follows the standard SCWE full-spectrum extract ranges used across all species in this guide. These mg/kg tiers apply specifically to whole-mushroom SCWE extracts and should not be compared with myceliated-grain powders or non-extracted mushroom products. Begin at the lower end of the tier and titrate gradually over 5–7 days, with additional caution in sensitive or medically compromised animals.

> *For extended dosing considerations – including species notes, titration strategies and clinical modifiers – practitioners can refer to* Section 2, point 3 *of this guide.*

8.4 Interesting Research - Key Studies Relevant to Golden Oyster and Ergothioneine in Animals

Golden oyster (*Pleurotus citrinopileatus*) is notable for its naturally high levels of ergothioneine, a sulfur-containing amino acid now recognised as a candidate 'longevity vitamin' and powerful cytoprotective antioxidant. Recent animal studies show that ergothioneine can extend lifespan, reduce frailty, support cognitive function, and protect reproductive cells from oxidative damage, while golden-oyster-derived lectins and polysaccharides demonstrate antitumour effects in murine models. Together, these data support the therapeutic potential of golden oyster-based preparations as part of integrative strategies targeting healthy ageing, metabolic resilience and oncology in veterinary patients.

1. Ergothioneine Promotes Longevity and Healthy Ageing in Male Mice, 2024

Daily oral ergothioneine (≈4-5 mg/kg) given in drinking water from young adulthood to natural death significantly extended lifespan and 'non-frailty span' in male C57BL/6J mice, while also improving survival and robustness in *C. elegans*. Treated mice showed less age-related decline in body weight, fat mass, locomotor performance and cognitive function, alongside lower inflammatory and senescence biomarkers and preservation of hippocampal neurogenesis. The authors highlight ergothioneine as a vitamin-like nutrient with multi-system anti-ageing effects and note prior data where golden-oyster-derived ergothioneine extracts improved memory and neurogenesis, underscoring translational relevance for neurocognitive and geriatric support in companion animals.

2. Ergothioneine Improves Healthspan in Aged Animals via H�S Signalling and NAD� Metabolism, 2025

In this mechanistic study, ergothioneine supplementation enhanced healthspan in aged *C. elegans* and rats, improving mobility, exercise endurance, muscle mass and muscle vascularisation, while reducing age-associated molecular damage. The work shows ergothioneine acts as an alternative substrate for cystathionine-γ-lyase (CSE), boosting hydrogen sulfide (H2S) production and widespread protein persulfidation, including activation of cytosolic glycerol-3-phosphate dehydrogenase (cGPDH) to increase NAD(+) levels. These findings provide a plausible mechanistic rationale for using ergothioneine-rich mushrooms such as golden oyster to support sarcopenia, metabolic resilience and mitochondrial function in ageing animals, even though direct canine or feline trials are not yet available.

3. Ergothioneine Supplementation Protects Porcine Oocytes and Embryos from Oxidative Stress, 2024

Using an in-vitro porcine model, supplementation of maturation media with ergothioneine (10-50 μM) during oocyte maturation improved intracellular antioxidant status, increasing glutathione (GSH) and reducing reactive oxygen species (ROS). Ergothioneine up-regulated Nrf2 and downstream antioxidant genes (e.g. NQO1, HMOX1), while decreasing KEAP1 expression, and enhanced cleavage and blastocyst rates after IVF without increasing apoptosis. Although this is a reproductive biotech setting, it strongly supports ergothioneine's role as a potent cellular antioxidant capable of protecting high-value cells from oxidative damage-relevant when considering ergothioneine-rich mushroom extracts for fertility support, reproductive health, or general oxidative-stress modulation in veterinary practice.

4. Pleurotus citrinopileatus Lectin and Antitumour Activity in Sarcoma-Bearing Mice, 2008

A homodimeric lectin purified from *Pleurotus citrinopileatus* exhibited potent antitumour effects in mice implanted with sarcoma-180. Intraperitoneal administration at 5 mg/kg for 20 days inhibited tumour growth by roughly 80%, and the lectin showed strong mitogenic activity on murine splenocytes, indicating robust immunostimulatory properties. In addition, the same lectin inhibited HIV-1 reverse transcriptase in vitro, suggesting broader bioactivity. While not a companion-animal trial, these data confirm that golden oyster contains non-ergothioneine bioactives (lectins) with measurable antitumour and immunomodulatory potential, supporting its consideration in oncology-adjunct formulations, with appropriate dosing, safety evaluation and veterinary oversight.

5. Pleurotus ostreatus - Veterinary Applications and Nutritional Value, 2021

Oyster mushrooms (*Pleurotus ostreatus*) contain an array of bioactive compounds including β-glucans, ergothioneine, lectins, and other polysaccharides that contribute to antioxidant, antimicrobial, immunomodulatory, and metabolic effects. While controlled veterinary studies remain limited, emerging evidence and clinical application reports highlight potential benefits for companion animals, particularly in supporting musculoskeletal health, gut microbiota balance, and immune resilience. Their high-quality protein, B-vitamins, vitamin D, and trace minerals such as selenium make oyster mushrooms suitable as adjuncts in holistic veterinary nutrition. Preparations derived from fruiting-body extracts are preferred to ensure maximal ergothioneine and polysaccharide bioavailability.

8.5 Summary

Golden Oyster is emerging as the longevity and neuroprotective mushroom in veterinary wellness, recognised for its naturally elevated levels of ergothioneine and its potential to support cellular resilience and healthy ageing. This sulphur-containing amino acid is increasingly regarded as a cytoprotective nutrient concentrated in tissues with high oxidative demand – including the liver, kidneys, brain and bone marrow. Through its antioxidant and mitochondrial-preserving activity, Golden Oyster may offer valuable support for animals experiencing chronic inflammation, environmental toxin exposure or age-related oxidative stress. When delivered as a full-spectrum extract that retains natural fibre and co-factors, its ergothioneine content provides a unique foundation for maintaining physiological integrity and long-term vitality.

Beyond its ergothioneine profile, Golden Oyster shares the broader therapeutic attributes of the Pleurotus genus, including β-glucan-mediated immune modulation, potential lipid-balancing effects and gentle prebiotic support for gut–immune interactions. These combined effects make it especially relevant for senior-animal wellness programmes, metabolic resilience, recovery pathways and general health span optimisation. Golden Oyster is particularly compelling when used alongside mushrooms with neurotrophic or metabolic properties, where its mitochondrial and antioxidant actions complement neuroregenerative, immune or metabolic pathways to enhance whole-system resilience in companion and performance animals.

> “Ergothioneine may prove to be a longevity vitamin essential for healthy ageing.”
> *Source:* Beelman et al., *Nutrition Journal* (2020)

Key Sources (Summary)

- Beelman et al., Penn State University ergothioneine research, 2019–2024
- Halliwell & Cheah, ergothioneine and cellular longevity reviews, 2013–2023
- Kawagishi et al., Pleurotus bioactive compound studies, 2004–2015
- Nammex technical monographs on ergothioneine-rich species
- Hobbs, C., *Medicinal Mushrooms: The Essential Guide*, 2017
- Traditional East Asian culinary and medicinal records on Pleurotus species

> “Ergothioneine is avidly retained in the body and accumulates at sites of tissue injury, where it may help to reduce oxidative damage. *Source:* Halliwell et al., *Biochemical and Biophysical Research Communications* (2018)”

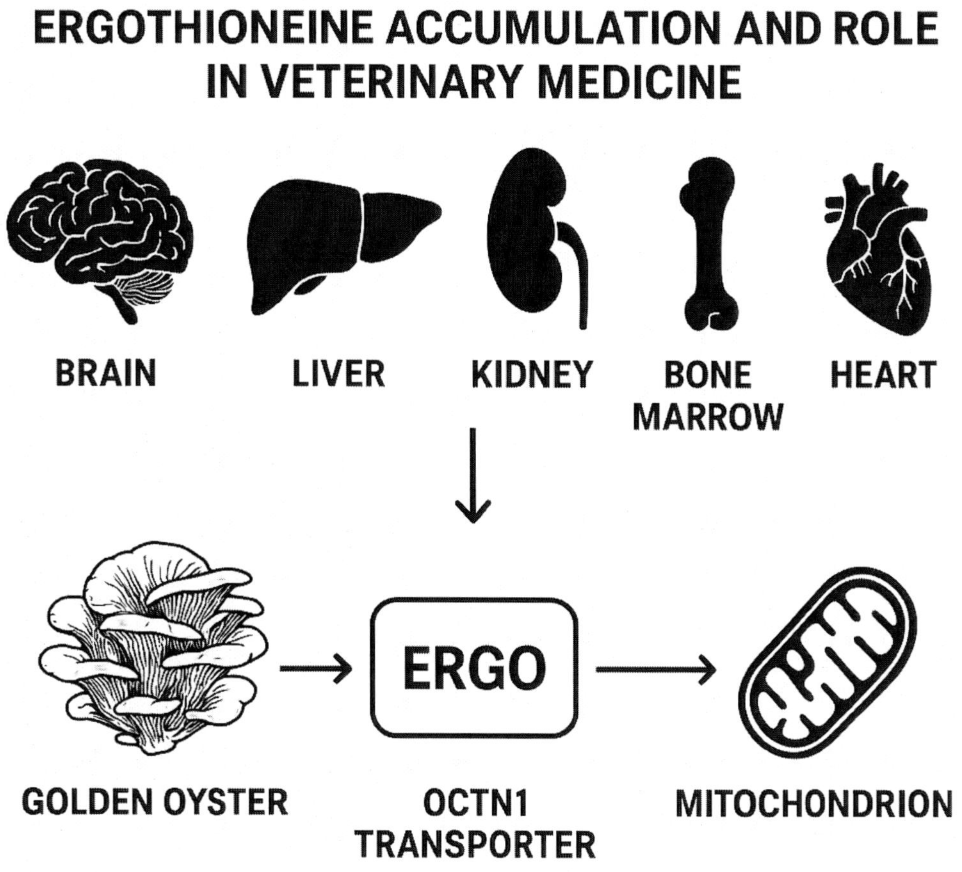

9

Livestock and Equine Health

INTRODUCTION

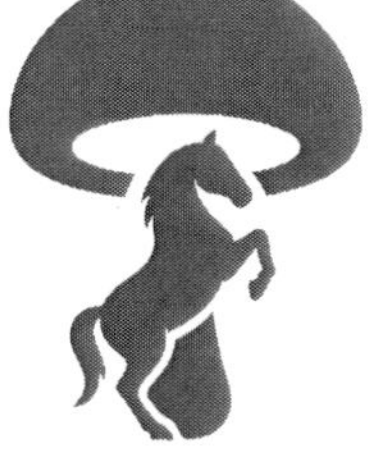

While functional mushrooms are now well established in companion-animal practice, their applications in equine and livestock health are expanding rapidly. As veterinary understanding of immunomodulation, gut-microbiome dynamics and oxidative stress deepens, mushrooms are emerging as safe, natural adjuncts for supporting performance, recovery and metabolic balance across species.

However, not all mushroom products are equivalent. Many equine and farm-animal supplements are made from myceliated grain rather than true fruiting-body extracts. These grain-based powders are dominated by alpha-glucans (starches) with relatively low levels of β-glucans and secondary metabolites, and their residual starch content may alter gut microbiota and metabolic control unfavourably in vulnerable animals.

In this guide, the focus is on full-spectrum fruiting-body extracts, produced via sub-critical water extraction (SCWE). This method preserves the whole biochemical matrix of the mushroom – β-glucans, triterpenes, polyphenols, ergothioneine, cordycepin and natural prebiotic fibre – without introducing grain-derived starches. These are the extract standards used in OMG Mushrooms formulations and form the basis for the Mycotherapy applications discussed in larger animals.

9.1 Applications in larger animals

9.1.1 Why use functional mushrooms in larger animals?

Functional mushrooms offer several cross-species benefits that are particularly relevant in equine and livestock practice.

Immune modulation and infection resilience

Mushroom β-glucans enhance macrophage and NK-cell activity in horses, pigs and poultry, contributing to more balanced immune responses against respiratory and enteric pathogens. Emerging reviews in veterinary literature describe improved immune markers and vaccine responsiveness in livestock and equines receiving Reishi- or Turkey Tail-derived polysaccharides.

Exercise recovery and oxidative stress

Cordyceps and Chaga extracts have been investigated for their capacity to reduce oxidative stress and post-exercise inflammatory markers in athletic animals. Pilot work in performance horses suggests that mushroom-enriched diets may support endurance, modulate muscle enzyme profiles and improve subjective recovery following intense training blocks.

Gut microbiome and nutrient utilisation

Turkey Tail and Maitake β-glucans support beneficial gut bacteria, increase short-chain fatty acid (SCFA) production and enhance gut-barrier function. Studies in pigs and cattle indicate that inclusion of mushroom polysaccharides can improve feed conversion efficiency, digestion and immune competence – outcomes that translate conceptually to equine and ruminant health.

Liver support and detoxification

Reishi and Shiitake triterpenes have demonstrated reductions in hepatic lipid accumulation and oxidative damage in large-animal models. Improvements in liver enzyme activity and reduced lipid peroxidation have been reported in swine supplemented with Ganoderma-based extracts, suggesting a role for mushrooms in metabolic and hepatoprotective support in production animals.

Stress adaptation and metabolic balance

Cordyceps and Maitake polysaccharides have been associated with modulation of cortisol and insulin pathways, supporting more stable stress and energy responses in working animals. Early evidence in horses under exercise stress points to reduced cortisol fluctuations and improved blood-glucose stability where mushroom supplementation is employed as part of a broader nutritional programme.

Although much of this work is preclinical or extrapolated from non-equine species, the mechanistic overlap is strong: immune modulation, oxidative balance, gut integrity, hepatic support and endocrine steadiness are central concerns across performance horses, breeding stock and intensively managed livestock.

> “Integrative medicine gives us more tools to help animals live healthier, longer lives.”
> *Source: Dr Gary Richter, DVM, The Ultimate Pet Health Guide (2017)*

9.1.2 Clinical relevance for integrative vets

For integrative veterinarians, functional mushrooms can:

- complement traditional care for performance horses, breeding animals and production livestock experiencing metabolic, inflammatory or infectious pressures
- provide terrain-focused support in immune-compromised or high-stress environments (transport, shows, intensive housing)
- enhance the value of vaccination and biosecurity programmes by supporting more competent immune responses
- offer non-antibiotic strategies for promoting gut and respiratory resilience in herd and flock settings

SCWE full-spectrum extracts are particularly suited to large animals, where digestive capacity, hindgut fermentation and variable microbiota can challenge absorption and consistency. By retaining both high-molecular-weight β-glucans and smaller secondary metabolites in a solvent-free format, SCWE extracts provide a predictable, pharmaconutrition-style tool for Mycotherapy in the paddock, stable or farm.

As with small animals, grain-based mycelium products are best avoided when seeking therapeutic outcomes. Their low β-glucan content and higher starch load are unlikely to deliver the desired immunological and metabolic benefits, and in insulin-dysregulated or laminitis-prone animals they may be counterproductive.

9.1.3 Equine Dosing Framework (SCWE Extracts)

General principles

Horses tolerate functional mushrooms well and metabolise polysaccharides efficiently. SCWE extracts allow lower-dose application due to higher concentration and improved solubility.

Baseline Equine Dosing

For a 500 kg horse:

Tier 1 (Wellness / Maintenance) - 2–4 g/day total mushroom extract (SCWE)

Tier 2 (Supportive / Metabolic / Inflammatory) - 4–7 g/day

Tier 3 (Intensive / Oncology / Chronic Immune Dysregulation) - 7–10 g/day *(Best under integrative veterinary supervision.)*

Notes

- Divide into 1–2 feeds
- Introduce gradually over 5–7 days
- Prioritise fruiting-body SCWE extracts (avoid myceliated grain)
- Adjust for metabolic status (EMS/PPID horses may benefit from the upper end of T2)
- **For laminitis, please see section 9.2 section**

9.2 Laminitis and Medicinal Mushrooms

Laminitis has been incorporated into this guide as an exception to the broader format because of its high prevalence in horses, its multifactorial systemic nature, and the emerging concern that myceliated-grain mushroom products - due to their residual starch and sugar content - may exacerbate metabolic instability in laminitic or insulin-dysregulated animals. Given the strong mechanistic overlap between laminitis pathophysiology and the documented actions of medicinal mushrooms, a focused Mycotherapy analysis is both clinically relevant and warranted.

Laminitis is a severe, multifactorial inflammatory disorder of the equine hoof laminae, often resulting in debilitating pain, lameness and long-term structural compromise. Modern understanding recognises laminitis not as a purely mechanical failure, but as a complex systemic syndrome involving chronic inflammation, dysregulated endocrine function, vascular disturbance, oxidative stress and gastrointestinal–immune imbalance. Within this framework, medicinal mushrooms provide a biologically plausible and clinically promising integrative adjunct. Their actions on inflammatory cytokines, insulin sensitivity, microcirculation, gut integrity and immune modulation mirror the central pathways responsible for laminitic pathology. While controlled equine trials are still lacking, the convergence of preclinical research, cross-species mechanistic evidence and growing veterinary anecdote supports the careful application of Mycotherapy as part of a laminitis strategy.

Anti-inflammatory and immunomodulatory actions

Persistent inflammation underlies laminar damage, pain and tissue breakdown. Across animal and mechanistic studies, medicinal mushrooms consistently demonstrate significant anti-inflammatory activity. Reishi (Ganoderma lucidum) contains triterpenoids with cortisone-like actions that reduce inflammatory signalling. Cordyceps species downregulate NF-κB expression and suppress pro-inflammatory cytokines such as TNF-α and IL-1β. Maitake, Lion's Mane and Agaricus blazei have been repeatedly shown to reduce oxidative stress and modulate both innate and adaptive immune responses.

These actions align directly with laminitis, where inflammatory mediators initiate laminar failure and amplify pain sensitivity. Integrative equine practitioners frequently report calmer inflammatory profiles and improved comfort in laminitis-prone horses receiving mushrooms such as Reishi, Turkey Tail and Shiitake. Dr Tom Schell, DVM, has described improved outcomes in horses with metabolic syndrome and laminitic tendencies when medicinal mushrooms were integrated into broader management - particularly in animals showing combined inflammatory and digestive fragility (anecdotal).

Metabolic modulation and insulin regulation

Endocrinopathic laminitis is strongly driven by hyperinsulinaemia and insulin resistance. Several mushrooms possess insulin-sensitising and glucose-regulating properties. Maitake polysaccharides (including D-fraction) enhance insulin receptor function and improve glycaemic balance. Reishi extracts reduce fasting glucose, improve endogenous insulin responses and counteract insulin resistance in rodent models. Ganoderma supplementation in high-fat-fed mice has prevented metabolic syndrome through modulation of the gut microbiota and improved glucose metabolism.

These mechanisms reinforce the relevance of Mycotherapy in horses with Equine Metabolic Syndrome (EMS) or Pituitary Pars Intermedia Dysfunction (PPID). Anecdotally, equine practitioners observe more stable metabolic behaviour, fewer laminitic relapses and improved weight regulation when Maitake, Reishi or multi-mushroom formulas are used. SCWE (sub-critical water extraction) strengthens this relevance: by retaining the full biochemical matrix - β-glucans, triterpenes, sterols, peptides and prebiotic fibre - SCWE provides high potency without the added starch present in myceliated-grain powders. For laminitic horses, where dietary sugar and starch must be minimised, avoiding grain-based mycelium is essential.

Vascular and microcirculatory relevance

Vascular dysfunction is a well-recognised contributor to laminitis. Hyperinsulinism can induce vasoconstriction and compromise digital blood flow, predisposing laminar tissues to ischaemia. Several mushrooms exert circulatory benefits that may support digital perfusion. Auricularia (wood ear mushroom) contains adenosine, a compound with vasodilatory, anti-thrombotic and anti-platelet-aggregating effects. Reishi displays mild anti-coagulant and vasomodulatory properties, and Cordyceps improves oxygen utilisation and peripheral circulation in animal models.

Although equine-specific vascular studies are unavailable, the pathways affected by these mushrooms - improved blood flow, reduced platelet aggregation, reduced oxidative vessel stress - are directly relevant to laminitis. Horse owners and integrative practitioners have anecdotally noted improved hoof warmth and steadier digital pulse quality in horses receiving mushrooms with circulatory influence.

Gut–immune–laminar interactions

The gastrointestinal microbiome and intestinal barrier play pivotal roles in laminitis. Grain overload, hindgut dysbiosis and endotoxin release can precipitate systemic inflammation and laminar injury. Mushrooms offer several supportive mechanisms in this domain. Pleurotus (oyster mushroom) exerts prebiotic and anti-inflammatory activity in the gut. Lion's Mane (Hericium erinaceus) enhances mucosal healing, supports epithelial repair and reduces oxidative stress in the gastrointestinal lining. Turkey Tail (Trametes versicolor) provides complex β-glucans and polysaccharopeptides that stabilise the gut–immune axis and support microbial balance.

These actions make mushrooms particularly suitable for horses with digestive fragility - a group at disproportionately high risk for laminitis. Practitioners report improvements in stool quality, reduced digestive sensitivity and more stable appetitive behaviour in horses receiving mushroom support. By strengthening the gut barrier and reducing endotoxin leakage, mushrooms may reduce the systemic inflammatory triggers that precipitate laminitic episodes.

Pre-clinical evidence and cross-species relevance

Although no equine clinical trials have evaluated mushrooms directly in laminitis, the preclinical literature is extensive and mechanistically relevant. Research indicates that medicinal mushrooms:

- reduce inflammatory cytokines and oxidative markers
- modulate insulin sensitivity and glucose transport
- improve lipid metabolism
- support microvascular stability and inhibit platelet aggregation
- repair gastrointestinal mucosa and modulate microbiota
- enhance mitochondrial function and metabolic resilience

These pathways correspond precisely to the multifactorial nature of laminitis.

Anecdotal equine experience

Within equine integrative medicine, medicinal mushrooms are increasingly used in horses with chronic laminitis, EMS-associated laminitic cycles, post-grain-overload instability and older horses with metabolic or gut sensitivities. Case impressions describe improved comfort, reduced flare frequency, steadier digital pulses and better metabolic consistency. European Mycotherapy practitioners routinely recommend combinations including Reishi, Maitake, Lion's Mane, Turkey Tail, Auricularia and Pleurotus for laminitis support.

Practical application in laminitis management

Medicinal mushrooms serve as adjunctive support within a holistic management plan that includes dietary carbohydrate restriction, weight control, appropriate farriery, cryotherapy, analgesia and endocrine stabilisation. In practice, mushrooms are provided as powdered whole fruiting bodies or SCWE extracts. Typical equine usage ranges from approximately 10–30 g daily of a combined multi-mushroom blend for a 500 kg horse, adjusted for concentration and clinical presentation. Horses generally tolerate mushrooms well, often requiring only a brief introduction period before reaching full dose.

A multi-mushroom approach is preferred due to the complementary actions of different species. A laminitis-supportive blend may include:

- **Reishi** – systemic immunomodulation, inflammatory control, hepatic support
- **Shiitake** – hepatic steadiness, mild antimicrobial support and gut balance
- **Maitake** – insulin sensitisation and metabolic regulation
- **Cordyceps** – vascular support, mitochondrial energy regulation and anti-inflammatory benefit
- **Lion's Mane** – gastrointestinal mucosal repair and gut–brain axis modulation
- **Pleurotus** – prebiotic fibre and gastrointestinal anti-inflammatory support
- **Agaricus blazei** – broad immunomodulation, particularly useful in horses with allergic or hyper-reactive immune tendencies
- **Auricularia** – microcirculation and anti-coagulant support

High-quality, whole-fruiting-body extracts are preferred. Myceliated-grain powders introduce starches that can destabilise metabolic conditions and are therefore inappropriate for laminitis-prone horses. Consistency of use is essential: mushrooms act as metabolic and immunological tonics, with improvements emerging gradually over weeks, although some horses show early changes in comfort or digestive steadiness.

Mushrooms are not a replacement for conventional care during an acute laminitis episode but are used alongside established therapies to support systemic regulation. Long-term, they may also contribute to prevention in high-risk horses by stabilising metabolic pathways, supporting gut integrity and moderating inflammatory and oxidative load.

Safety considerations

Medicinal mushrooms are generally safe for equine use. Precautions include monitoring in horses with known fungal allergies, and awareness of mild anti-coagulant effects in species such as Auricularia and Reishi. Introducing each mushroom slowly helps identify sensitivities, and monitoring insulin and glucose dynamics is advisable in Equine Metabolic Syndrome (EMS) or Pituitary Pars Intermedia Dysfunction (PPID) horses.

Conclusion

In summary, while conventional therapy remains paramount for laminitis, medicinal mushrooms offer a promising complementary approach grounded in anti-inflammatory, metabolic, circulatory and gut-supportive mechanisms. Modern research confirms that mushrooms such as Reishi, Maitake, Cordyceps, Lion's Mane, Shiitake and others contain bioactive compounds that reduce inflammatory cytokines, enhance insulin sensitivity, improve circulation and support gut health - all of which counteract the fundamental pathways involved in laminitis. Equine practitioners and herbalists are increasingly incorporating Mycotherapy to quell inflammation, support metabolic control and strengthen immune resilience during laminitic recovery. Though controlled equine trials are still forthcoming, the strength of preclinical evidence and the positive anecdotal outcomes provide a compelling rationale for integrating medicinal mushrooms into laminitis protocols.

Medicinal mushrooms align with a 'whole-horse' approach, supporting not just the hoof but the entire metabolic and immune terrain of the animal. They reinforce regeneration, strengthen immune competence and moderate the systemic pressures that drive laminitis. Future equine-specific studies will deepen understanding, but current knowledge suggests that mushrooms offer a meaningful, biologically grounded tool in reducing laminitis incidence and supporting horses on their path to recovery.

9.3 Overall Summary

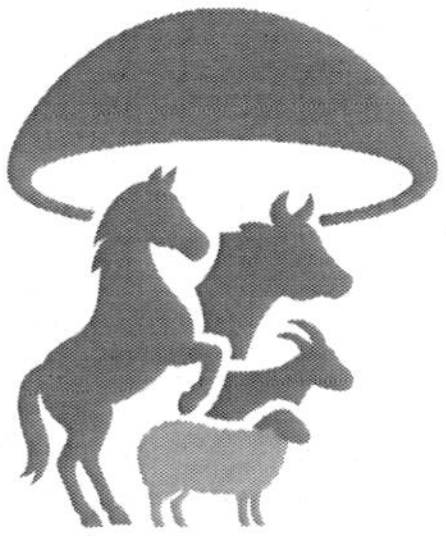

Functional mushrooms are not confined to small-animal practice. Their role in equine and livestock health is supported by an emerging body of international research demonstrating improved performance, metabolic stability, immune competence and oxidative resilience in a range of species. Within this context, ganoderma-, turkey tail-, maitake-, cordyceps- and pleurotus-based extracts provide integrative vets with flexible tools for supporting the health of performance horses, breeding animals and production herds.

With SCWE full-spectrum extracts, practitioners can extend Mycotherapy beyond the clinic to larger animals while maintaining the same standards of purity, efficacy and biochemical integrity that underpin functional mushroom use in companion animals. In high-risk equine cases such as laminitis, attention to product quality and avoidance of myceliated-grain powders is critical, ensuring that therapeutic Mycotherapy supports, rather than challenges, metabolic and vascular stability.

> " Nature provides us with remarkable tools for healing - our job is to recognise and use them wisely. *Source: The Royal Treatment (2013) Dr Barbara Royal, DVM, CVA* "

9.4 Research

1. Influence of *Ganoderma lucidum* on Blood Biochemistry and Immunocompetence in Horses

In one of the earliest controlled equine trials, *Ganoderma lucidum* supplementation was found to be safe and to significantly enhance immune responsiveness. Horses receiving *G. lucidum* showed elevated percentages of CD5(+), CD4(+), and CD8(+) T-lymphocytes and produced higher antibody titres following antigen challenge. The study demonstrated that Reishi may augment both cell-mediated and humoral immunity without adverse effects on haematology or serum biochemistry - supporting its use as an equine immune modulator.

2. Biological Effects of β-D-Glucans from Natural Sources on Equine Health (2025)

This review highlights the role of β-glucans - including those derived from mushrooms, improving equine immune competence, gut microbiota composition, and overall health. The paper outlines how β-glucan supplementation modulates inflammatory pathways, enhances vaccine response, and supports recovery in performance horses. It provides a scientific rationale for integrating mushroom-derived polysaccharides within equine nutrition and veterinary protocols.

3. Effects of *Ganoderma lucidum* Fermentation Products on Growth and Immunocompetence in Weanling Pigs

Feeding *G. lucidum* fermentation products to piglets improved growth rates, nutrient utilisation, and immune responses. The supplemented group exhibited higher antibody titres against pseudorabies, reduced blood glucose, and increased lymphocyte proliferation. These outcomes indicate that Reishi-derived β-glucans can enhance resilience and immune system maturity in young pigs during post-weaning stress, suggesting promising applications for herd health management.

4. *Ganoderma lucidum* Powder and Immunity in Broiler Chickens

A controlled study in broiler chickens compared basal diets, antibiotic growth promoters, and *G. lucidum* powder. Birds receiving 0.2 % *G. lucidum* showed improved weight gain, feed conversion, and gut microbiota balance, with increased lactic-acid bacteria and thymus weight. Unlike antibiotic controls, mushroom supplementation did not suppress immunoglobulin levels. These findings support *G. lucidum* as a natural, non-antibiotic feed additive for immune and gut health in poultry.

9.4.1 Key Sources (Medicinal Mushrooms and Laminitis)

Hetland et al. (2021); Paterson (2008); Chen et al. (2019); Chang et al. (2015); Konno et al. (2002); Diling et al. (2019); Jayakumar et al. (2006); Boh et al. (2007); Standish et al. (2012); Brennan & Gormally (2018); Schell (2017); Patterson-Kane & Karikoski (2019).

SECTION FOUR

Extended Insights for Veterinary Practice

Extended chapters exploring each mushroom in depth

Functional mushrooms have long held a place in traditional healing systems; however, modern chemistry and veterinary physiology now reveal the full complexity of their actions. While the 'Clinical Briefs' in Section 3 provide concise, practitioner-ready summaries, the extended chapters explore each mushroom species in far greater depth – examining their taxonomy, biochemical architecture and the mechanistic pathways through which they influence immune, metabolic, neurological and gastrointestinal health. These chapters are designed to give veterinarians a scientific foundation for understanding how and why medicinal mushrooms exert their effects across multiple physiological systems.

Each profile integrates historical usage, contemporary research and veterinary relevance. Detailed descriptions of β-glucans, triterpenes, phenolics, diterpenes, polysaccharopeptides and other bioactive compounds help contextualise their clinical significance. Mechanistic pathways such as cytokine modulation, oxidative balance, mitochondrial support, autonomic regulation and microbiome interactions are explained with reference to current peer-reviewed studies. For practitioners managing complex or chronic cases, this depth of understanding supports more precise therapeutic reasoning and more confident formulation decisions.

Practical considerations specific to veterinary practice, including extraction methodology, the importance of fruiting-body integrity, dose reasoning, safety cautions and species variability across dogs, cats, horses and livestock are provided. Where relevant, the profiles highlight emerging areas of research, unresolved questions and future directions that may influence how functional mushrooms are integrated into veterinary care... Together, these extended chapters provide the scientific foundation of this guide and serve as a reference for practitioners seeking an evidence-supported understanding of medicinal mushrooms in Mycotherapy for animals.

> "Fungi make worlds, digest worlds, and bind worlds together. *Source: Entangled Life (2020) Merlin Sheldrake, PhD*"

1

REISHI (Ganoderma lucidum)

1.1 Introduction to Reishi – *The Calming Guardian / Mushroom of Immortality*

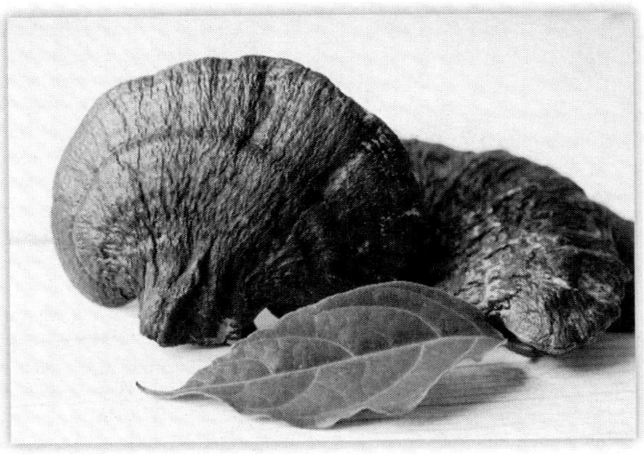

Reishi (Ganoderma lucidum), long celebrated in East Asian medical traditions as the 'mushroom of spiritual potency, mushroom of immortality and the calming mushroom,' a symbol of vitality and longevity, represents one of the oldest continuously used medicinal fungi. In classical Chinese medical texts, Reishi was regarded as a sovereign tonic capable of nourishing qi, strengthening the lungs, calming the spirit (shen) and promoting long life. Although these descriptions were articulated in human terms, Reishi was also used for working animals, including horses and hunting dogs, to enhance stamina, calm agitation and support recovery from exertion.

In modern Mycotherapy, Reishi occupies a unique therapeutic space where immune regulation, neuroendocrine balance, hepatic protection and stress resilience intersect. It is neither a stimulant nor a suppressive agent; rather, it works by restoring physiological equilibrium. This property makes it particularly relevant for animals whose conditions arise from chronic inflammatory load, oxidative stress, environmental pressures, ageing or long-term medication.

Contemporary biochemical research has identified a broad range of constituents that underpin Reishi's traditional reputation, including β-glucans, proteoglucans, terpenes, triterpenoid acids, sterols, polyphenols and peptide–glycan complexes. These compounds influence multiple systems simultaneously, giving Reishi its characteristic profile as a whole-system modulator. For veterinary clinicians, this means Reishi is not confined to isolated symptom categories but instead contributes to foundational terrain support, improving resilience, metabolic stability and immune vigilance across species.

Reishi's therapeutic actions accumulate gradually. It is rarely used for acute intervention but shines in chronic care, senior care, behavioural dysregulation, chronic inflammation and integrative oncology. Its value lies in promoting the steady recovery of balance, enabling the animal's internal systems to function with less friction and greater stability.

1.2 Taxonomy, Morphology and Extract Science

Ganoderma lucidum represents a complex species aggregate rather than a single uniform organism. The name 'Reishi' is frequently applied to multiple species, including G. lucidum, G. lingzhi and G. tsugae, each with distinct triterpene signatures and morphological characteristics. This taxonomic variability has direct clinical implications because the therapeutic properties associated with Reishi arise predominantly from the dense, lacquered fruiting body rather than mycelium.

Commercial supplements formed from mycelium grown on grain are chemically distinct from true fruiting body extracts. Grain-grown mycelium contains elevated starch, reduced β-glucan levels and lacks the full triterpene spectrum responsible for many of Reishi's most clinically relevant actions. In veterinary Mycotherapy, where dosing must be accurate and consistent, fruiting body extracts are therefore essential.

The fruiting body is exceptionally tough and woody, a feature that reflects the density of its chitin–glucan matrix and the concentration of bound triterpenes. Traditional preparations required prolonged decoction to extract these compounds. Modern extraction techniques vary widely in their capacity to capture Reishi's full biochemical profile. Alcohol extracts disproportionately emphasise lipophilic triterpenes but lose polysaccharides. Hot-water extracts favour polysaccharides but neglect important triterpenes and sterols.

Sub-critical water extraction (SCWE) offers a superior solution for veterinary use because it extracts both hydrophilic and lipophilic compounds without solvents, yielding a full-spectrum preparation that preserves natural fibre, proteoglucans, triterpenes, polyphenols and sterols in physiologically appropriate ratios. This method retains the structural matrix that underpins Reishi's broad regulatory action, making SCWE extracts particularly suitable for long-term use in companion animals.

In veterinary Mycotherapy, extract fidelity is critically important. Full-spectrum SCWE preparations maintain the mushroom's natural biochemical ecology, including polysaccharides, triterpenes, proteoglucans, minor sterols and the native prebiotic fibre that shapes gut–immune communication. By avoiding the compositional distortion associated with dual-extraction tinctures and grain-grown mycelium products, SCWE provides a physiologically coherent extract that more faithfully reflects the complexity of the whole fruiting body. For clinical use, particularly in chronic inflammatory, gastrointestinal or hepatic conditions, this structural fidelity offers a practical advantage by aligning closely with the biological pathways upon which Reishi's therapeutic effects depend.

> In modern Mycotherapy, Reishi occupies a unique therapeutic space where immune regulation, neuroendocrine balance, hepatic protection and stress resilience intersect.

1.3 Bioactive Constituents – Mechanistic Relevance to Veterinary Physiology

Reishi's therapeutic breadth reflects the extraordinary complexity of its bioactive matrix. Unlike narrow-acting botanicals whose benefits can be attributed to a single dominant compound, Reishi expresses a multi-layered pharmacology in which polysaccharides, triterpenes, proteoglucans, sterols and antioxidant molecules converge to produce broad regulatory effects. This biochemical diversity explains why Reishi consistently influences immunity, inflammation, hepatic function, respiratory stability, behavioural calm and tissue resilience across species. Understanding these constituents in depth reveals how Reishi interfaces with veterinary physiology and why whole-mushroom SCWE extracts offer a more coherent therapeutic representation of its natural mechanisms.

The β-glucans and proteoglucans present in Reishi are central to its immunological influence. These compounds interact with pattern-recognition receptors including Dectin-1, Toll-like receptor 2 (TLR-2) and complement receptor 3 (CR3), priming macrophages, neutrophils and dendritic cells for more effective surveillance. Thus, this priming does not provoke inflammatory excess but instead improves recognition accuracy and response calibration. In practical terms, animals exhibit more efficient pathogen defence while maintaining a calm inflammatory baseline. Proteoglucans contribute an additional layer of modulation by shaping cytokine tone and supporting steady-state immune balance within the gastrointestinal tract, respiratory system and peripheral tissues.

Reishi's triterpenes form a second major pharmacological pillar. These compounds, including the ganoderic and lucidenic acid groups, are responsible for many of Reishi's hallmark clinical actions. They moderate nuclear factor kappa B (NF-kB) signalling, inhibit cyclo-oxygenase 2 (COX-2) and inducible nitric oxide synthase (iNOS), and reduce production of key inflammatory cytokines such as interleukin 6 (IL-6), tumour necrosis factor alpha (TNF-α) and interleukin 1 beta (IL-1β). This is particularly relevant for animals with chronic dermatitis, airway inflammation, musculoskeletal discomfort or gastrointestinal reactivity. Triterpenes also influence mast-cell behaviour by reducing histamine release and stabilising hyperresponsive tissue environments, an action that complements clinical management of allergies, pruritus and chronic inflammatory skin conditions. Beyond these regulatory roles, triterpenes exhibit anti-fibrotic properties through attenuation of stellate-cell activation and demonstrate anti-angiogenic effects that contribute to their value in supportive oncology. These findings are predominantly preclinical, but they present a consistent mechanistic pattern that aligns closely with long-standing traditional use.

Sterols, including ergosterol and related molecules, contribute supportive rather than primary actions. They interface with cellular membrane stability, assist lipid regulation and may provide modest benefits to cardiovascular efficiency in dogs, horses and senior animals experiencing metabolic strain. While their influence is subtler than that of triterpenes or polysaccharides, their presence completes the broader biochemical profile that gives Reishi its tonic reputation.

Reishi also contains a wide array of phenolic compounds and antioxidant peptides. These molecules protect cellular membranes, stabilise mitochondrial function, reduce lipid peroxidation and prevent the accumulation of oxidative injury common in ageing, chronic illness or prolonged medication use. Their actions complement Reishi's anti-inflammatory pathways and provide tissue-level resilience in senior or medically vulnerable animals. When extracted via SCWE, these antioxidant compounds remain embedded within the natural fibre matrix, preserving the synergistic interaction that supports gastrointestinal integrity and immune signalling.

Peptide–glycan complexes round out Reishi's bioactive network. Their dual influence on immunological modulation and antioxidant efficiency reinforces the mushroom's whole-system orientation, providing broad but gentle support that suits the long-term integrative strategies used in veterinary practice. Collectively, these constituents explain why Reishi operates not as a stimulant or suppressant but as a regulator of physiological balance, restoring steady-state function across multiple biological domains.

> Reishi's therapeutic breadth reflects the extraordinary complexity of its bioactive matrix.

1.4 Immune System Modulation

Reishi's reputation as an immune regulator is firmly established within both traditional medicine and modern research. Unlike agents that provoke sharp immunostimulatory cascades, Reishi exerts a measured, cumulative effect that enhances immune vigilance while simultaneously preventing unnecessary inflammatory escalation. This distinction is crucial in veterinary practice, where many chronic diseases involve a combination of low-grade inflammation, immune fatigue or inappropriate hypersensitivity rather than simple immune weakness. Reishi's immunological influence is guided by regulatory intelligence rather than brute stimulation, making it suitable for long-term use in animals with chronic conditions, age-related decline or stress-associated immune disturbance.

The primary influence on innate immunity arises from the activity of Reishi's β-glucans, which prime macrophages and dendritic cells for more effective recognition of pathogens and cellular debris. This priming does not overstimulate; instead, it enhances the ability of sentinel immune cells to respond appropriately to microbial or inflammatory challenges. In canine research, dietary supplementation with Ganoderma lucidum has been associated with improved phagocytic function and increased expression of major histocompatibility complex class II (MHC-II), a marker of enhanced antigen-presenting capacity. These findings, though modest in scale, reinforce the practical clinical use of Reishi for animals experiencing recurrent infections, immune exhaustion, slow recovery from illness or the normal decline in surveillance capacity that accompanies ageing.

Beyond the innate branch, Reishi influences adaptive immune dynamics in a manner that promotes equilibrium across T-helper (Th1 and Th2) responses and enhances regulatory T-cell activity. Preclinical studies consistently show that Reishi reduces excessive Th2 signalling, which is frequently associated with allergic disease, while supporting a more balanced Th1 profile. This recalibration is particularly beneficial in animals with atopic tendencies, chronic respiratory sensitivities or gastrointestinal inflammation driven by immune imbalance. Rather than suppressing immune overactivity, Reishi smooths the oscillations between over- and under-reactive states, allowing the system to respond with greater precision.

A key aspect of Reishi's contribution to allergic and inflammatory conditions stems from the behaviour of its triterpenes, which stabilise mast cells and reduce histamine release. Chronic pruritus, dermatological flare cycles and inflammatory skin patterns often involve mast-cell hyperreactivity, and Reishi's moderating effect can reduce the intensity and frequency of these episodes. Integrative veterinarians frequently observe calmer, more predictable skin responses when Reishi is introduced alongside appropriate nutritional, dermatological or environmental interventions.

Reishi also plays an important role in supporting immune resilience in older animals. Immunosenescence is characterised by diminished natural killer (NK)-cell activity, reduced adaptive sensitivity and declining regulatory function. Reishi's polysaccharides and triterpenes help restore immune tone in this context, offering a level of support that may translate into improved vitality, cleaner recovery from mild infections, steadier inflammatory patterns and improved appetite or energy. While these findings are based largely on preclinical research and practitioner observation, the convergence of evidence supports Reishi's tonic role in senior care.

Clinical nuance remains important. While Reishi's actions are primarily regulatory, animals with complex autoimmune disease or those receiving immunosuppressive medications require careful monitoring. In most cases, the modulating influence is beneficial, but adjustments may be necessary to avoid unintended interaction with prescribed therapies. For the majority of companion animals, however, Reishi's balanced influence on immunity offers a reliable and gentle means of supporting long-term physiological resilience.

> Reishi's reputation as an immune regulator is firmly established within both traditional medicine and modern research.

1.5 Inflammation and Oxidative Stress Pathways

Chronic inflammation and oxidative stress lie at the centre of many clinical presentations in small-animal and equine practice, from dermatitis and degenerative joint disease to chronic enteropathies, hepatic burden and long-term pharmacological exposure. Reishi exerts a broad regulatory influence across these processes, not by suppressing inflammation outright but by modulating the molecular signals that sustain inflammatory cycles. Its actions are multi-layered, involving triterpenes, polysaccharides, antioxidant compounds and fibre-bound complexes that collectively recalibrate inflammatory tone and restore physiological steadiness.

A principal mechanism underpinning Reishi's anti-inflammatory effect is the inhibition of nuclear factor kappa B (NF-kB). Ganoderic acids prevent the degradation of NF-kB's inhibitory proteins, thereby reducing downstream transcription of pro-inflammatory cytokines such as tumour necrosis factor alpha (TNF-α), interleukin 1 beta (IL-1β) and interleukin 6 (IL-6). This pathway has been consistently documented in preclinical models and provides a compelling explanation for Reishi's ability to calm persistent inflammatory behaviour across dermatological, gastrointestinal and musculoskeletal systems. In practice, animals with chronic skin irritation, relapsing gut inflammation or ongoing tissue discomfort often exhibit steadier inflammatory patterns after sustained Reishi supplementation.

Reishi also acts upon enzymatic drivers of inflammation. Its triterpenes suppress cyclo-oxygenase 2 (COX-2) and inducible nitric oxide synthase (iNOS), reducing the biochemical mediators that contribute to tissue irritation, swelling and inflammatory pain. These pathways are relevant to chronic joint discomfort, soft-tissue inflammation and airway hyperreactivity, conditions in which oxidative load and inflammatory mediators maintain a cycle of discomfort. Although Reishi does not replace NSAIDs or other anti-inflammatory medications, its regulatory influence can complement medical therapy and help reduce the amplitude of inflammatory flare episodes.

Another hallmark of Reishi's profile is its effect on mast cells and histamine-mediated responses. The triterpene fraction stabilises mast cells and reduces the release of histamine and related mediators. This is particularly important in companion animals with environmental allergies, food sensitivities or mixed allergic–inflammatory syndromes. By moderating mast-cell reactivity rather than suppressing it pharmacologically, Reishi encourages a calmer baseline response to environmental triggers. Integrative practitioners often observe reduced pruritus intensity, fewer flare triggers and steadier skin comfort when Reishi is incorporated into chronic dermatological support plans.

Reishi's antioxidant influence reinforces its anti-inflammatory actions. Chronic inflammation generates oxidative stress, which in turn perpetuates inflammatory signalling. Reishi interrupts this cycle by increasing the activity of endogenous antioxidant enzymes such as superoxide dismutase, catalase and glutathione peroxidase. These preclinical findings translate clinically into improved resilience for senior animals, working dogs and those with chronic inflammatory or metabolic burden. Reduced oxidative load is reflected in improvements in coat quality, stamina, behavioural steadiness and recovery after exertion or illness.

Mitochondrial protection forms an additional layer of support. Reishi reduces lipid peroxidation, maintains mitochondrial membrane integrity and improves energy efficiency at the cellular level. These actions are particularly relevant in ageing animals or those recovering from systemic inflammation, where mitochondrial decline can contribute to reduced stamina, cognitive fatigue or persistent inflammatory behaviour. Many clinicians note an increase in vitality and stamina in older dogs when Reishi is used consistently over several weeks.

Reishi may also exert anti-fibrotic effects. Preclinical studies show inhibition of stellate-cell activation and reduced collagen deposition in hepatic tissue, with emerging evidence suggesting similar actions in pulmonary pathways. These mechanisms carry significance for animals with chronic liver strain or respiratory inflammation, where fibrosis contributes to long-term functional decline. Although these findings are early, they align with Reishi's long-standing traditional use for liver and respiratory support and offer promising avenues for integrative care.

When extracted using Sub-critical water extraction, Reishi preserves the broad matrix of triterpenes, polysaccharides and antioxidant molecules required for these anti-inflammatory and antioxidant actions. SCWE preparations maintain the fibre-bound compounds that influence gut–immune communication and systemic inflammatory stability, offering a whole-food extract whose structure more closely reflects the mushroom's natural regulatory complexity.

In summary, Reishi addresses inflammation and oxidative stress not through isolated suppression but through systemic recalibration. By modulating cytokine signalling, stabilising mast-cell behaviour, enhancing antioxidant capacity and supporting mitochondrial health, Reishi provides a gentle yet comprehensive tool for long-term management of chronic inflammatory and oxidative conditions in veterinary practice.

> Reishi addresses inflammation and oxidative stress not through isolated suppression but through systemic recalibration.

1.6 Gastrointestinal, Microbiome and Metabolic Health

The gastrointestinal tract represents both a digestive organ and one of the body's most active immunological interfaces. In dogs and cats, a significant proportion of immune cells reside along the mucosal surface, where antigen sampling, microbial dialogue and inflammatory signalling shape systemic health. Reishi exerts a meaningful influence across this landscape through its polysaccharides, proteoglucans, fibre-bound complexes, triterpenes and antioxidant compounds, each contributing to a more stable and resilient gastrointestinal environment. Its actions are neither rapid nor suppressive; instead, they unfold gradually, supporting the restoration of mucosal balance, microbial diversity and metabolic steadiness in animals prone to chronic gastrointestinal disturbance.

Reishi's effects on gastrointestinal inflammation are among its most well-documented preclinical actions and hold particular relevance for veterinary medicine. Chronic enteropathies, dietary sensitivities and immune-mediated colitis frequently involve persistent up-regulation of inflammatory cascades, many of which are modulated by Reishi's triterpenes. Numerous laboratory models show inhibition of nuclear factor kappa B, reduced expression of interleukin 6, tumour necrosis factor alpha and interleukin 1 beta, and the suppression of inducible nitric oxide synthase and cyclo-oxygenase 2. These shifts help calm mucosal irritation and limit oxidative injury to the epithelial surface. In experimental colitis, Reishi extracts have been shown to normalise tissue architecture and reduce inflammatory infiltration, findings that mirror clinical impressions from integrative veterinarians who observe improved stool consistency, fewer flare episodes and greater comfort in animals with chronic gastrointestinal sensitivities receiving Reishi as part of a broader management plan.

The stability of the gut barrier is critical to gastrointestinal and systemic health, particularly in animals with chronic inflammation, allergic disease or hepatic burden. Oxidative stress contributes to increased intestinal permeability, disrupting tight-junction integrity and allowing translocation of endotoxin and other metabolites into the portal circulation. Reishi's antioxidant peptides and polyphenols help counter this process by reducing lipid peroxidation and supporting the activity of endogenous antioxidant enzymes along the mucosal lining. Its polysaccharide and proteoglucan fractions also play a role in maintaining epithelial resilience, supporting tighter junctional structure and reducing the cyclical inflammatory load that accompanies chronic permeability dysfunction. Though veterinary-specific studies remain limited, the mechanistic basis for these actions is well supported in rodent models and in vitro systems, and aligns closely with the improvements often noted by clinicians after several weeks of consistent Mycotherapy.

A central component of Reishi's influence on the gastrointestinal system lies in its prebiotic activity. Full-spectrum preparations produced through SCWE retain the mushroom's native fibre matrix, including indigestible polysaccharides that nourish beneficial microbes and promote the production of short-chain fatty acids such as butyrate. These fatty acids provide fuel for colonocytes, support intestinal barrier function, reduce local inflammation and interact with the gut–immune axis in ways that influence systemic immunity. Research in canine nutrition demonstrates that medicinal mushroom supplementation can increase microbial richness and beneficial taxa without compromising nutrient digestibility. While these studies utilised mixed mushroom formulations rather than Reishi alone, the polysaccharide composition of Reishi supports similar expectations. By enhancing microbial balance, Reishi contributes not only to gastrointestinal comfort but also to wider metabolic and immune stability, reflecting the bidirectional communication between gut flora and systemic physiology.

The gut–liver axis provides another important justification for Reishi's use in chronic gastrointestinal disease. Dysbiosis, intestinal permeability and mucosal inflammation increase hepatic load by allowing inflammatory mediators and bacterial metabolites to enter the portal circulation. Reishi's combined effects on the gut barrier, microbial ecology and inflammatory tone can help reduce this burden, offering secondary hepatic support in animals with chronic enteropathy, toxin exposure or long-term medication use. Its influence on metabolic regulation further reinforces this connection. Preclinical models show improved glucose tolerance, reduced lipid accumulation and enhanced insulin sensitivity following Reishi supplementation, suggesting a modulatory effect on metabolic pathways commonly disrupted in overweight, senior or endocrine-disordered animals. These findings provide mechanistic plausibility for the clinical impression that Reishi supports metabolic steadiness and energy consistency in animals with overlapping gastrointestinal and metabolic conditions.

Reishi also appears to exert a stabilising influence on appetite, nausea and digestive comfort. Many integrative practitioners note that animals experiencing chronic stress, inflammatory disease or oncology treatment show steadier eating habits and less episodic nausea when Reishi is incorporated into their care plan. These effects likely arise from its combined anti-inflammatory and antioxidant actions within the gastrointestinal tract, as well as its broader regulatory influence on the hypothalamic–pituitary–adrenal axis, mitochondrial function and inflammatory signalling. Improvements tend to emerge gradually rather than acutely, reflecting Reishi's slow-building, cumulative nature.

In clinical practice, Reishi is rarely used as a stand-alone intervention for gastrointestinal disorders. It performs best as part of a comprehensive plan informed by diagnostic assessment, dietary adjustments, stress reduction, appropriate medical therapy and, where suitable, additional Mycotherapy support such as Lion's Mane, Shiitake or Turkey Tail. Its cumulative regulatory nature means that benefits are usually seen over two to six weeks, as mucosal stability improves, microbial ecosystems rebalance and inflammatory cascades settle. The objective is not to suppress symptoms but to rebuild gastrointestinal resilience through balanced modulation of inflammation, oxidative stress and microbial ecology.

Reishi's role in gastrointestinal, microbiome and metabolic health embodies its broader identity as a whole-system modulator. By supporting mucosal integrity, encouraging beneficial microbial patterns, calming inflammatory activation and assisting hepatic–metabolic balance, it helps create a more stable internal environment for recovery. This positions Reishi as a valuable tool in the long-term management of chronic enteropathies, mixed gastrointestinal–allergic syndromes, stress-related digestive patterns and metabolic conditions with a gastrointestinal component. When delivered as a full-spectrum, fibre-retaining SCWE extract, its prebiotic, immunological and antioxidant contributions are maintained in a form most compatible with physiological processes, offering animals gentle, sustained and clinically meaningful support.

> Reishi's effects on gastrointestinal inflammation are among its most well-documented preclinical actions and hold particular relevance for veterinary medicine.

1.7. Cardiovascular and Respiratory Physiology

Reishi has a long-standing reputation as a tonic for both the cardiovascular and respiratory systems, a view deeply rooted in traditional East Asian medicine. Although the historic language of qi, vitality and lung nourishment differs from contemporary biomedical terminology, modern research provides compelling mechanistic parallels. The triterpenes, sterols, polysaccharides and antioxidant compounds found in Ganoderma lucidum exert demonstrable effects on vascular tone, endothelial function, lipid metabolism, airway smooth muscle and respiratory inflammatory pathways. These actions are particularly relevant for senior animals, performance animals, those exposed to chronic environmental irritants and individuals experiencing low-grade cardiopulmonary strain associated with age or systemic disease.

Reishi supports cardiovascular function through several complementary mechanisms. In preclinical studies, ganoderic acids and related sterols promote vasodilation by influencing nitric oxide availability and improving endothelial responsiveness. These effects encourage smoother vascular tone and may reduce peripheral resistance, thereby supporting more efficient circulation. While controlled veterinary trials are limited, these mechanistic findings align with the experiences of integrative practitioners who report improved stamina, better exercise tolerance and more stable recovery patterns in older dogs or working animals supplemented with Reishi. Such observations remain anecdotal but are consistent across multiple practitioners and species.

Reishi also contributes to cardiovascular stability via its influence on lipid metabolism. In animal models, Reishi supplementation has been associated with reductions in total cholesterol and triglycerides, alongside improved regulation of sterol pathways. These outcomes are thought to arise from its combined effects on hepatic function, reduced oxidative stress and modulation of metabolic enzyme activity. Although dogs and cats differ from humans in their susceptibility to atherosclerotic change, dyslipidaemia does occur in overweight animals, in endocrine disorders or in metabolic inflammation. In such contexts, Reishi's lipid-modulating and hepatoprotective actions may help reduce metabolic burden and support overall vitality.

One of the most clinically relevant aspects of Reishi's cardiovascular influence is its antioxidant protection of cardiac tissue. The heart is highly vulnerable to oxidative injury due to its continuous metabolic demand. Reishi's phenolic antioxidants, triterpenes and peptide complexes reduce oxidative stress within cardiomyocytes and support mitochondrial integrity. Preclinical studies consistently demonstrate enhanced mitochondrial stability and reduced oxidative markers in cardiac tissue following Ganoderma supplementation. These findings have clear translational relevance for senior pets with age-related cardiac workload, performance dogs requiring increased oxygen utilisation and animals experiencing chronic inflammatory conditions that exert secondary strain on cardiovascular tissues.

> One of the most clinically relevant aspects of Reishi's cardiovascular influence is its antioxidant protection of cardiac tissue.

In animals with early or subclinical cardiac compromise, for example dogs with low-grade murmurs or cats with mild hypertrophic changes, Reishi may provide gentle supportive benefit by reducing inflammatory and oxidative load. It is not a primary cardiac therapy and should never be used as a replacement for essential pharmacological intervention, but its regulatory influence may complement conventional management. Caution is advisable in animals receiving antihypertensives or vasodilators, since mild additive effects are theoretically possible, although such interactions remain largely theoretical rather than clinically documented.

Reishi's relevance to respiratory physiology reflects a similarly multi-layered profile. In traditional medicine, it was regarded as a 'lung tonic', used to ease breathing, strengthen respiratory endurance and calm cough. Modern research provides plausible explanations for these observations. Several triterpenes modulate airway smooth muscle and promote bronchodilation, improving airflow and reducing respiratory tension. Preclinical studies demonstrate reduced airway resistance and improved oxygen utilisation following Ganoderma extract administration, findings that may be clinically relevant for brachycephalic dogs experiencing chronic airway strain, athletic dogs working at high respiratory load or older animals with reduced pulmonary compliance.

Inflammatory regulation within respiratory tissue provides a second key mechanism. Reishi suppresses cyclo-oxygenase 2 (COX-2), inducible nitric oxide synthase (iNOS) and pro-inflammatory cytokines such as interleukin 6 (IL-6) and tumour necrosis factor alpha (TNF-α). These findings support Reishi's inclusion in animals with chronic environmental allergies, respiratory hypersensitivity or inflammatory airway patterns. While controlled veterinary respiratory trials remain limited, integrative practitioners frequently report calmer breathing patterns, reduced cough sensitivity and improved respiratory comfort in animals receiving Reishi as part of broader multimodal care.

A further relevant mechanism is Reishi's influence on mucosal immune activity within the respiratory system. The β-glucans and proteoglucans present in full-spectrum extracts interact with immune cells at the respiratory interface, supporting appropriate responses to inhaled antigens and reducing excessive inflammatory reactivity. This influence dovetails with Reishi's mast-cell stabilising properties, helping to reduce histamine-driven airway irritation in sensitive animals. Such effects are particularly useful in animals with recurrent allergic airway disease, chronic upper respiratory inflammation or mixed dermatological–respiratory allergic syndromes.

These actions position Reishi as a supportive adjunct in a range of cardiovascular and respiratory contexts. It is not a replacement for bronchodilators, cardiac medications or essential diagnostic evaluation but rather a background regulator that enhances tissue resilience and inflammatory balance. In veterinary practice, Reishi may be considered for senior dogs with reduced cardiovascular stamina, overweight animals with circulatory or respiratory strain, working dogs requiring improved oxidative resilience, brachycephalic animals with chronic airway tension, or animals recovering from respiratory infection where post-inflammatory sensitivity persists.

Because cardiovascular and respiratory tissues are highly sensitive to oxidative and inflammatory stress, whole-mushroom SCWE extracts may be particularly valuable in these cases. SCWE preserves Reishi's triterpenes, sterols, polysaccharides and antioxidant compounds in their natural ratios, maintaining the integrity of the molecular architecture responsible for its vascular and airway regulatory effects. For animals with chronic cardiopulmonary load, this whole-matrix fidelity provides a gentle and physiologically coherent form of long-term support.

Reishi has a long-standing reputation as a tonic for both the cardiovascular and respiratory systems, a view deeply rooted in traditional East Asian medicine.

1.8. Neurological and Behavioural and Stress-Response Modulation

Reishi has long been regarded as a mushroom that supports emotional steadiness, restorative sleep and mental resilience. Traditional descriptions characterise it as a 'spirit-calming' tonic, and modern research has begun to clarify the physiological basis for these observations. Its influence extends across the neuroendocrine system, inflammatory pathways within the central nervous system, oxidative balance, mitochondrial stability and autonomic regulation. In veterinary behavioural medicine, where chronic stress, age-related cognitive change and inflammatory influences on behaviour are increasingly recognised, Reishi offers a gentle and multi-layered supportive role.

A central mechanism underlying Reishi's behavioural effects is its modulation of the hypothalamic–pituitary–adrenal (HPA) axis. Chronic stress disrupts cortisol rhythm, contributes to immune dysregulation and creates patterns of behavioural reactivity that are difficult to resolve through training alone. Preclinical studies demonstrate that Reishi can attenuate stress-induced cortisol elevation and support a more stable endocrine trajectory. These effects are not attributable to sedation, nor do they blunt the animal's natural awareness. Instead, they reflect a reduction in the inflammatory and oxidative "noise" that destabilises HPA-axis signalling during chronic stress exposure.

In clinical practice, this presents as improved stress recovery, calmer reactivity thresholds and more predictable behavioural patterns in animals facing sustained environmental pressures. Dogs with noise or storm sensitivity, separation-related behaviours, post-surgical adrenal stress or chronic illness often show modest but meaningful improvements in steadiness when Reishi is incorporated as part of a broader behavioural support strategy. Its role is cumulative, with benefits emerging gradually as neuroendocrine stability improves.

Reishi's contribution to neurological health also encompasses its influence on neuroinflammation. Chronic inflammation within the central nervous system is increasingly recognised as a factor in cognitive decline, behavioural dysregulation and neurodegenerative processes in ageing animals. Reishi's triterpenes reduce microglial overactivation, suppress pro-inflammatory cytokines within neural tissue and protect neuronal membranes from oxidative injury. These actions, though predominantly preclinical, align closely with patterns observed in senior animals receiving Reishi, where improvements in cognitive engagement, reduced nocturnal restlessness and steadier mood are frequently reported.

Mitochondrial protection forms another important layer of Reishi's neurological activity. The mushroom's antioxidant peptides and phenolic compounds stabilise mitochondrial membranes, reduce lipid peroxidation and support energy availability in neuronal tissue. This is particularly relevant for older dogs experiencing early cognitive changes or animals recovering from chronic inflammatory disease, where mitochondrial fragility contributes to reduced mental stamina and irritability. By supporting mitochondrial efficiency, Reishi helps maintain clearer cognitive function and smoother behavioural responses.

Sleep regulation represents an additional domain in which Reishi provides subtle yet significant benefit. Historical use describes Reishi as promoting restful sleep without sedation, and modern interpretations suggest that this arises from its influence on autonomic balance and inflammatory tone rather than any direct hypnotic action. Integrative practitioners commonly observe improvements in sleep–wake patterns in senior dogs, anxious pets and animals experiencing fragmented sleep due to pain or cognitive dysregulation. These changes accumulate over weeks and contribute to more stable daytime behaviour, as restorative sleep supports both neurological and immune function.

Reishi's behavioural relevance extends beyond the central nervous system to the gut–brain axis, where its influence on gastrointestinal inflammation, mast-cell activity and microbial stability can indirectly affect behavioural outcomes. Animals with combined gastrointestinal sensitivity and anxiety often demonstrate notable improvements in overall calmness when inflammatory triggers within the gut are reduced. This dual influence on both neurological and gastrointestinal regulatory systems highlights Reishi's unique profile as a whole-system behavioural support agent.

In veterinary behavioural practice, Reishi is best understood as an adjunct. It does not replace behavioural modification, environmental management or pharmacological intervention when required. Instead, it enhances the animal's physiological capacity to respond appropriately to those interventions by lowering inflammatory load, stabilising neuroendocrine rhythm and improving mitochondrial resilience. It is especially valuable in animals whose behavioural dysregulation arises from chronic inflammation, endocrine strain, gastrointestinal disturbance or age-related neurological decline.

Reishi may be considered in cases involving chronic anxiety, noise sensitivity, storm reactivity, cognitive ageing, behavioural tension linked to chronic disease or recovery after stress-intensive medical events. When paired with Lion's Mane, which offers complementary neurotrophic support, Reishi provides a regulatory foundation that protects neural tissue, stabilises inflammatory pathways and promotes emotional balance. Sub-critical water extraction enhances this profile by preserving the full spectrum of triterpenes, polysaccharides and fibre-bound compounds that contribute to Reishi's neuroimmune regulation.

Across these domains, Reishi's behavioural actions reflect a consistent theme: steadiness, not sedation. By modulating the physiological systems that underlie behavioural expression, Reishi creates a more stable internal environment in which training, enrichment, environmental modification and caregiver support can be more effective. This cumulative stability makes Reishi a valued component of integrative behavioural medicine for both companion and senior animals.

> Reishi has long been regarded as a mushroom that supports emotional steadiness, restorative sleep and mental resilience.

1.9. Oncology and Adjunctive Cancer Support

Reishi has a long-standing reputation as a supportive agent in oncology, rooted in both traditional use and modern biochemical investigation. Although it is not a primary anticancer therapy nor a substitute for conventional veterinary oncology, its broad physiological influence makes it highly valuable as an adjunct in animals undergoing cancer treatment or living with chronic neoplastic disease. Its benefits arise not from a single targeted pathway but from a constellation of regulatory effects that together help maintain physiological stability during periods of profound metabolic, inflammatory and oxidative stress. In this context, Reishi functions less as a tumour-directed agent and more as a terrain-modifying intervention that supports immune competence, tissue resilience and overall wellbeing.

A key aspect of Reishi's oncology relevance lies in its influence on immune surveillance. Cancer progression is heavily shaped by the competence of innate and adaptive immune responses, and Reishi's polysaccharides and β-glucans play a central role in improving this surveillance. Preclinical studies show enhanced activity of macrophages, natural killer cells and dendritic cells, each of which contributes to the recognition and containment of abnormal cellular proliferation. Laboratory evidence demonstrates that Reishi polysaccharides encourage dendritic-cell maturation, improve antigen presentation and enhance cytotoxic activity, offering a strong mechanistic rationale for their integration into supportive oncology care. Although direct veterinary clinical trials remain limited, the consistency of these findings across models strengthens their translational relevance for companion animals.

In parallel with its immune-modulating effects, Reishi exerts several actions on tumour biology in preclinical settings. Its ganoderic acids demonstrate the ability to induce apoptosis via mitochondrial pathways, inhibit DNA synthesis, suppress malignant cell proliferation and interfere with signalling mechanisms associated with metastatic behaviour. These outcomes are laboratory based and should not be interpreted as evidence of tumour regression in clinical patients; nevertheless, they offer insight into how Reishi may ease the biological burden that tumours place on an animal. Notably, some studies describe selective cytotoxicity, where malignant cells are more strongly affected than healthy tissue, suggesting a nuanced and targeted biochemical influence, though this remains preclinical.

Another dimension of support arises from Reishi's anti-angiogenic and anti-metastatic properties. Several triterpenes within Ganoderma lucidum reduce vascular endothelial growth factor (VEGF) expression, limiting the development of new blood vessels required for tumour growth. Additional findings show modulation of matrix metalloproteinases involved in tissue invasion, offering a plausible explanation for slower metastatic momentum in some laboratory settings. These effects have yet to be replicated in controlled veterinary trials, yet they integrate logically with the broader pharmacological behaviour of Reishi, reinforcing its potential value in multi-modal oncology strategies.

> Perhaps the most consistently observed benefit of Reishi within veterinary oncology is not its influence on tumour biology but its capacity to support animals undergoing chemotherapy and radiation.

Perhaps the most consistently observed benefit of Reishi within veterinary oncology is not its influence on tumour biology but its unique capacity to support animals undergoing chemotherapy and radiation. These treatments place immense oxidative and inflammatory strain on the body, often depleting antioxidant reserves, impairing mitochondrial function and generating secondary metabolic challenges. However, Reishi's antioxidant peptides, anti-inflammatory mechanisms and glutathione-promoting effects offer a protective buffer against these stressors. Preclinical studies show reduced oxidative damage during chemotherapeutic exposure, preservation of endogenous antioxidant capacity and potential protection of bone marrow progenitor cells. In veterinary practice, integrative clinicians frequently report steadier appetite, improved energy, calmer demeanour and better overall tolerance of conventional treatments in animals receiving Reishi concurrently, although these observations remain anecdotal and require case-by-case assessment.

Beyond its mechanistic and adjunctive treatment roles, Reishi contributes meaningfully to quality-of-life care. Cancer is not solely a localised pathology; it affects the entire metabolic landscape, generating chronic inflammation, oxidative load, immune exhaustion and changes in behaviour, appetite and sleep quality. Reishi's regulatory influence across multiple physiological domains allows it to stabilise some of these secondary processes. Improvements in appetite consistency, stress tolerance, nocturnal restlessness and general vitality are often reported by integrative practitioners and owners alike, forming a supportive terrain that helps animals maintain resilience throughout the course of their disease or treatment. These effects are cumulative and subtle rather than rapid or dramatic, aligning with Reishi's nature as a regulatory, whole-system tonic.

From a clinical perspective, Reishi may be considered in animals with solid tumours associated with chronic inflammation, immune-exhausted patients, animals undergoing chemotherapy or radiation, senior animals with concurrent chronic disease and palliative or comfort-focused care plans. It is especially valuable in cases where systemic inflammation or metabolic strain accelerates disease progression. However, its integration requires veterinary oversight, especially in patients receiving immunosuppressive or immunomodulatory drugs whose therapeutic objectives must not be unintentionally counteracted. Similarly, animals on medications affecting vascular tone or hepatic metabolism should be monitored closely to ensure additive effects are avoided, given Reishi's gentle vasomodulatory and hepatic-supportive properties.

Overall, Reishi's role in veterinary oncology is best described as supportive, regulatory and resilience-enhancing. It does not replace surgery, chemotherapy or radiation but instead reinforces the physiological foundations upon which these treatments depend. By stabilising immune function, reducing inflammatory and oxidative load, supporting mitochondrial health and improving comfort, Reishi provides a meaningful adjunct to integrative oncology practice. Its benefits unfold gradually, reflecting the accumulative nature of Mycotherapy, but when used consistently and thoughtfully it contributes significantly to the wellbeing and quality of life of animals facing cancer.

> A key aspect of Reishi's oncology relevance lies in its influence on immune surveillance.

1.10. Endocrine and Neuroendocrine Stability

Reishi's influence on the endocrine system is subtle, cumulative and regulatory rather than stimulatory. This makes Reishi a valuable tool for addressing the chronic physiological imbalances that underlie many behavioural, metabolic and inflammatory conditions in companion animals. While it is not an endocrine drug and should not be positioned as a replacement for hormone-based therapies, its effects on the hypothalamic–pituitary–adrenal (HPA) axis, inflammatory signalling and mitochondrial resilience contribute meaningfully to improved endocrine stability in animals living under prolonged stress or systemic inflammatory load.

One of Reishi's most relevant endocrine actions is its modulation of the HPA axis. Chronic stress disrupts cortisol rhythm, destabilises immune competence and alters gastrointestinal and behavioural function. Preclinical research consistently demonstrates that Reishi can attenuate stress-induced hypersecretion of cortisol, support a more stable diurnal pattern and reduce downstream inflammatory activation triggered by sustained HPA dysregulation. These effects appear to arise from a combination of antioxidant support, cytokine modulation and mitochondrial protection rather than any direct hormone-like action. In practice, this often equates to steadier behaviour, improved resilience to environmental triggers and more predictable physiological recovery from stressors such as separation, storms, veterinary procedures or illness.

Reishi also influences endocrine pathways through its broad anti-inflammatory behaviour. Persistent inflammatory signalling affects thyroid regulation, pancreatic function and adrenal load, altering the hormonal milieu in ways that compound chronic disease. By calming nuclear factor kappa B activation, reducing cytokines such as interleukin 6 and tumour necrosis factor alpha, and supporting endogenous antioxidant systems, Reishi helps moderate the inflammatory backdrop that disrupts endocrine communication. This regulatory influence may be relevant in animals with inflammatory-driven metabolic instability, early thyroid imbalance, chronic skin disease or gastrointestinal–endocrine overlap.

Although direct veterinary studies examining Reishi's effects on insulin regulation or thyroid physiology are limited, preclinical models indicate improved glucose tolerance, enhanced insulin signalling and reduced lipid accumulation. These effects align with the clinical impression that Reishi can support metabolic steadiness in overweight, senior or endocrine-disordered animals, particularly when metabolic changes are driven by chronic inflammation, oxidative stress or gut–liver dysregulation. Its influence in these scenarios is not that of a glucose-lowering agent, but rather of a systemic modulator that reduces the physiological stressors contributing to metabolic imbalance.

Reishi's contribution to endocrine stability is further supported by its effects on mitochondrial function. Endocrine tissues are metabolically active and highly sensitive to oxidative injury; by supporting mitochondrial resilience, Reishi helps maintain normal signalling and cellular endurance in tissues affected by chronic inflammatory or metabolic demand. This may contribute to improved stamina, calmer behaviour and less volatility in animals whose endocrine function is compromised by chronic disease or prolonged stress.

Overall, Reishi's role in endocrine and neuroendocrine stability reflects its broader identity as a regulatory mushroom. It does not exert isolated, hormone-specific effects but instead restores balance to interconnected physiological systems whose dysregulation underlies many chronic veterinary conditions. In this way, Reishi offers valuable support for animals experiencing chronic stress, behavioural instability, metabolic tension and inflammatory–endocrine overlap, providing a foundation upon which medical and behavioural interventions can build.

1.11 Behavioural and Neurological Support

Reishi's traditional description as a 'spirit-calming' mushroom finds strong resonance in modern neurophysiological research. Its effects on behaviour and neurological function arise from its capacity to regulate inflammatory signalling within the central nervous system, support mitochondrial stability, modulate the HPA axis and reduce oxidative injury across neural tissues. In veterinary medicine, these pathways are increasingly recognised as central contributors to anxiety, cognitive decline, stress responsiveness and behavioural dysregulation in dogs and cats.

Neuroinflammation is a foundational mechanism in many behavioural and cognitive disorders. Microglial activation, oxidative stress and the overproduction of inflammatory cytokines disrupt neuronal communication, alter synaptic plasticity and contribute to anxiety patterns and cognitive decline. Reishi exerts measurable effects on these pathways in preclinical models, reducing microglial activation, suppressing pro-inflammatory mediators such as interleukin 6 and tumour necrosis factor alpha and protecting neuronal mitochondria from oxidative injury. These findings support the clinical rationale for pairing Reishi with Lion's Mane in cognitive ageing, neuroinflammatory syndromes and behavioural conditions involving chronic stress or neurological vulnerability.

Reishi also plays a meaningful role in stress adaptation, which has direct implications for behavioural health. Chronic or unresolved stress contributes to heightened reactivity, noise sensitivity, storm-related anxiety, separation-associated distress and a range of maladaptive coping behaviours. By moderating the HPA axis and supporting more stable cortisol rhythms, Reishi helps calm the physiological substrate of stress-related behaviours. Its influence is regulatory rather than sedating; animals become steadier and more adaptable rather than subdued. This distinction is crucial in behavioural medicine, where excessive sedation can hinder learning, habituation or environmental processing.

Cognitive wellbeing is another area where Reishi's cumulative effects may be valuable. Senior animals frequently develop patterns of nocturnal restlessness, disorientation, disrupted sleep architecture and anxiety associated with cognitive change. Reishi's ability to reduce oxidative stress, support neuronal mitochondrial function and modulate neuroinflammation provides plausible mechanisms for improving comfort and maintaining cognitive performance in ageing dogs and cats. Integrative practitioners often observe calmer night-time behaviour, more settled sleep and improved engagement in daily routine after sustained use, though these observations remain anecdotal and require thoughtful monitoring.

Reishi's contributions to behavioural health also intersect with gastrointestinal and endocrine regulation. Animals with stress-linked digestive disturbance, chronic gastrointestinal sensitivity or inflammatory-driven anxiety patterns often respond well to Reishi due to its combined effects on the gut–brain axis, mucosal stability and neuroendocrine balance. By reducing inflammatory and oxidative load across multiple systems, Reishi decreases the overall physiological strain that contributes to behavioural reactivity.

In veterinary practice, Reishi is frequently incorporated into behavioural support plans alongside environmental modification, behaviour therapy, nutritional interventions. Its effects accumulate gradually, typically emerging over several weeks, and are best understood as a stabilising influence that enhances the animal's capacity for adaptation, learning and recovery. Reishi is not a replacement for appropriate behavioural pharmacology when required, but it provides a supportive physiological foundation that can improve outcomes and enhance quality of life in animals experiencing behavioural and neurological challenges.

> Reishi's traditional description as a 'spirit-calming' mushroom finds strong resonance in modern neurophysiological research.

1.12. Veterinary Pharmacology and Drug Interaction Considerations

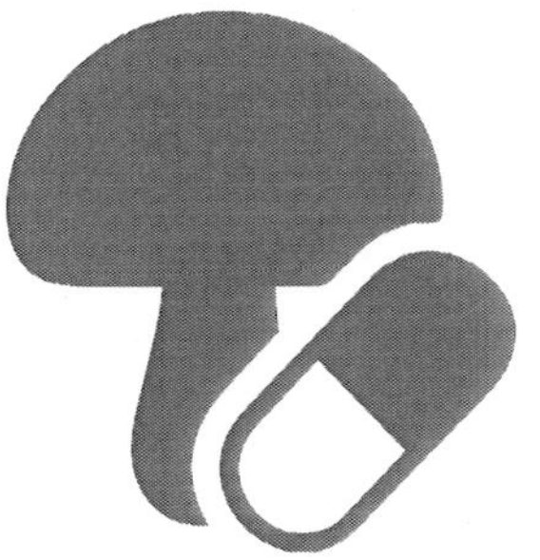

Reishi's pharmacology is complex and multidimensional, reflecting the diversity of its polysaccharides, triterpenes, proteoglucans, antioxidant peptides and fibre-bound compounds. For veterinary clinicians, understanding how these molecules are absorbed, metabolised and interact with commonly prescribed medications is essential for the safe and effective integration of Reishi into clinical practice. Although species-specific pharmacokinetic studies in dogs and cats remain limited, useful insights can be drawn from preclinical models, human pharmacology and accumulated experience within integrative veterinary medicine. Collectively, this evidence supports the view that Reishi behaves as a gentle, regulatory agent whose benefits accumulate gradually, yet whose pharmacological nuances warrant thoughtful consideration in complex or medically fragile patients.

Absorption and bioavailability

Reishi's diverse bioactive constituents follow different absorption pathways, which helps explain its broad, layered pharmacological profile. Polysaccharides and proteoglucans exhibit limited direct systemic absorption but exert significant biological influence through interaction with the gut-associated lymphoid tissue, with immune receptors such as Dectin-1 and Toll-like receptor 2, and through modulation of the gut microbiome. Their primary actions occur locally within the gastrointestinal tract and immune system, where they contribute to immune signalling rather than systemic pharmacokinetics.

Triterpenes behave differently. Being lipophilic, their absorption is more efficient than that of polysaccharides, although still modest overall. Sub-critical water extraction of the whole mushroom enhances triterpene dispersion and may improve uptake relative to simple hot-water extracts, likely due to preservation of the natural fibre matrix, hydrophilic–lipophilic balance and proteoglucan complexes that contribute to physiological transport. Once absorbed, triterpenes undergo hepatic metabolism and exert gradual pharmacodynamic effects, which accords with the clinical observation that Reishi's influence unfolds slowly over several weeks.

Hepatic metabolism and detoxification pathways

Reishi interacts with hepatic detoxification systems, including phase I and phase II pathways. Preclinical studies demonstrate modulation of cytochrome P450 enzymes, although the direction and magnitude of this effect vary depending on the specific extract and dose. Reishi also influences conjugation pathways, including glucuronidation and glutathione-dependent reactions, supporting hepatic resilience in animals exposed to chronic inflammation or polypharmacy.

These effects create both therapeutic opportunity and a need for clinical attentiveness. Reishi may help buffer the hepatic oxidative load associated with long-term use of NSAIDs, anticonvulsants, corticosteroids or chemotherapy agents. Conversely, in animals receiving narrow-therapeutic-index drugs, small changes in metabolic rate may theoretically be relevant. Although clinically significant interactions in dogs or cats have not been documented, veterinarians are advised to monitor liver enzymes and drug response when introducing Reishi into complex medication regimens.

Effects on platelet function and coagulation

A consistent pharmacological feature of Reishi is its mild antiplatelet activity. Triterpenes such as ganoderic acids can inhibit platelet aggregation and influence intracellular calcium signalling, contributing to a subtle anticoagulant effect. In healthy animals, this is rarely clinically significant. However, the effect becomes relevant when animals are receiving anticoagulant or antiplatelet medications, have clotting disorders or are approaching surgery. In these circumstances, clinicians may elect to reduce the dose or temporarily discontinue Reishi for several days prior to procedures, reintroducing it gradually during recovery. In thrombocytopenic patients or those with haemostatic fragility, use should be cautious and closely monitored.

Immunological interactions

Reishi's influence on the immune system is regulatory rather than stimulatory, a distinction that is central to its safe integration with immunomodulatory medications. It does not provoke inappropriate immune activation, nor does it typically counteract medical immunosuppression. However, in patients receiving potent immunosuppressive drugs, high doses of Reishi could theoretically modulate immune tone in a direction inconsistent with therapeutic intent. This concern is largely theoretical and unsupported by clinical evidence, yet it remains prudent to exercise careful monitoring when combining Reishi with corticosteroids, calcineurin inhibitors or immunomodulatory oncology agents such as checkpoint inhibitors. Collaboration with the attending oncologist or internal medicine specialist is strongly advised in these scenarios.

Interactions with sedatives, anxiolytics and behavioural medications

Reishi exerts a calming, regulatory effect on the neuroendocrine system, particularly the hypothalamic–pituitary–adrenal axis, but does not possess sedative pharmacology. It does not potentiate the effects of anxiolytics, gabapentin or behavioural medications in a clinically significant manner.

Instead, its influence contributes to overall steadiness, improved stress recovery and more stable behaviour, effects that align favourably with behaviour modification programmes and pharmacological interventions. These outcomes are best considered synergistic rather than interactive, reflecting complementary mechanisms rather than drug-level potentiation.

Interactions relevant to endocrine disorders

Reishi's regulatory effects on insulin sensitivity and glucose handling, as demonstrated in preclinical metabolic studies, warrant mild caution in diabetic patients. Although hypoglycaemic effects are modest, they may theoretically enhance the glucose-lowering effects of insulin or oral hypoglycaemics. For this reason, veterinarians should begin with a low dose in diabetic animals and monitor blood glucose during the initial weeks of supplementation. Adjustments to medication should be made only under clinical supervision. Reishi does not mimic thyroid or adrenal hormones, and no evidence suggests direct endocrine disruption; its effects are best understood as reductions in inflammatory and oxidative load that indirectly assist endocrine homeostasis.

Gastrointestinal absorption interactions

Reishi's natural fibre matrix, retained in SCWE full-spectrum extracts, may influence the absorption of orally administered medications. This effect is generally mild but may be relevant for drugs requiring precise pharmacokinetics or those best absorbed on an empty stomach. Oral antibiotics, certain anticonvulsants and drugs with narrow absorption windows may be given at times separate from Reishi to minimise theoretical interference. In most clinical situations, staggering administration by one to two hours is sufficient.

Overall pharmacological perspective for veterinary clinicians

Reishi's pharmacology is best characterised as gentle, regulatory and supportive. Unlike pharmaceuticals that exert singular, high-intensity effects, Reishi interacts with multiple systems in ways that promote equilibrium rather than disruption. The majority of clinically meaningful considerations involve mild antiplatelet effects, hepatic enzyme modulation, metabolic regulation, immune tone balancing and fibre-related influences on gastrointestinal absorption. When integrated thoughtfully into patient care, Reishi combines safely with most veterinary medications and supports resilience in animals facing chronic disease, treatment-related stress or physiological imbalance. Its safe use hinges on gradual introduction, patient-specific monitoring and collaborative veterinary oversight, particularly in oncology or complex internal medicine cases.

Reishi's pharmacology is best characterised as gentle, regulatory and supportive.

1.13. Clinical Application in Veterinary Practice

Reishi occupies a unique role in integrative veterinary medicine, functioning not as a single-purpose intervention but as a multi-system regulator that supports long-term physiological stability. Its cumulative activity across inflammatory, oxidative, neuroendocrine and immune pathways positions it as a foundational agent in cases where chronic dysregulation underlies clinical expression. Rather than producing rapid symptomatic shifts, Reishi steadies the biological terrain, contributing to improved comfort, resilience and adaptive capacity over weeks to months. Its integration into clinical practice is most effective when guided by an understanding of its mechanistic breadth and the long-standing experiential evidence reported by integrative veterinarians.

Dermatological and allergic conditions

Inflammatory and allergic skin conditions remain among the most common presentations in small-animal practice, and they frequently involve mast-cell degranulation, histamine release, dysregulated interleukin signalling and chronic T-helper imbalance. Reishi addresses these pathways through the combined actions of its triterpenes, which stabilise mast cells and reduce histamine release, and its polysaccharides, which help regulate T-helper (Th1 and Th2) activity. Excessive Th2 skewing is a hallmark of many allergic disorders, and Reishi's capacity to moderate this pattern provides a mechanistic basis for its use in chronic dermatology.

In clinical settings, Reishi is rarely used alone but provides important background support within multimodal allergy management. Over sustained administration, practitioners frequently observe calmer skin cycles, fewer inflammatory flares and reduced pruritic intensity. These responses are not immediate; they reflect downstream effects on immune tone, barrier stability and inflammatory signalling. When paired with dietary interventions, allergen avoidance strategies, omega-3 fatty acids and pharmacological therapies where appropriate, Reishi helps to reduce the severity and volatility of chronic allergic presentations.

Gastrointestinal sensitivities and chronic enteropathies

Chronic gastrointestinal disorders are intrinsically tied to inflammatory, microbial and neuroendocrine imbalance. Reishi's effects within the gastrointestinal tract draw on several well-characterised mechanisms: the down-regulation of nuclear factor kappa B, suppression of cytokines such as interleukin 6 and tumour necrosis factor alpha, inhibition of inducible nitric oxide synthase and cyclo-oxygenase 2, stabilisation of epithelial barrier integrity and reduction of oxidative injury. These pathways contribute to a calmer mucosal environment and improved tolerance to dietary variation and environmental stress.

The retention of Reishi's natural fibre matrix in SCWE enhances its prebiotic influence. This fibre supports microbial diversity, encourages short-chain fatty acid production and interacts with the gut–immune axis in a manner that promotes gastrointestinal stability. Clinically, many animals with intermittent gastrointestinal discomfort, stress-responsive diarrhoea or chronic enteropathy show steadier stool consistency and reduced flare episodes after several weeks of consistent supplementation. Reishi is most effective when integrated into a broader plan involving diet modification, microbiome support, appropriate medication and additional Mycotherapy species such as Shiitake or Chaga in more complex cases.

Hepatic strain and chronic medication use

Many veterinary patients experience cumulative hepatic load due to long-term medications, chronic inflammation or ageing. Reishi's hepatoprotective profile, supported by preclinical evidence, includes inhibition of inflammatory cytokines, protection against lipid peroxidation, modulation of hepatic enzyme systems and support for endogenous antioxidant pathways such as glutathione. These mechanisms position Reishi as a valuable adjunct where hepatic metabolism is under prolonged strain.

In practice, animals on non-steroidal anti-inflammatory drugs, anticonvulsants, chemotherapeutic protocols or endocrine medications may experience more stable hepatic enzyme trends and improved overall vitality when Reishi is introduced gradually. It does not replace conventional hepatic support agents such as S-adenosylmethionine, N-acetylcysteine or phosphatidylcholine, but acts synergistically by modulating the upstream oxidative and inflammatory pressures that contribute to hepatocellular stress. Clinicians often observe steadier appetite, improved stamina and better tolerance of medication regimens in senior or chronically medicated animals receiving Reishi consistently.

Behavioural dysregulation and stress-responsive conditions

Reishi's regulatory influence on the hypothalamic–pituitary–adrenal axis, combined with its anti-inflammatory actions within the central nervous system, makes it a valuable adjunct in animals experiencing chronic stress, anxiety patterns or behavioural dysregulation. Unlike sedatives, Reishi does not blunt cognitive function or suppress behaviour. Instead, it modulates the physiological drivers of chronic stress, promoting steadiness, stress recovery and emotional resilience.

Veterinarians often integrate Reishi into care plans for dogs with separation-related concerns, noise sensitivity, storm-associated reactivity, hospitalisation stress or behaviour changes secondary to chronic disease. Improvements are subtle but meaningful, typically appearing as calmer demeanour, improved coping capacity and greater tolerance for environmental stressors. These benefits are maximised when combined with environmental modification, behaviour-modification programmes and, where appropriate, pharmacological support.

Senior animal support and healthy ageing

Ageing animals experience complex physiological shifts, including declining immune surveillance, chronic low-grade inflammation, increased oxidative load, mitochondrial inefficiency and early cognitive changes. Reishi's capacity to modulate these interconnected processes makes it particularly well suited to geriatric veterinary care.

Clinical experience suggests improvements in stamina, appetite stability, nocturnal restlessness and general engagement with daily routine when Reishi is incorporated into senior care. Its pairing with Lion's Mane is especially valued in early cognitive change, combining Reishi's neuroprotective and anti-inflammatory actions with Lion's Mane's neurotrophic influence. Over time, many senior animals demonstrate improved sleep–wake patterns, behavioural steadiness and increased resilience to routine disruptions or environmental challenges.

> Ageing animals experience complex physiological shifts and Reishi's capacity to modulate these makes it particularly well suited to geriatric veterinary care.

Respiratory vulnerability and airway reactivity

Reishi's influence on airway physiology has relevance in chronic respiratory vulnerability, brachycephalic airway strain, age-related pulmonary stiffness and mixed allergic–respiratory syndromes. Its triterpenes exert smooth-muscle modulating effects, reducing airway irritability, while its anti-inflammatory actions help to calm chronic mucosal inflammation. Although not a replacement for bronchodilators or corticosteroids, Reishi provides a stabilising backdrop that may reduce the frequency or severity of recurrent respiratory episodes. Clinicians occasionally report improved respiratory comfort in dogs recovering from respiratory infections or living with chronic airway inflammation.

Integrative oncology and long-term cancer care

Reishi's role in oncology centres on quality of life, immune competence and resilience during conventional treatment. It does not replace chemotherapeutic or surgical interventions, but supports the physiological terrain in which these treatments operate. By modulating inflammation, buffering oxidative stress and assisting immune surveillance, Reishi can help animals maintain appetite, comfort and day-to-day stability during oncology protocols.

Its use as an adjunct therapy is well-recognised in human integrative oncology, where organisations such as the American Cancer Society list Reishi and Turkey Tail as supportive therapies within evidence-informed care frameworks. While direct veterinary evidence remains limited, these human data – together with mechanistic studies demonstrating effects on immune signalling, mitochondrial stability and inflammatory pathways – offer a credible rationale for its cautious, integrative use.

In veterinary practice, Reishi is best viewed as terrain support: a means of reinforcing systemic resilience, improving treatment tolerability and helping sustain quality of life throughout the cancer-care continuum.

Complex or multi-systemic cases

Multi-systemic veterinary conditions often involve overlapping inflammation, endocrine tension, chronic pain, gastrointestinal instability and immune dysregulation. Reishi's wide-ranging actions allow it to contribute meaningfully to these complex presentations, particularly when combined with other Mycotherapy species that complement its strengths. Lion's Mane may be included for neurological support, Turkey Tail for immune–gastrointestinal modulation or Chaga for high-level antioxidant reinforcement. In such cases, dosing must remain individualised, with gradual introduction and careful monitoring, particularly in animals with advanced disease, multi-organ involvement or extensive polypharmacy.

Integration with other functional mushrooms

Reishi pairs exceptionally well with a number of functional mushrooms due to its unique combination of triterpenoids, β-glucans, sterols and immunoregulatory compounds. Its calming influence on the HPA axis, cardiovascular steadiness, hepatic support and immune-balancing effects allow it to function as a core 'anchor mushroom' in many integrative veterinary protocols. The following pairings illustrate how Reishi enhances multi-system resilience when combined with other species.

- **With Turkey Tail** - This combination strengthens immune surveillance, oncology resilience and microbiome-associated immune modulation. Turkey Tail's diverse β-glucan profile primes innate and adaptive immune pathways, while Reishi provides triterpenoid-mediated inflammatory modulation and stress-system stabilisation. Together, they support animals undergoing integrative oncology care, chronic immune dysregulation or age-related immune decline. This pairing is particularly valuable when a gentle yet comprehensive immune-support strategy is required.
- **With Lion's Mane** -Reishi's adaptogenic, calming and anti-inflammatory effects complement Lion's Mane's neurotrophic influence on the CNS and gut–brain axis. This pairing offers both neuroprotective and neuroregenerative support, helping to stabilise behavioural reactivity, cognitive ageing and stress-linked gastrointestinal fragility. Reishi's influence on autonomic balance enhances Lion's Mane's capacity to support nerve regeneration, making this pairing highly suitable for senior animals, cognitive dysfunction syndromes and stress-exacerbated neurological presentations.
- **With Cordyceps** -Cordyceps contributes respiratory resilience, mitochondrial energy optimisation and enhanced oxygen utilisation, while Reishi modulates cardiovascular tone, inflammatory responsiveness and oxidative stress. The combined effect is a balanced, steady-state improvement in energy, performance and recovery. This pairing is particularly beneficial in working dogs, performance animals, animals recovering from chronic fatigue states, or those requiring support through exercise-induced oxidative stress and metabolic strain.
- **With Chaga** - Reishi and Chaga together provide a powerful antioxidant and hepatic-supportive combination. Chaga's polyphenols, melanin complexes and SOD-like activity offer robust oxidative-stress buffering, while Reishi adds hepatoprotective triterpenes and im-

munoregulatory balance. This synergy supports animals with chronic inflammation, dermatological or allergic patterns, metabolic imbalance or hepatic workload due to medication, environmental toxins or ageing. The pairing is also helpful in animals with mast-cell activation tendencies, stress-driven inflammatory cycles or immune hypersensitivity.

- **With Golden Oyster** - Golden Oyster's ergothioneine-rich profile adds a potent mitochondrial and cellular-protection dimension to Reishi's calming and regulatory effects. Reishi stabilises inflammatory pathways and autonomic tone, while Golden Oyster enhances cytoprotection, redox balance and cellular longevity. Together, they support healthy ageing, improve recovery from oxidative stress, and bolster resilience in animals exposed to environmental or physiological stressors. This pairing works especially well in senior animals, chronic inflammatory states, stress-reactive conditions and metabolic frailty.

> Synergistic pairings or triads of mushrooms can act across multiple physiological pathways, broadening the supportive effect and contributing to a full-spectrum, terrain-based Mycotherapy strategy

1.14. Safety, Contraindications and Monitoring

Reishi is widely regarded as one of the safest medicinal mushrooms for long-term use in companion animals, supported by an extensive record of traditional application and a favourable profile in contemporary nutritional, toxicological and pharmacological literature. Its safety derives partly from its regulatory rather than stimulatory nature, and partly from the inherent balance of its polysaccharides, triterpenes, sterols and fibre-bound compounds. Despite this reassuring background, its use in veterinary practice still requires thoughtful, case-specific assessment. Safety in Mycotherapy is influenced not only by the mushroom's inherent properties but also by extraction method, dose titration, concurrent medication and the physiological status of the patient. Understanding these dimensions allows clinicians to integrate Reishi confidently while minimising risk in medically fragile animals.

General tolerability and gastrointestinal sensitivity

Most dogs and cats tolerate Reishi well, particularly when it is introduced gradually at the lower end of the therapeutic tier. The most common minor reaction is transient digestive sensitivity, typically manifesting as soft stools, mild flatulence or brief appetite fluctuation during the initial adjustment period. These effects usually resolve spontaneously within several days and reflect the microbiome's natural response to an increase in complex polysaccharides and prebiotic fibre. They are less frequently observed with full-spectrum Sub-critical water extracts, as these maintain the mushroom's fibre–proteoglucan matrix in a physiologically familiar form that integrates more smoothly into gastrointestinal signalling. Gradual titration over five to seven days is generally sufficient to avoid discomfort in sensitive or senior animals.

Platelet function and bleeding considerations

Reishi's triterpenes exhibit mild antiplatelet effects in preclinical pharmacology, largely through inhibition of platelet aggregation and modulation of intracellular calcium dynamics. In healthy animals this effect is subtle and rarely clinically relevant. However, it becomes important in situations where coagulation balance is already fragile. Animals receiving antiplatelet or anticoagulant drugs, such as aspirin, clopidogrel, heparin or warfarin analogues, may experience additive effects, and should therefore be monitored for bruising, bleeding tendencies or prolonged clotting times. Similar caution applies in thrombocytopenia, congenital coagulopathies, hepatic insufficiency affecting clotting-factor production and the peri-operative period. Temporary withholding of Reishi several days before elective surgery is prudent in high-risk individuals, even though serious bleeding events are rare.

Considerations in immune-mediated disease

Reishi's influence on the immune system is regulatory rather than stimulatory, tending to restore balance across innate and adaptive branches rather than driving heightened immune activity. Yet in patients where immune suppression is critical to disease management, such as autoimmune haemolytic anaemia, immune-mediated thrombocytopenia or immune-mediated polyarthritis, even subtle shifts in immune tone can be clinically significant. In such cases Reishi can still be considered, but only with careful oversight. At low doses it is unlikely to provoke disease escalation, and some clinicians report improved stability when oxidative and inflammatory load is reduced. Nonetheless, the decision to introduce Reishi in immune-mediated disease should always be individualised, with clear monitoring criteria in place.

Hepatic considerations

Reishi's hepatoprotective effects are well established in preclinical research, including inhibition of lipid peroxidation, reduced stellate-cell activation, improved antioxidant capacity and modulation of phase I and phase II detoxification pathways. These properties make Reishi a valuable adjunct in animals exposed to long-term medication or chronic inflammatory burdens. However, fragile hepatic patients require careful consideration. In advanced hepatic insufficiency, impaired bile flow or pronounced synthetic dysfunction, even gentle nutraceutical interventions may place additional metabolic demand on compromised hepatocytes. In this context, clinicians should begin with conservative dosing, titrate slowly and monitor liver enzymes, albumin, clotting parameters and overall clinical stability. Most animals tolerate Reishi well, but vigilance is essential where hepatic reserve is limited.

Renal considerations

Unlike certain mushrooms with naturally high oxalate content, Reishi does not pose a specific renal risk when used appropriately. Nevertheless, animals with advanced kidney disease often have altered metabolic capacity, reduced nutrient tolerance and fluctuating hydration status. Senior cats, in particular, may require very gradual introduction to avoid gastrointestinal sensitivity. While significant renal adverse effects from Reishi are not reported, clinicians should still monitor these patients closely, especially if appetite, hydration or electrolyte balance is fragile.

Endocrine and metabolic disorders

Reishi influences metabolic physiology through mild improvements in glucose handling, lipid regulation and oxidative balance, as shown in preclinical models. In diabetic animals receiving insulin or oral hypoglycaemic agents, these effects may modestly enhance glucose control, creating the possibility of additive hypoglycaemia. For this reason, blood-glucose monitoring should be performed more frequently during the first one to two weeks of introduction, and any medication adjustments should be made only under veterinary guidance.

Animals with adrenal, thyroid or pituitary disorders may benefit indirectly from Reishi's regulatory influence on oxidative stress and inflammatory load. However, Reishi does not mimic endocrine hormones and should not be viewed as a substitute for primary endocrine therapy. Its role is supportive, helping create a more stable metabolic environment while conventional treatment remains the principal therapeutic driver.

Interactions with pharmaceuticals

Reishi interacts with hepatic detoxification pathways, including cytochrome P450 enzymes and conjugation systems, though the direction and magnitude of these effects vary across extracts and doses. Clinically significant drug interactions have not been widely reported in veterinary practice, yet theoretical interactions exist for medications with narrow therapeutic indices, such as phenobarbital, digoxin, certain chemotherapeutics, specific cardiac drugs and immunomodulatory oncology agents. In such cases, gradual introduction, dose stability and periodic monitoring are advisable until the animal's response is clearly established. Full-spectrum SCWE extracts offer greater biochemical predictability compared with alcohol-based dual extracts, which may introduce variable solubility and pharmacokinetic behaviour due to residual ethanol.

Reishi does not potentiate sedatives or anxiolytics in a pharmacological sense, but its influence on the hypothalamic–pituitary–adrenal axis may contribute to an overall calmer behavioural profile. This synergistic effect is generally favourable rather than concerning, and does not meaningfully alter dosing requirements for behavioural medication.

Pregnancy, lactation and paediatric animals

Evidence regarding Reishi use in pregnancy or lactation remains extremely limited across species. While no reproductive toxicity has been identified, the absence of controlled data warrants a conservative approach. Pregnant or lactating animals should only receive Reishi when there is clear clinical justification and under direct veterinary supervision. Paediatric animals generally tolerate Reishi well, but neonates or immunologically immature individuals require cautious titration due to their developing gastrointestinal and immune systems.

Extraction quality and safety considerations

Extraction quality strongly influences safety and tolerability. Sub-critical water extraction produces a full-spectrum preparation that preserves hydrophilic and lipophilic constituents, including polysaccharides, triterpenes, proteoglucans, sterols and the native fibre structure. This method avoids ethanol residues and prevents the starch dilution commonly found in grain-grown mycelium products, both of which can alter gastrointestinal and immune responses.

In veterinary Mycotherapy, the biochemical fidelity of the extract matters deeply. SCWE extracts maintain the molecular ecology of the whole fruiting body, producing more stable physiological effects and reducing the risk of unpredictable reactions that occasionally accompany solvent-extracted or fractionated products. For chronic inflammatory, hepatic, gastrointestinal or multi-systemic cases, this structural coherence aligns closely with the regulatory pathways upon which Reishi's therapeutic value depends.

Monitoring and clinical oversight

Safe integration of Reishi in veterinary practice relies on thoughtful monitoring that matches the needs of the individual patient. Assessment of stool quality, appetite and gastrointestinal comfort during the first ten days allows early identification of dose-related sensitivity. Behaviour and sleep patterns should be reviewed over the first month, particularly in animals receiving Reishi for stress modulation or cognitive support. In hepatic or renal patients, periodic blood work provides essential information about organ stability. Animals receiving anticoagulants should be observed for signs of altered clotting, and oncology patients benefit from structured quality-of-life tracking to evaluate Reishi's contribution to comfort and resilience.

Above all, the guiding principles are gradual introduction, individualised dosing and consistent clinical observation. When integrated in this way, Reishi's safety profile remains excellent, and its long-term regulatory benefits can be realised fully within a medically sound framework.

1.15 Clinical Relevance Summary

Reishi's therapeutic value in veterinary medicine lies in its cumulative, terrain-modifying influence rather than acute or symptom-driven effects. It strengthens physiological resilience across multiple systems, creating conditions in which healing, comfort and stable homeostasis can occur more readily. For animals with chronic inflammatory disease, metabolic load, immune imbalance or long-term oxidative stress, Reishi provides a regulatory framework that supports more predictable and sustained clinical progress.

In dermatological and allergic conditions, its mast-cell stabilising activity and capacity to balance T-helper dynamics complement dietary management and pharmacological interventions, often resulting in reduced flare intensity and smoother recovery cycles over time. In gastrointestinal inflammatory disease, the combined effects on mucosal integrity, immune signalling and microbiome equilibrium help restore digestive comfort and support long-term gut resilience.

Senior patients and animals receiving chronic medications frequently benefit from Reishi's hepatoprotective and mitochondrial-supportive properties, which may manifest as steadier stamina, improved demeanour and more stable clinical parameters. Within integrative oncology, Reishi serves as a supportive agent that enhances quality of life, buffers treatment-associated strain and reinforces immune vigilance without interfering with conventional oncology protocols when used judiciously.

Caution remains appropriate in immune-mediated disease, advanced hepatic insufficiency and cases involving complex polypharmacy. Slow titration and attentive monitoring ensure that Reishi's regulatory benefits are realised safely. Overall, Reishi functions as a gentle but profoundly stabilising contributor to long-term integrative care, reinforcing the physiological ground upon which recovery, resilience and healthy ageing depend.

1.16 Evidence Quality Commentary

Reishi (Ganoderma lucidum) occupies a distinctive position within veterinary Mycotherapy because of its unusually broad research foundation. Its evidence base is neither sparse nor anecdotal, yet nor is it dominated by species-specific clinical trials. Instead, it sits in the middle of the translational spectrum, supported by strong mechanistic research, extensive preclinical validation, emerging animal studies and a large, consistent body of practitioner observations across species. For veterinarians seeking to apply Reishi responsibly, understanding *where* the evidence is strongest, *where* it is developing and *where* clinical judgment is required is central to safe, effective integration.

The most robust data underpin Reishi's immunomodulatory and anti-inflammatory actions. Multiple independent laboratories have demonstrated that its β-glucans, proteoglucans and triterpenes modulate cytokine signalling, regulate nuclear factor kappa B (NF-κB), suppress cyclo-oxygenase-2 (COX-2) and inducible nitric oxide synthase (iNOS), influence mast-cell stability and enhance innate immune surveillance. These findings, which collectively form one of the strongest mechanistic portfolios in medicinal mycology, are highly relevant to canine and feline physiology, as the pathways involved are deeply conserved across mammalian species. In practice, this translates to reliable, cumulative regulatory support in chronic inflammatory, allergic and immune-impaired conditions.

Oxidative stress regulation and hepatic protection are also supported by moderate to high-quality evidence. Reishi's antioxidant peptides, triterpenes and polyphenols have repeatedly demonstrated protection against lipid peroxidation, cellular oxidative injury and hepatic stress in metabolic, toxic and inflammatory models. Although veterinary-specific hepatic trials remain limited, these mechanistic findings align closely with the clinical reality faced by practitioners managing older animals, polypharmacy cases and chronic inflammatory disease. In these contexts, Reishi's gradual stabilisation of biochemical parameters is consistent with its documented molecular actions.

Behavioural modulation, stress physiology support and HPA-axis regulation represent domains where mechanistic evidence is developing but clinical observations are strong and consistent. Preclinical findings show that Reishi can modulate cortisol secretion, reduce neuroinflammation, support mitochondrial resilience in neuronal tissue and improve stress-related metabolic markers. While these effects have yet to be confirmed in companion animal trials, veterinarians frequently report improved emotional steadiness, smoother sleep–wake patterns and reduced reactivity in anxious or stressed animals when Reishi is incorporated into behaviour or senior-care plans. These observations, although anecdotal, demonstrate remarkable congruence with underlying biochemical pathways, lending them contextual credibility.

Evidence supporting gastrointestinal and microbiome benefits is moderate and primarily derived from preclinical colitis models, in vitro epithelial studies and translational data from canine nutrition research using medicinal mushroom blends. These studies support Reishi's capacity to improve mucosal integrity, reduce inflammatory cytokine output, promote beneficial microbial taxa and support short-chain fatty acid production. The coherence between mechanistic, preclinical and clinical anecdotal findings in gastrointestinal cases makes this a promising, though still developing, area of veterinary application.

Oncology represents a particularly nuanced domain. Reishi's anticancer actions - including apoptosis induction, angiogenesis inhibition, immune-enhanced tumour surveillance and suppression of metastatic signalling - are strongly supported in preclinical tumour models. However, these effects should not be interpreted as evidence of direct tumour regression in clinical veterinary patients. Rather, Reishi's strongest oncology value lies in supporting the terrain: enhancing resilience, mitigating treatment-associated oxidative and inflammatory load, supporting appetite and comfort, and improving immunological tone. Practitioners repeatedly report improved quality-of-life metrics in animals undergoing chemotherapy, radiation or palliative care, and these observations correlate closely with Reishi's documented molecular actions.

Respiratory and cardiovascular evidence is still emerging. Preclinical studies indicate potential benefits in vascular function, airway smooth-muscle modulation and pulmonary inflammatory control, but species-specific veterinary trials are limited. These actions nonetheless provide a rationale for including Reishi in chronic airway sensitivity, age-related cardiovascular strain and respiratory–allergic overlap when used as part of a broader integrative plan.

Clinical veterinary trials remain limited across all domains. This is not unique to Reishi but reflects the state of medicinal mushroom research globally. In this context, practitioner experience becomes a meaningful supplementary layer of evidence. It does not replace clinical trials, but it offers pattern recognition across thousands of animals treated over many years. Importantly, these real-world observations consistently reinforce the mechanistic and preclinical foundations described above, rather than contradicting them.

This spectrum of evidence is summarised in the following table:

Domain	Evidence Strength	Primary Evidence Type
Immunomodulation	High	Preclinical, animal models, canine studies
Anti-inflammatory activity	High	Preclinical, mechanistic consistency
Antioxidant and hepatic support	Moderate to high	Preclinical, translational rationale
Behavioural and stress regulation	Moderate	Preclinical, strong anecdotal evidence
Gastrointestinal support	Moderate	Preclinical, canine nutrition studies
Oncology adjunct use	Moderate	Preclinical, strong practitioner consensus
Respiratory and cardiovascular support	Emerging	Preclinical, extrapolated physiology
Clinical veterinary trials	Limited	Small number, emerging field

When the mechanistic findings, preclinical evidence, practitioner experience and the evidence-quality summary are considered together, Reishi emerges as a scientifically grounded, low-risk, multi-system supportive agent within integrative veterinary practice. Its actions develop slowly and depend on consistent administration, reflecting its role as a regulator rather than a symptom-suppressing intervention. This cumulative, terrain-focused mechanism is especially valuable in chronic inflammatory disease, immune dysfunction, geriatric medicine, behavioural dysregulation and oncology support, where long-term stability is a defining clinical goal.

Within this framework, extract fidelity becomes essential. Reishi's wide-ranging actions arise from the interplay of triterpenes, polysaccharides, proteoglucans, sterols and fibre-bound constituents that function synergistically within their native biochemical matrix. Sub-critical water extraction (SCWE) preserves this complexity by retaining both hydrophilic and lipophilic compounds, as well as the prebiotic fibre that shapes gut–immune interactions and moderates absorption. This contrasts with solvent-based tinctures, which isolate specific fractions, and grain-grown mycelium products, which dilute active compounds with starch. For clinicians, full-spectrum whole-food extracts produced via SCWE provide a physiologically coherent preparation that aligns more closely with the regulatory pathways described throughout this monograph.

When combined with careful dosing, attentive monitoring and integration within a broader multimodal plan, Reishi offers a stable, predictable and evidence-aligned contribution to veterinary care. Its value lies not in dramatic or acute effects but in its capacity to restore balance, protect physiological integrity and support long-term resilience across multiple interconnected systems.

> Reishi emerges as a scientifically grounded, low-risk, multi-system supportive agent within integrative veterinary practice.

1.17 Veterinary Considerations and Therapeutic Relevance

Reishi is most effective when understood as a slow, steady contributor to systemic resilience rather than an acute, symptom-focused intervention. In animals with chronic inflammatory conditions, metabolic strain or long-standing oxidative stress, Reishi provides a regulatory foundation within which recovery processes can operate more efficiently.

In dermatological and allergic patterns, its mast-cell stabilising activity and influence on T-helper balance complement dietary modification and conventional treatments. Over time, many clinicians observe reduced flare intensity, smoother recovery cycles and a decline in secondary infections when Reishi is incorporated into long-term management. Similarly, in gastrointestinal inflammatory disease, its combined anti-inflammatory, antioxidant and prebiotic effects support improved mucosal comfort and more stable stool patterns, particularly when used alongside appropriate dietary interventions and targeted pharmaceuticals.

Senior patients and those receiving chronic medications often benefit from Reishi's hepatic and mitochondrial protective effects. In such cases, improvements tend to emerge gradually as enhanced stamina, brighter demeanour, improved coat quality or more stable biochemical parameters. Within integrative oncology, Reishi is primarily used to support quality of life, maintain immune vigilance and buffer the physiological stress associated with treatment. While not a standalone anticancer agent, its regulatory immune effects, anti-inflammatory contribution and support for metabolic stability make it a valuable adjunct in appropriately supervised care plans.

Caution remains appropriate in animals with immune-mediated disease, advanced hepatic insufficiency or complex medication regimens. In such contexts, gradual titration and veterinary oversight ensure safe and predictable integration. Overall, Reishi functions as a terrain-modifying agent, strengthening the physiological foundation upon which healing, resilience and long-term stability depend.

> Reishi is most widely recognised in veterinary practice for its role as an adjunct in oncology, where it supports immune steadiness, resilience and overall quality of life during conventional treatment.

1.18 Conclusion – Integrative Significance and Extraction Considerations

Reishi holds a singular position within integrative veterinary medicine as a whole-system regulator whose influence extends steadily across inflammatory, immunological, neuroendocrine, gastrointestinal, hepatic and behavioural pathways. Its value does not lie in rapid symptomatic change, but in its ability to restore physiological steadiness in animals living with chronic inflammatory load, metabolic tension, age-related decline or long-term oxidative stress. This cumulative, terrain-centred mechanism makes Reishi particularly well suited to the chronic, multifactorial presentations commonly encountered in veterinary practice, where single-pathway interventions often fall short of addressing the broader biological context.

Across clinical domains, Reishi consistently supports patterns of improved resilience: calmer inflammatory behaviour, steadier gastrointestinal function, enhanced stress recovery, more predictable immune tone, stronger liver tolerance to medication and clearer cognitive engagement in senior animals. These outcomes align closely with the mushroom's mechanistic architecture, in which β-glucans, proteoglucans, triterpenes, antioxidant peptides, sterols and fibre-bound compounds interact to modulate cytokine activity, stabilise mast cells, protect mitochondrial function and support neuroendocrine rhythm. Because these pathways are deeply conserved across mammalian species, Reishi's effects translate predictably into companion-animal physiology despite the limited number of controlled veterinary trials.

Reishi also integrates seamlessly with other functional mushrooms, serving as a stable anchor within multi-species protocols. When paired with Lion's Mane it contributes a regulatory foundation that enhances neurotrophic and gut–brain support; with Turkey Tail it strengthens immune–gastrointestinal synergy for integrative oncology and chronic immune dysregulation; with Cordyceps it provides a counterbalance of inflammatory moderation and cardiovascular steadiness to complement respiratory and mitochondrial support. Its compatibility with Chaga and Golden Oyster extends this synergy into oxidative resilience, hepatic stability and cellular longevity. Across these combinations, Reishi's role is consistently that of a mediator and harmoniser, enhancing the coherence of the overall Mycotherapy strategy.

Extraction fidelity is central to the safe and effective use of Reishi in veterinary care. Its therapeutic breadth is dependent on the intact biochemical matrix of the fruiting body, where hydrophilic and lipophilic compounds coexist in naturally balanced ratios. Sub-critical water extraction preserves this full-spectrum architecture - polysaccharides, triterpenes, proteoglucans, sterols, phenolics and the native prebiotic fibre - without the solvent residues or selective fractionation seen in dual extracts and with none of the starch dilution inherent to grain-grown mycelium. This structural coherence ensures physiological predictability, smoother gastrointestinal integration and a regulatory profile that reflects the mechanistic pathways described throughout this monograph.

Ultimately, Reishi functions as a slow-building but deeply stabilising contributor to long-term veterinary wellbeing. Its role is not to replace pharmaceuticals, behavioural therapy or diagnostic investigation, but to reinforce the physiological ground upon which those interventions depend. When introduced gradually, monitored with clinical insight and integrated thoughtfully into multimodal care, Reishi offers a safe, coherent and evidence-aligned means of supporting resilience, comfort and healthy ageing across a wide range of chronic conditions. Its legacy as a longevity and vitality mushroom retains full relevance in modern veterinary medicine - expressed not through dramatic effects, but through steady, cumulative restoration of systemic balance.

> Reishi holds a singular position within integrative veterinary medicine as a whole-system regulator whose influence extends steadily across inflammatory, immunological, neuroendocrine, gastrointestinal, hepatic and behavioural pathways.

Reishi key sources (summary)

Boh et al., 2013; Gao et al., 2003; Wasser, 2014; Chu et al., 2012; Lai & Yu, 2010; Shi et al., 2014; Park & Kim, 2020; Meng et al., 2021; Kim & Park, 2014; Memorial Sloan Kettering Cancer Center, 2024; Bosch et al., 2015. **Full professional reference list available in the Master References section.**

> “The bioactive compounds in medicinal mushrooms present significant promise for supporting immune function in cancer care. *Source: Integrative Oncology research commentary Dr. Gordon Saxe, MD, PhD (Integrative Oncology Researcher)*”

2 | TURKEY TAIL (Trametes versicolor)

2.1. Introduction to Turkey Tail – *The Immune Defender*

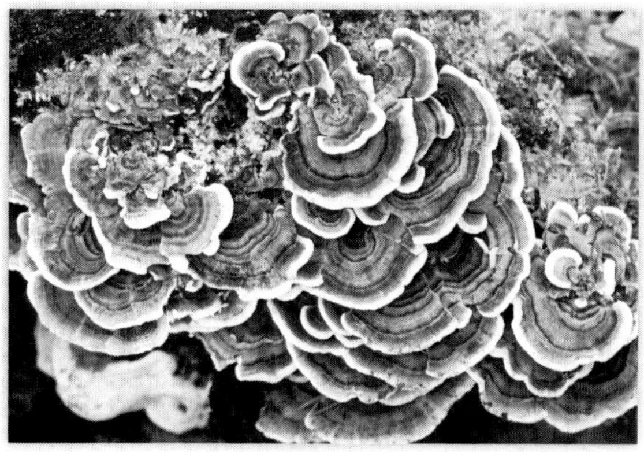

Turkey Tail (Trametes versicolor) is one of the world's most extensively researched medicinal mushrooms, distinguished by its striking multicoloured fan-shaped fruiting body and its long-standing role in immune health. In both traditional and modern medicinal systems, Turkey Tail is prized for its ability to strengthen host defences, modulate inflammatory responses and support resilience during chronic illness. Its reputation is strongly supported by decades of rigorous scientific investigation, including some of the most advanced immunological research undertaken on any medicinal mushroom.

In veterinary Mycotherapy, Turkey Tail stands out as a primary immunological modulator with broad applicability across species. Its polysaccharopeptides, beta-glucans, proteoglucans and triterpene-adjacent compounds influence both innate and adaptive immunity through multiple pathways, making it one of the most effective mushrooms for supporting immune surveillance, regulating dysregulated immune signalling and supporting the gut–immune interface.

Turkey Tail is especially relevant in cases of chronic infection, immune depletion, convalescence, age-related immune decline, gastrointestinal dysbiosis and integrative oncology. Yet, its influence extends well beyond immune stimulation: Turkey Tail provides terrain-level support for gut-associated lymphoid tissue (GALT), modulates inflammatory cascades, protects cellular integrity and supports metabolic resilience in chronically stressed or medically vulnerable animals.

Because Turkey Tail's efficacy depends heavily on extraction quality and the preservation of its fibre–polysaccharide matrix, whole-food SCWE extracts offer the most physiologically faithful representation of its therapeutic potential, a point revisited later in this monograph in a strictly scientific context.

> In veterinary Mycotherapy, Turkey Tail stands out as a primary immunological modulator with broad applicability across species.

2.2 Taxonomy, Morphology and Extraction Science

Trametes versicolor is a highly adaptive basidiomycete found worldwide in temperate forests. Its taxonomy is well defined compared with other medicinal mushrooms, allowing for consistent biochemical characterisation. The mature fruiting body is tough, high in chitin and rich in layered polysaccharides, reflecting its evolutionary role as a wood-decaying fungus and its biological synergy with lignin-rich substrates.

In medicinal use, fibre-rich fruiting bodies are essential. Myceliated grain lacks the polysaccharopeptide structures, beta-glucan complexity and proteoglucan arrays that underpin Turkey Tail's immunological and gut-microbiome effects. This makes fruiting-body-only extracts a non-negotiable requirement in clinical Mycotherapy.

Extraction Science and Clinical Implications

Turkey Tail's most studied immune-supportive molecules, including the well-characterised polysaccharopeptide (PSP) and polysaccharide-K (PSK), are tightly bound to a structural matrix of chitin, proteoglucans and fibre. Extraction technique directly determines whether these compounds retain their functional three-dimensional architecture and whether they remain biologically active.

Traditional decoctions capture a fraction of these compounds but may not fully solubilise key proteoglucan complexes or the deeper fibre-bound beta-glucans. Alcohol-based extracts emphasise lipophilic compounds but lack the immunologically significant hydrophilic fractions.

Sub-critical water extraction (SCWE) offers a more clinically coherent solution. SCWE provides a full-spectrum preparation that maintains the structural continuity of Turkey Tail's polysaccharopeptides, beta-glucans, proteoglucans and fibre-bound complexes. By utilising water at controlled temperature and pressure, SCWE extracts both hydrophilic and mildly lipophilic compounds without solvents, retaining the mushroom's natural fibre matrix. This biochemical fidelity is particularly relevant in veterinary Mycotherapy, as it preserves the molecular patterns that interact with gut-associated lymphoid tissue and innate immune receptors. In contrast, grain-grown mycelium or dual-extraction tinctures cannot replicate the immunological depth of the whole fruiting body. For chronic gastrointestinal, immune-regulatory or oncology applications, SCWE therefore offers a more physiologically aligned extract.

2.3. Bioactive Constituents – Molecular Drivers of Therapeutic Action

Turkey Tail's therapeutic profile arises from a highly complex array of bioactive compounds that interact with immune, gastrointestinal and metabolic pathways in ways that are unusually well characterised for a medicinal mushroom. Its most studied constituents are the polysaccharopeptides PSP and PSK, which combine protein fractions with structurally diverse beta-glucans to create molecules capable of influencing both innate and adaptive immunity. These compounds are embedded within a fibre-dense matrix of chitin, proteoglucans, polysaccharides and minor sterols, forming a biochemical ecosystem in which each component supports or amplifies the others.

PSP and PSK have attracted considerable scientific attention because they engage pattern-recognition receptors, including toll-like receptors and Dectin-1, initiating regulatory cascades that enhance immune surveillance while moderating inflammatory excess. Their protein-bound structure appears essential for their capacity to shape immune function, a feature that cannot be replicated in alcohol tinctures or myceliated grain products, which lack these compounds almost entirely.

Alongside these immunological agents, Turkey Tail contains a substantial portfolio of phenolic antioxidants that support cellular resilience during chronic illness, infection or oxidative stress. These compounds contribute to the mushroom's ability to protect epithelial tissues, stabilise mucosal surfaces and support mitochondrial function during periods of physiological strain.

The natural fibre matrix itself plays a significant therapeutic role. This structural component acts as a prebiotic substrate within the gut, influencing microbial diversity, short-chain fatty acid production and gastrointestinal immune tone. Because fibre architecture is easily disrupted by extraction methods that fragment or strip the polysaccharide framework, the preservation of this matrix through whole-food SCWE extraction is particularly relevant for clinical use. Together, these constituents form a highly integrated therapeutic system that underpins Turkey Tail's distinctive role in veterinary care.

2.4. Immune System Modulation – Restoring Coordination and Surveillance

Turkey Tail is one of the most comprehensively studied mushrooms in the field of immune regulation, and its influence across both innate and adaptive immunity is highly relevant to veterinary practice. Rather than acting as a crude stimulant, Turkey Tail modulates immune function with noteworthy precision. It enhances immune vigilance where required, yet reduces inappropriate inflammatory escalation, making it suitable for animals with impaired immunity, chronic infection, age-related immune decline or long-standing inflammatory disease.

Its principal immunological activity originates from polysaccharopeptides such as PSP and PSK and a range of structurally diverse beta-glucans and proteoglucans. These compounds interact with immune cells at multiple points of contact. On the innate side, **preclinical** work shows that Turkey Tail can activate macrophages, increase dendritic cell maturation and enhance natural killer cell responsiveness. These changes improve the animal's ability to recognise pathogens and abnormal cells during early immune engagement. Although direct veterinary trials remain limited, translational research and practitioner experience both indicate improved resilience in animals prone to recurrent infections or slow recovery during convalescence.

Within adaptive immunity, Turkey Tail supports T-cell coordination and the resilience of the broader lymphocyte population. Polysaccharopeptides have been shown in **cellular and animal**

models to enhance cytotoxic T-cell function and encourage more efficient antigen processing by dendritic cells. These shifts contribute to more efficient responses to chronic immune challenges, including persistent viral conditions, chronic inflammation and situations where immune signalling becomes fragmented or fatigued. PSP and PSK have also been shown to influence T-helper cell behaviour and regulatory T-cell balance, helping to maintain an immune environment that is responsive without being inflammatory.

Cytokine modulation represents another crucial dimension of Turkey Tail's activity. **Preclinical research** demonstrates suppression of excess interleukin 6, tumour necrosis factor alpha and interleukin 1 beta during inflammatory episodes, while preserving or enhancing interferon pathways necessary for viral defence and immune coordination. This dual mode of action makes Turkey Tail particularly well suited for veterinary patients with chronic inflammatory or immune-mediated conditions, where the goal is not to amplify immune activity indiscriminately but to restore a stable and functional immune rhythm.

Ageing animals also benefit meaningfully from Turkey Tail's immune-restorative properties. Natural immunosenescence leads to diminished innate and adaptive function, weaker vaccine responses and reduced capacity to respond to microbial or inflammatory challenges. Turkey Tail's complex beta-glucans and protein-bound polysaccharides help restore aspects of innate immunity and improve coordination within adaptive pathways. Although veterinary-specific ageing studies are still emerging, mechanistic parallels and clinical impressions suggest Turkey Tail is one of the most reliable mushrooms for senior immune support.

Across species, Turkey Tail supports a more intelligent and coordinated immune response, appropriate for long-term integrative care. Its regulatory influence provides a counterbalance to chronic inflammation, immune fragmentation and the metabolic strain associated with prolonged illness. For dogs and cats with chronic infections, cancer, immune dysregulation or age-related immune decline, Turkey Tail offers a safe, scientifically grounded tool to support resilience and steady immune function.

> Turkey Tail is one of the most comprehensively studied mushrooms in the field of immune regulation, and its influence across both innate and adaptive immunity is highly relevant to veterinary practice.

2.5. Anti-inflammatory Pathways and the Gut–Immune Axis

Turkey Tail's modulation of inflammation cannot be separated from its intimate interaction with the gastrointestinal tract. A substantial proportion of its therapeutic effect arises not from systemic suppression of inflammatory mediators but from its capacity to regulate inflammatory initiation at the mucosal surface. The gut represents the largest immune organ in the body, and Turkey Tail engages this interface in a manner that promotes stability and coordination.

At the molecular level, **preclinical studies** show that Turkey Tail suppresses activation of NF-kB, one of the primary transcription factors driving inflammatory cascades. By reducing the activity of NF-kB, the mushroom limits the expression of cytokines such as interleukin 6, interleukin 1 beta and tumour necrosis factor alpha. These cytokines are pivotal in a wide range of chronic veterinary conditions, including gastrointestinal inflammation, atopic disease, musculoskeletal pain and systemic inflammatory syndromes. The ability to modulate, rather than blunt, these pathways places Turkey Tail among the most adaptable anti-inflammatory mushrooms for long-term veterinary support.

The gut–immune axis amplifies these benefits. Turkey Tail interacts with gut-associated lymphoid tissue through its polysaccharopeptides and fibre-bound beta-glucans, shaping immune behaviour at the very point where immune signalling begins. This results in improved immune coherence, reduced inappropriate inflammatory escalation and enhanced mucosal resilience. Over time, these effects translate clinically into improved digestive comfort, enhanced stool quality and steadier responses to dietary or environmental stressors.

Because inflammatory states in the gut often contribute to systemic imbalance, Turkey Tail's influence at the mucosal level frequently produces improvements in distant tissues, including the liver, skin and joints. Its actions are cumulative and require sustained administration, but the pattern of response, particularly in animals with chronic gastrointestinal sensitivity, is remarkably consistent.

2.6. Gastrointestinal Resilience and Microbiome Health

Turkey Tail is one of the most reliable mushrooms for restoring gastrointestinal balance in veterinary patients, largely due to its capacity to modulate the microbiome and reinforce mucosal integrity. Its natural fibre matrix and polysaccharopeptide-rich composition create a terrain in which beneficial microbial taxa can thrive, and where the inflammatory signals that initiate digestive discomfort are progressively reduced.

Within the gastrointestinal tract, Turkey Tail supports epithelial health by moderating the inflammatory mediators responsible for mucosal injury. **Preclinical research** demonstrates that its polysaccharopeptides reduce inflammatory cell infiltration and strengthen tight-junction proteins, limiting the permeability that contributes to hepatic strain, endotoxin translocation and immune dysregulation. These effects help stabilise the gut lining in animals with chronic enteropathy, inflammatory bowel disease-like syndromes or diet-related gastrointestinal sensitivity.

> Turkey Tail is one of the most reliable mushrooms for restoring gastrointestinal balance in veterinary patients,

Equally significant is Turkey Tail's influence on microbial diversity. Its complex fibre acts as a fermentable substrate for beneficial bacteria, supporting increased production of short-chain fatty acids such as butyrate. These metabolites nourish epithelial cells, reduce mucosal inflammation and support more efficient immune signalling. In veterinary practice, this translates into steadier stools, improved nutrient assimilation and a more predictable response to dietary interventions.

The liver also benefits from these gastrointestinal improvements. Reduced gut permeability and improved microbial stability decrease the burden of inflammatory metabolites reaching the hepatic portal circulation. As a result, Turkey Tail is frequently included in comprehensive care for animals experiencing hepatic strain, particularly those undergoing long-term pharmacological treatment.

Sub-critical water extraction plays a meaningful role in preserving these gastrointestinal benefits. SCWE retains the structural fibre and proteoglucan complexes that a whole-food extract requires in order to exert predictable effects on the gut–immune axis. Extracts lacking this fibre matrix do not provide comparable mucosal support, making SCWE particularly well aligned with gastrointestinal therapeutic goals.

2.7. Oncology and Adjunctive Cancer Support

Turkey Tail holds a well-recognised position in integrative oncology owing to its immunologically active polysaccharopeptides (PSP and PSK) and its long history of evaluation in human cancer care. Although veterinary-specific trials remain limited, the adjunctive use of Turkey Tail in human oncology is widely acknowledged, including by organisations such as the American Cancer Society, which lists it as a supportive therapy within evidence-informed integrative frameworks. This external validation provides useful translational relevance for veterinary practitioners seeking safe, non-pharmacological terrain support during conventional cancer treatment.

Its influence on both innate and adaptive immunity is well documented. Preclinical research demonstrates enhanced activity of macrophages, dendritic cells, natural killer cells and cytotoxic T lymphocytes – immune functions central to early tumour recognition and control of abnormal cellular proliferation. For animals experiencing immune depletion, chronic oncological burden or recurrent infections, this immunomodulatory influence may contribute to more stable physiological responses during treatment.

Turkey Tail also helps regulate the inflammatory environment in which tumours develop. Chronic inflammation drives angiogenesis, tissue breakdown and metabolic dysregulation. By moderating inflammatory mediators and strengthening antioxidant defence, Turkey Tail supports a more balanced terrain, potentially improving tolerance to chemotherapy, radiation or palliative protocols. These benefits are frequently reported in clinical practice and align with its mechanistic evidence, though they should not be interpreted as direct anti-tumour effects.

Gastrointestinal sensitivity, appetite fluctuation and metabolic fatigue are common challenges for oncology patients. Turkey Tail's prebiotic fibre and polysaccharopeptides can help stabilise digestive comfort, support appetite and promote immune steadiness throughout the treatment cycle. These improvements are subtle and cumulative, reinforcing its role as a supportive, terrain-focused adjunct rather than a primary intervention.

Extraction fidelity is critical in oncology settings. PSP and PSK are not extracted through alcohol tinctures and are minimal or absent in myceliated grain products. SCWE full-spectrum extraction preserves the full complement of polysaccharopeptides, β-glucans, phenolics and prebiotic compounds without degrading sensitive structures, making it the most clinically appropriate preparation for oncology patients with already compromised physiology.

Turkey Tail holds a well-recognised position in integrative oncology owing to its immunologically active polysaccharopeptides (PSP and PSK) and its long history of evaluation in human cancer care.

2.8. Hepatic Protection and Metabolic Support

Although not traditionally highlighted for its hepatic effects, Turkey Tail provides meaningful support to the liver through its interaction with inflammation, oxidative stress and the gut–liver axis. The liver is constantly exposed to microbial metabolites, dietary by-products and inflammatory mediators originating from the gastrointestinal tract. By reducing mucosal inflammation and stabilising microbial balance, Turkey Tail indirectly lowers hepatic burden and supports more consistent metabolic function.

Its antioxidant compounds further protect hepatocytes from oxidative injury, particularly in animals undergoing long-term drug therapy or those experiencing chronic systemic inflammation. **Preclinical studies** demonstrate improvements in markers of oxidative stress and inflammatory load in liver tissue when animals receive Turkey Tail extracts, suggesting that the mushroom may help preserve hepatic stability under conditions of metabolic strain.

Turkey Tail also contributes to broader metabolic resilience by supporting mitochondrial energy production, moderating inflammatory cytokines and enhancing the short-chain fatty acid profile generated within the gut. These multi-level effects are subtle but cumulative, and contribute to improved energy, steadier appetite and general vitality in chronically ill or ageing animals.

Within integrative practice, Turkey Tail is often combined with Reishi for hepatic modulation, with Chaga for antioxidant reinforcement and with Shiitake for support of lipid metabolism. When extraction is performed via SCWE, the resulting whole-food extract retains the proteoglucans, polysaccharides and fibre-bound compounds necessary for predictable hepatic and metabolic influence without solvent residues or excess starch.

2.9. Neurological and Behavioural Relevance

Turkey Tail's most recognised actions lie within immunological and gastrointestinal domains, yet its influence extends to neurological and behavioural health through mechanisms that are increasingly relevant in veterinary medicine. A growing body of research emphasises the profound interconnectedness between the gut microbiome, immune signalling and the central nervous system. Turkey Tail acts upon this axis in ways that support emotional stability, behavioural resilience and overall neurological well-being.

Through its regulation of inflammatory mediators, Turkey Tail reduces systemic cytokines that can cross or influence the blood–brain barrier. Chronic elevations of interleukin 6, interleukin 1 beta and tumour necrosis factor alpha are associated with neuroinflammation, cognitive decline and behavioural dysregulation in multiple species. By moderating these pathways, Turkey Tail provides an indirect but meaningful reduction in the neuroinflammatory load that can exacerbate anxiety, irritability and cognitive decline in companion animals.

The mushroom's influence on the microbiome further reinforces this effect. Improvements in microbial diversity and short-chain fatty acid production support the synthesis of neuroactive molecules, including serotonin precursors, and improve vagal signalling between the gut and the brain. **Preclinical studies** indicate that changes in gut microbial metabolism can reduce behavioural markers of stress, improve cognitive performance and enhance adaptability to environmental pressure. While species-specific veterinary trials are limited, these mechanistic insights align closely with the clinical observations of integrative practitioners who note that Turkey Tail can support calmer demeanour, improved digestive–behavioural synchrony and greater stress tolerance in animals with chronic gastrointestinal or inflammatory conditions.

Although Turkey Tail does not stimulate neurotrophic factors directly, its capacity to reduce inflammatory interference in neuronal signalling makes it a useful co-therapy in senior animals, those recovering from chronic illness or those experiencing behavioural symptoms linked to gastrointestinal discomfort. When paired with Lion's Mane, the mushroom frequently forms part of a broader neurological support strategy, with Turkey Tail providing the regulatory and gastrointestinal foundation upon which neurotrophic interventions can act more effectively.

2.10. Veterinary Pharmacology and Drug Interactions

Turkey Tail expresses a gentle and broadly compatible pharmacological profile, characterised by low toxicity, physiological adaptability and predictable behaviour when used alongside common veterinary medications. Its primary actions arise from its polysaccharopeptides (PSK and PSP), β-glucans, proteoglucans and fibre-bound compounds, each of which interacts with the gastrointestinal and immune systems in ways that tend to support rather than interfere with pharmaceutical treatment. Nonetheless, thoughtful integration remains an essential clinical responsibility, particularly in animals with complex internal medicine needs or polypharmacy.

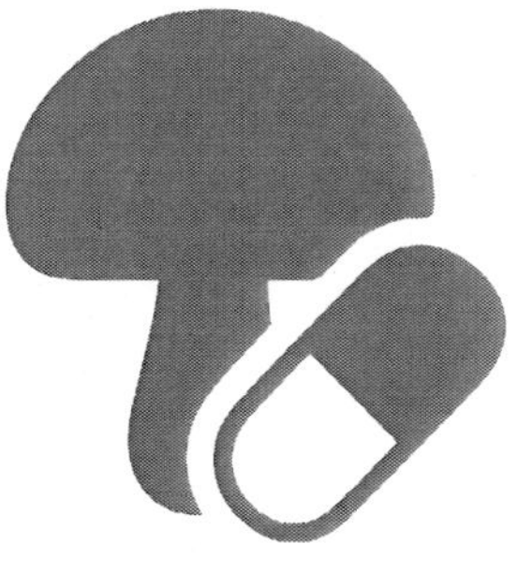

Immune-modulatory interactions

Turkey Tail's regulatory influence on innate and adaptive immunity can, in some circumstances, intersect with immunosuppressive medication. Its polysaccharopeptides enhance antigen presentation, macrophage tone and aspects of T-helper regulation. These actions do not produce immune overstimulation, but they may theoretically counterbalance the intended effects of corticosteroids, ciclosporin or other immunosuppressants when used at higher therapeutic doses. In practice, many clinicians report stable co-administration when Turkey Tail is introduced conservatively and adjusted according to the patient's medical goals, yet each case must be evaluated individually, particularly in autoimmune disease.

Interactions with anti-inflammatory agents

Turkey Tail frequently complements non-steroidal anti-inflammatory drugs and corticosteroids by contributing a background reduction in inflammatory mediators within the gastrointestinal, dermatological and systemic environments. Its influence on the gut–immune axis may indirectly reduce inflammatory load. Although no significant pharmacokinetic conflicts have been documented, animals with pre-existing gastrointestinal fragility warrant careful monitoring, as synergistic anti-inflammatory effects may unmask underlying sensitivity.

Hepatic metabolism and polypharmacy considerations

Because many pharmaceuticals exert hepatic strain over time, Turkey Tail's influence on the gut–liver axis can support metabolic resilience during chronic pharmacological therapy. Animals receiving anticonvulsants, chemotherapeutic drugs, corticosteroids or long-term analgesics may benefit from Turkey Tail's gentle stabilising effect on mucosal immunity, microbial balance and hepatic inflammatory tone. While this support is typically favourable, monitoring liver enzymes in medically fragile patients remains best practice.

Extraction quality and pharmacological predictability

Sub-critical water extraction (SCWE) improves pharmacological clarity by eliminating solvent residues and preserving the mushroom's natural fibre and polysaccharopeptide matrix. SCWE preparations avoid the metabolic unpredictability associated with alcohol tinctures and the starch-heavy distortion of myceliated grain products. In elderly animals, those with hepatic compromise or individuals receiving complex medication regimes, this biochemical fidelity offers a safer and more consistent therapeutic profile.

2.11. Clinical Application

Overview and therapeutic positioning

Turkey Tail is one of the most versatile functional mushrooms in veterinary Mycotherapy, recognised for its broad-spectrum β-glucans, polysaccharopeptides (PSP/PSK), prebiotic fibre and gut–immune axis modulation. Its primary actions centre on mucosal immunity, balanced immune surveillance, gastrointestinal stability and long-term inflammatory regulation. Turkey Tail is not intended as a rapid symptomatic agent; rather, it acts as a slow, steady terrain-modulating species that reinforces physiological resilience over time. It is especially valuable in chronic immune fragility, gastrointestinal dysbiosis, integrative oncology protocols and age-related immune decline.

Gastrointestinal regulation and mucosal integrity

Turkey Tail is widely used in veterinary practice for chronic enteropathies, intermittent diarrhoea, dysbiosis and stress-responsive gastrointestinal upset. Its prebiotic polysaccharides promote microbial diversity and short-chain fatty acid production, supporting mucosal healing and stabilising the gut–immune interface. Over time, practitioners observe improved stool quality, steadier appetite and reduced relapse in animals with chronic digestive vulnerability. Its gentle, fibre-rich profile makes it well tolerated across a broad range of species.

Immune modulation and chronic inflammatory conditions

Turkey Tail's diverse β-glucan architecture and PSP-associated pathways support both innate and adaptive immune function without overstimulation. This makes it a valuable tool for animals with recurrent infections, chronic inflammatory cycles, immune exhaustion or age-related drift in immune competency. Its ability to regulate immune patterning also benefits dermatological reactivity and allergic tendencies, particularly when combined with species such as Reishi or Chaga.

Oncology support and immune surveillance

Turkey Tail has a long-established role in integrative oncology. Its polysaccharopeptides contribute to improved immune surveillance, enhanced NK-cell activity and moderated inflammatory responses. It supports quality of life, appetite, digestive stability and energy resilience in animals undergoing cancer treatment. When integrated with whole-food SCWE extracts, Turkey Tail's contribution to mitochondrial buffering and metabolic calm further assists animals experiencing treatment-related physiological load.

Respiratory and stress-linked conditions

In animals with respiratory vulnerability - including chronic inflammation, airway irritation or post-infectious fragility - Turkey Tail's immune-balancing and mucosal-stabilising effects offer supportive benefit. Because immune and mucosal pathways influence airway behaviour, Turkey Tail can help reduce flare frequency and restore steadier baseline function. Its gentle influence on stress-immune crosstalk also supports animals whose immune fragility worsens under environmental or emotional stress.

Long-term terrain support and preventative care

As a terrain-focused mushroom, Turkey Tail works cumulatively rather than acutely. Consistent daily administration promotes long-term stability in gastrointestinal, immune and inflammatory networks. It integrates seamlessly into preventative wellness strategies for senior animals, those recovering from chronic illness, and individuals prone to recurrent digestive or immunological disturbances.

Integration with other functional mushrooms

Turkey Tail integrates seamlessly into multi-mushroom veterinary protocols due to its diverse β-glucan architecture, polysaccharopeptides (PSP/PSK), microbiome-modulating actions and broad immunoregulatory influence. It pairs particularly well with mushrooms that offer complementary effects across immunity, oncology, metabolism and gut–brain physiology. These combinations expand Turkey Tail's already substantial clinical value, especially in chronic, immune-mediated or oncology-centred care.

- **With Reishi** - Turkey Tail and Reishi form one of the most clinically relevant pairings in integrative veterinary practice. Turkey Tail contributes robust immune-priming activity through PSP/PSK-associated pathways and β-glucan signalling, supporting NK-cell activity, macrophage behaviour and adaptive immune tone. Reishi brings triterpenoid-mediated inflammatory balance, autonomic steadiness and antiviral influence. Together, they provide a stabilising combination for chronic infection risk, oncology protocols, age-related immune decline and cases requiring moderated but reliable immune engagement. This pairing is particularly valuable for animals undergoing long-term integrative care or recovering from chronic immune suppression.

- **With Chaga** - Chaga deepens Turkey Tail's antioxidant and cellular-protective profile. While Turkey Tail modulates immune patterning and microbiome stability, Chaga contributes high polyphenol content, melanin complexes, trace minerals and SOD-like activity that buffer oxidative stress at a mitochondrial and tissue level. This pairing is suited to animals experiencing chronic inflammation, allergy tendencies, hepatic workload, dermatological instability or environmental toxin exposure. For oncology support, the duo provides both immune surveillance enhancement and redox-balancing defence, helping moderate treatment-related oxidative burden.

- **With Maitake** -Turkey Tail and Maitake together offer a potent blend of immune-system reinforcement, metabolic support and oncology-directed synergy. Maitake's influence on insulin signalling, metabolic regulation and NK-cell responsiveness complements Turkey Tail's PSP-mediated immune effects. This pairing is valuable for animals with metabolic vulnerability (overweight, endocrine shifts, age-related insulin fluctuations), chronic inflammatory disease or those requiring layered immune defence during oncology care. The combination also supports gut–immune crosstalk through their shared prebiotic fibre contributions when extracted via whole-mushroom SCWE methods.

- **With Lion's Mane** - Lion's Mane adds a neurotrophic and gut–brain axis dimension to Turkey Tail's immune-microbiome network. Turkey Tail improves microbial balance and short-chain fatty acid production, while Lion's Mane supports neuronal regeneration, enteric nervous system stability and stress-modified gastrointestinal function. This synergy benefits animals with cognitive decline, behavioural fragility, chronic gut dysbiosis or stress-linked immune suppression. Turkey Tail's immune modulation helps stabilise systemic resilience, while Lion's Mane enhances neurological and gastrointestinal integration.
- **With Golden Oyster** - Golden Oyster contributes an ergothioneine-rich cytoprotective and mitochondrial-supportive layer to Turkey Tail's immune effects. ERGO enhances antioxidant defence, protects DNA and mitochondrial membranes, and buffers metabolic stress – complementing Turkey Tail's β-glucan-driven immune priming. This pairing supports long-term cellular health, healthy ageing trajectories, recovery from oxidative load and resilience during chronic disease management. It is particularly relevant for senior animals, those undergoing oncology treatment, or those with chronic inflammatory patterns where both immune balance and deep cellular protection are required.

> Synergistic pairings or triads of mushrooms can act across multiple physiological pathways, broadening the supportive effect and contributing to a full-spectrum, terrain-based Mycotherapy strategy.

Species Specific Consideration with Turkey Tail

Dogs

Dogs frequently benefit from Turkey Tail in cases of gastrointestinal sensitivity, chronic enteropathies, immune exhaustion, atopic tendencies and age-related decline. Its influence on the gut–immune–skin axis also makes it a useful supportive agent in animals with recurrent skin or ear issues linked to immune imbalance or dysbiosis, including those with secondary yeast overgrowth. Clinicians and owners have reported anecdotal improvements when Turkey Tail is paired with Reishi, reflecting their combined effects on immune modulation, inflammatory tone and mucosal and dermal resilience. Dogs recovering from infection or immune fragmentation often show steadier vitality, improved stool regularity and enhanced immune tone over several weeks. Turkey Tail also plays a prominent role as supportive care in integrative oncology, where its polysaccharopeptides contribute to immune surveillance and comfort during treatment.

Turkey Tail also plays a prominent and well-recognised role as supportive care in integrative oncology. Its polysaccharopeptides (PSP/PSK) have been studied for their immune-modulating and immune-surveillance effects, and its influence on appetite, vitality and digestive steadiness can support quality of life during treatment. In recent years, its profile has broadened further, in part due to widespread public awareness generated by *The Forever Dog*, which highlighted Turkey Tail's supportive role in cancer-related care. Within clinical practice, veterinarians frequently integrate Turkey Tail alongside Reishi or Chaga to provide a broader spectrum of immune balance, antioxidant protection and metabolic calm for dogs undergoing conventional or integrative cancer protocols.

Cats

In feline practice, Turkey Tail is valued for its gentle prebiotic activity, gut–immune stabilisation and suitability for inflammatory airway or mucosal disorders. Cats with chronic herpesvirus flare-ups, gingivostomatitis, intermittent diarrhoea or immune frailty may respond particularly well. Its neutral sensory profile improves acceptance compared with stronger-flavoured mushrooms like Reishi.

Horses

Equine use focuses on immune modulation, respiratory resilience and gastrointestinal stability. Its fibre-rich composition aligns naturally with hindgut physiology. Horses with inflammatory airway conditions, recurrent infections or stress-responsive gastrointestinal fragility may benefit, though dosing must be carefully tailored to body weight, metabolic condition and sensitivity.

Small Mammals, Birds and Exotics

Turkey Tail may be cautiously integrated into supportive care where chronic inflammation, immune suppression or digestive instability are present. Given species-specific metabolic differences, conservative dosing and veterinary oversight are essential, but its broad safety profile supports thoughtful use across select exotic and small-animal species.

2.12. Safety, Contraindications and Monitoring

Turkey Tail is widely recognised as a safe and well-tolerated medicinal mushroom with a strong historical and translational safety record. Its suitability for long-term administration arises from its physiologically coherent action on the gut–immune axis and its low metabolic burden, yet thoughtful clinical oversight remains essential, particularly in complex or fragile patients.

General tolerability

Mild digestive adjustment is the most common minor reaction seen upon introduction, especially in animals with sensitive gastrointestinal systems. Transient soft stools, mild gassiness or small shifts in appetite usually resolve as the gut microbiome adjusts to the increased fibre and polysaccharopeptide content. A slow titration over five to seven days is advisable for sensitive individuals.

Immune-mediated disease and immunosuppression

Animals receiving immunosuppressive therapy require careful assessment before introducing Turkey Tail. While the mushroom modulates immune tone rather than stimulating it, its polysaccharopeptides may influence the clinical goal of immunosuppression if used at higher doses. Conservative introduction, low-tier dosing and close clinical monitoring are prudent in autoimmune or severe inflammatory disease.

Hepatic and renal considerations

Although Turkey Tail imposes minimal hepatic strain, animals with advanced hepatic insufficiency, severe cholestasis or multi-organ compromise benefit from cautious titration and periodic laboratory monitoring. Renal considerations are generally modest compared with high-oxalate mushrooms, but senior animals with reduced physiological reserve should be monitored during introduction.

Pregnancy, lactation and paediatric use

Controlled research is lacking in pregnant or lactating animals. While no reproductive toxicity has been reported, conservative clinical practice favours avoiding routine use during pregnancy unless the benefit is clearly justified. Young animals can receive Turkey Tail when clinically indicated, but gradual titration and close observation are recommended.

Extraction quality and clinical safety

SCWE extracts provide a solvent-free, fibre-intact preparation with predictable biochemical composition. Alcohol-based tinctures introduce residual ethanol unsuitable for long-term or high-dose administration, while grain-grown mycelium products dilute active compounds with starch and lack the polysaccharopeptide integrity that underpins Turkey Tail's effects. In medically vulnerable patients, SCWE preparations offer superior predictability and lower risk of digestive or metabolic disturbances.

Monitoring

Regular monitoring enhances both safety and therapeutic clarity. Clinicians should observe stool quality, appetite, demeanour and coat condition during the first fortnight, with laboratory assessment (e.g., hepatic enzymes, inflammatory markers) performed as appropriate in chronic disease cases or oncology protocols.

2.13. Evidence Quality Commentary

Turkey Tail is supported by one of the most extensive bodies of medicinal mushroom research globally, especially in the domains of immunology, mucosal defence and oncology. Its polysaccharopeptides PSK and PSP rank among the most researched natural immunomodulators, with decades of biochemical, preclinical and translational study forming a clear mechanistic foundation.

In veterinary contexts, the strength of the evidence lies in its consistency across mechanistic models. Preclinical studies repeatedly demonstrate enhancement of innate immune function, stabilisation of cytokine patterns and support for mucosal immunity. These findings translate logically to common veterinary challenges such as chronic enteropathy, immune exhaustion, allergic inflammation and recovery from infection.

Species-specific clinical trials remain limited, but the combined weight of mechanistic evidence, translational relevance from rodent and in vitro studies, and substantial practitioner experience provides a reliable framework for clinical integration. As with Reishi, the mushroom's strongest evidence supports its regulatory role rather than acute disease modification. It functions as a terrain-level agent, strengthening the underlying physiological systems that determine long-term health and resilience.

Extraction fidelity is central to interpreting this evidence. Research on PSK and PSP is based on whole-mushroom, fibre-containing extracts rather than myceliated grain products or alcohol tinctures. SCWE preparations most closely replicate the structural and biochemical characteristics used in foundational studies, preserving the polysaccharopeptide complexes and fibre-bound constituents that drive Turkey Tail's effects.

TURKEY TAIL (TRAMETES VERSICOLOR) – Evidence Quality Commentary Table

This spectrum of evidence is summarised in the following table:

Domain	Evidence Strength	Primary Evidence Type
Immunomodulation and immune recovery	High	Preclinical, animal models, human clinical adjunct trials
Oncology adjunct use	Moderate to high	Human clinical (PSK/PSP), preclinical, practitioner reports
Gut–microbiome and gastrointestinal support	Moderate	Preclinical, rodent and canine microbiome studies
Antioxidant and anti-inflammatory activity	Moderate	Preclinical, mechanistic in vitro and in vivo
Antiviral and respiratory support	Emerging	Preclinical viral models, extrapolated human clinical use
Hepatic and detoxification support	Emerging	Preclinical, mechanistic rationale
Metabolic and energy regulation	Emerging	Preclinical, limited targeted studies
Clinical veterinary trials	Limited	Small-scale canine studies and early pilot investigations

When mechanistic data, preclinical studies, human oncology experience and practitioner observations are considered together, Turkey Tail emerges as a scientifically credible, low-risk adjunct within integrative veterinary practice. Its polysaccharopeptides and β-glucan-rich fractions are strongly associated with immune modulation, improved immune surveillance and support for animals under significant physiological load, particularly in oncology and chronic immune dysregulation.

Within this context, extract fidelity is critical. The most clinically relevant effects arise from fruiting-body preparations that preserve the native matrix of polysaccharopeptides, β-glucans, phenolics and prebiotic fibres. SCWE full-spectrum extracts maintain this complexity while excluding grain-derived starch, providing a dependable option for terrain-focused Mycotherapy. For veterinarians, Turkey Tail is best positioned as a steady, long-term support agent – particularly in oncology, convalescence and immune-compromised states – rather than as a stand-alone or rapid-acting intervention.

2.14. Conclusion – Integrative Significance and Extraction Considerations

Turkey Tail's relevance in veterinary Mycotherapy arises from its capacity to restore balance across immune, gastrointestinal and metabolic systems. Its polysaccharopeptides enhance immune intelligence, its fibre-rich matrix supports mucosal resilience and microbial diversity, and its antioxidant and anti-inflammatory actions help stabilise chronic physiological disturbances.

Because these effects depend on the mushroom's full biochemical matrix, extract fidelity is critical. Turkey Tail's synergistic interplay of PSK, PSP, β-glucans, proteoglucans, phenolic antioxidants and fibre-bound compounds is only preserved in whole-food preparations. Sub-critical water extraction maintains this natural complexity, producing a solvent-free, structurally coherent extract that mirrors the biochemical architecture upon which modern research is based.

When integrated with thoughtful dosing, careful monitoring and a comprehensive veterinary plan, Turkey Tail functions as a predictable, evidence-aligned contributor to long-term health. Its strength lies not in acute symptomatic change but in its cumulative ability to support resilience, balance and physiological stability across species.

> Turkey Tail's relevance in veterinary Mycotherapy arises from its capacity to restore balance across immune, gastrointestinal and metabolic systems.

Key sources (summary)

Adachi et al., 1987; Jin et al., 2012; Bao & Lin, 2019; Kawagishi et al., 2008; Mizuno, 2012; Chu et al., 2017; Lull et al., 2005; Ooi & Liu, 2000; Zhou & Zhang, 2019; Smith et al., 2002; Li et al., 2020; Hobbs, 2021; Wasser, 2014. **Full professional reference list available in the Master References section.**

> Viruses and bacteria shape life, but fungi shape civilisation. *Source: Public scientific commentary (1960s) Dr. Andre Lwoff (Nobel Prize in Medicine)*

3 LION'S MANE (Hericium erinaceus)

3.1 Introduction to Lion's Mane – *The Brain Booster* and Gut Warrior

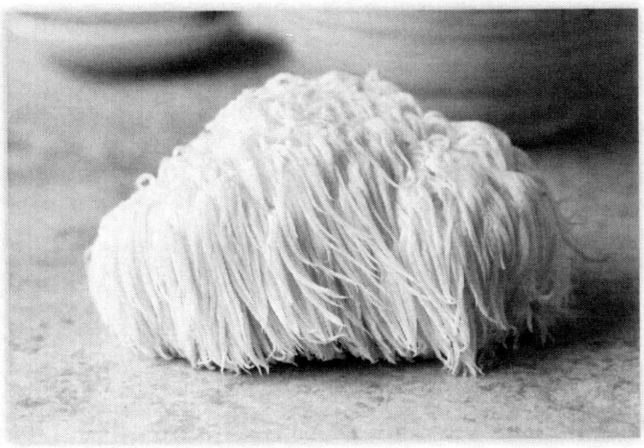

Lion's Mane (Hericium erinaceus) has gained international recognition for its unique neurotrophic properties, distinguished from all other medicinal mushrooms by its rare capacity to influence nerve growth factor (NGF) and brain-derived neurotrophic factor (BDNF). Historically used in traditional East Asian medicine as a tonic for digestion, vitality and mental clarity, it has now emerged as one of the most studied mushrooms in the fields of neuroprotection, cognitive ageing and gut–brain axis biology. This convergence of traditional knowledge and modern neurobiology places Lion's Mane at a unique intersection of veterinary neurology, behavioural medicine and geriatric care.

Modern research has confirmed that Lion's Mane contains a specialised class of diterpenoids (erinacines and hericenones) capable of activating pathways associated with neuronal regeneration, synaptic plasticity and myelin repair. These effects have been documented in models of cognitive decline, neuroinflammation, nerve injury and traumatic brain injury. Although veterinary-specific trials remain limited, Lion's Mane is increasingly adopted within integrative veterinary practice for age-related cognitive decline, stress-responsive behavioural issues, gastrointestinal fragility linked to neuroinflammatory patterns and adjunctive support in neurological recovery.

For clinical reliability, extract fidelity is essential. Only fruiting-body preparations contain both hericenones and the complex fibre–proteoglucan matrix that shapes Lion's Mane's gut–immune signalling. Sub-critical water extraction (SCWE) preserves this biochemical architecture by capturing both hydrophilic polysaccharides and lipophilic neuroactive constituents without solvent residues or mycelial starch. As with all Mycotherapy, the goal is not acute symptomatic change, but rather gradual restoration of physiological balance and long-term neural resilience.

3.2 Bioactive Constituents – Mechanistic Relevance to Veterinary Physiology

> Lion's Mane (Hericium erinaceus) has gained international recognition for its unique neurotrophic properties, distinguished from all other medicinal mushrooms by its rare capacity to influence nerve growth factor (NGF) and brain-derived neurotrophic factor (BDNF).

Lion's Mane expresses a unique ensemble of neuroactive and immunologically relevant compounds that together create its broad therapeutic profile. While often framed simply as a 'brain mushroom', its physiology extends beyond neuronal repair to include gastrointestinal integrity, immune modulation and metabolic regulation. Understanding these constituents is central to anticipating its actions across different veterinary contexts, particularly in senior animals or those with neuroinflammatory conditions.

The best-known compounds are the hericenones and erinacines, two families of diterpenoids capable of influencing nerve growth factor (NGF) and brain-derived neurotrophic factor (BDNF) pathways. Hericenones occur primarily in the fruiting body and contribute to enhanced synaptic plasticity, cognitive processing and hippocampal resilience in preclinical models. Erinacines, although more abundant in mycelial biomass, have mechanistic overlap, particularly in relation to neurite outgrowth and mitochondrial optimisation. SCWE fruiting-body extracts naturally carry diterpenoid fractions relevant to NGF modulation without the undesirable starch matrix introduced by myceliated-grain preparations. These compounds, alongside phenolic antioxidants and steroidal constituents, form the neurological backbone of Lion's Mane's therapeutic profile.

Equally important are the β-glucans and fibre-bound proteoglucans that define the mushroom's immunological and gastrointestinal actions. These polysaccharides modulate macrophage behaviour, influence microglial tone and regulate cytokines in ways that affect both systemic and central nervous function. Their interaction with gut-associated lymphoid tissue (GALT) helps stabilise mucosal immunity and contributes to improved communication across the gut–immune–brain axis. The natural fibre matrix, preserved through Sub-critical water extraction, plays a foundational role here, shaping microbial fermentation, supporting short-chain fatty acid production and promoting gastrointestinal tolerance in sensitive animals.

Lion's Mane also contains a range of phenolic antioxidants, terpenoids and secondary metabolites that contribute to vascular stability, metabolic balance and protection against oxidative injury. These compounds are not individually dominant but act in concert, reinforcing the mushroom's profile as a cumulative, regulatory and system-wide support rather than a narrowly targeted intervention. When delivered as a whole-food SCWE extract, Lion's Mane maintains a biochemical fidelity that allows these compounds to interact synergistically, providing predictable physiological effects across multiple body systems.

3.3 Immune Modulation and Neuroimmune Signalling

Lion's Mane exerts a gentle yet meaningful regulatory influence on both the peripheral immune system and central neuroimmune pathways. Unlike strongly immunostimulatory mushrooms such as

Turkey Tail, Lion's Mane operates through moderation rather than amplification, making it well suited to animals with chronic stress, behavioural reactivity or neuroinflammatory backgrounds. Its most clinically relevant actions arise from the way it harmonises immune signalling with neurological function, particularly in the ageing patient.

At the level of the central nervous system, Lion's Mane helps temper excessive microglial activation, a process implicated in cognitive decline, anxiety patterns, neuropathic discomfort and degenerative neurological change. Preclinical studies consistently show down-regulation of inflammatory mediators within neuronal tissue, including interleukin-6 (IL-6), tumour necrosis factor alpha (TNF-α) and inducible nitric oxide synthase (iNOS). This reduction in neuroinflammatory pressure contributes to improved neuronal resilience, steadier behavioural responses and enhanced cognitive processing over time. These findings are especially relevant to dogs with cognitive dysfunction, older cats with irritability or fragmented sleep, and animals recovering from neurological injury or compromise

Beyond the brain, Lion's Mane influences systemic immune behaviour through its β-glucans, proteoglucans and naturally occurring fibres. These constituents interact with immune receptors along the gastrointestinal tract and within mucosal tissues, promoting balanced macrophage activity, appropriate T-helper cell responses and moderated cytokine signalling. Rather than pushing the immune system toward heightened activity, Lion's Mane supports a more calibrated immune tone that reduces inappropriate inflammatory escalation. This regulatory influence is one reason why clinically observable improvements often occur in animals with overlapping gastrointestinal and behavioural sensitivities.

The gut–immune–brain axis represents a particularly important domain of activity. Lion's Mane has been shown to reshape microbial composition, favouring short-chain fatty acid–producing taxa that enhance epithelial integrity and reduce gut-derived inflammatory load. Improvements in vagal communication and serotonergic balance have been documented in preclinical models, offering mechanistic explanation for the calmer demeanour, improved digestive regularity and reduced stress reactivity reported by integrative veterinary practitioners. These interactions highlight Lion's Mane's suitability for animals presenting with intertwined digestive, behavioural and cognitive symptoms, particularly when environmental or emotional stress exacerbates gastrointestinal disturbance.

> Lion's Mane exerts a gentle yet meaningful regulatory influence on both the peripheral immune system and central neuroimmune pathways

3.4 Neurological and Behavioural Medicine

Lion's Mane has earned particular attention in veterinary neurology because it interacts with pathways fundamental to neuronal repair, synaptic resilience and behavioural stability. Its diterpenoid compounds, especially the hericenones and erinacines, influence nerve growth factor (NGF) and brain-derived neurotrophic factor (BDNF), both of which are central to neuroplasticity, cognitive processing and recovery from neural stress. These actions are supported by a growing body of preclinical research demonstrating enhanced neurite extension, mitochondrial protection and reduced neuroinflammatory load in diverse experimental models.

For ageing animals, especially dogs showing early signs of cognitive dysfunction, Lion's Mane offers a gentle means of supporting neurological architecture. Preclinical studies consistently demonstrate improvements in hippocampal signalling, reductions in microglial overactivation and enhanced antioxidant defence within neural tissue. Clinically, this translates into steadier sleep–wake patterns, improved environmental engagement and more consistent behavioural responses when administered over several weeks. The mushroom's actions are cumulative rather than immediate, aligning with patterns commonly observed in cognitive support interventions.

Within behavioural medicine, Lion's Mane contributes to regulation of the hypothalamic–pituitary–adrenal axis and autonomic tone. Although not sedative, its modulation of neuroinflammatory signalling and vagal communication appears to support calmer affect and improved stress recovery. These actions have relevance for dogs experiencing age-related anxiety, cats with chronic behavioural tension, and animals displaying reactivity exacerbated by gastrointestinal sensitivity or environmental instability. Emerging veterinary-focused studies, including open-label assessments combining Lion's Mane with mild anxiolytic botanicals, describe improvements in behavioural steadiness, reduced noise sensitivity and enhanced adaptability to routine variations. These observations are anecdotal but align closely with mechanistic research showing serotonergic and dopaminergic modulation.

Lion's Mane is also of interest in conditions involving structural or functional neuronal compromise. Experimental models of peripheral nerve injury, spinal cord damage and epileptiform activity demonstrate enhanced neuronal regeneration, reduced oxidative injury and improved mitochondrial stabilisation with Lion's Mane supplementation. While direct veterinary trials are limited, these mechanistic findings support its cautious inclusion in recovery plans for patients with intervertebral disc disease, neuropathic discomfort, degenerative myelopathy or chronic spinal irritation-always adjunctive to primary veterinary treatment.

In practice, Lion's Mane performs best as part of a multimodal neurological plan, particularly when paired with mushrooms offering complementary anti-inflammatory or neuroprotective actions, such as Reishi or Golden Oyster. Its role is not to replace conventional interventions but to provide a stable neurotrophic foundation upon which rehabilitation, behavioural therapy and appropriate medication can more effectively build.

For ageing animals, especially dogs showing early signs of cognitive dysfunction, Lion's Mane offers a gentle means of supporting neurological architecture

3.5 Gastrointestinal, Microbiome and Gut–Brain Axis

Lion's Mane exerts a broad and clinically meaningful influence on gastrointestinal function, microbial ecology and the bidirectional communication that defines the gut–brain axis. Although it is widely recognised for its neurotrophic properties, emerging evidence demonstrates that many of its neurological benefits originate within the gastrointestinal tract, where polysaccharides, β-glucans, hericenones and erinacines interact with mucosal immune networks, microbial populations and epithelial integrity. For veterinary patients with chronic enteropathy, stress-responsive digestive disturbance or combined gastrointestinal–behavioural patterns, Lion's Mane provides a regulatory framework that supports long-term digestive resilience.

Central to its gastrointestinal relevance is its modulation of key inflammatory mediators associated with mucosal irritation and enteric immune activation. These include interleukin-6 (IL-6), tumour necrosis factor-alpha (TNF-α) and cyclo-oxygenase-2 (COX-2)–three of the principal drivers of chronic gut inflammation and epithelial oxidative stress. Preclinical studies demonstrate that Lion's Mane down-regulates these pathways, resulting in reduced mucosal injury, improved epithelial recovery and a more stable inflammatory profile across the gastrointestinal tract. These findings carry particular significance for animals with chronic inflammatory bowel patterns, stress-triggered flares or gastrointestinal discomfort associated with immune hypersensitivity.

> Lion's Mane exerts a broad and clinically meaningful influence on gastrointestinal function, microbial ecology and the bidirectional communication that defines the gut–brain axis.

Lion's Mane also supports gut barrier integrity through its influence on tight-junction proteins and its protection of epithelial cells from oxidative damage. Oxidative stress is a major contributor to increased intestinal permeability, which in turn allows translocation of microbial products and inflammatory metabolites into systemic circulation. By enhancing endogenous antioxidant defences and reducing lipid peroxidation, Lion's Mane contributes to a stronger mucosal barrier and a more consistent gastrointestinal environment. Clinically, integrative veterinarians frequently observe improvements in stool quality, reduced variability in bowel function and more predictable gastrointestinal patterns after several weeks of consistent use.

The mushroom's prebiotic activity plays an equally important role. The indigestible polysaccharides and natural fibre present in full-spectrum extracts–particularly those produced via sub-critical water extraction (SCWE)–provide a fermentable substrate that enriches beneficial microbial populations. **Recent canine research confirms that Lion's Mane can shift the microbial landscape toward more favourable patterns in aged dogs, including increased Bacteroidetes abundance, reduced Firmicutes/Bacteroidetes ratios and meaningful reductions in inflammatory or dysbiosis-associated taxa such as *Campylobacter*, *Streptococcus* and *Tyzzerella*.** These microbial changes have downstream consequences for immune regulation, metabolic balance and emotional stability, all of which are mediated through the gut–brain axis. Short-chain fatty acids produced by microbial fermentation further support epithelial health, modulate mucosal inflammation and influence neurochemical pathways associated with mood and cognitive resilience.

Lion's Mane's gastrointestinal effects also intersect with its behavioural and neurological benefits. The gut–brain axis is highly responsive to changes in microbial composition and mucosal signalling, particularly in animals with stress-responsive digestion or chronic anxiety patterns. By reducing enteric inflammation, stabilising microbial balance and supporting epithelial protection, Lion's Mane contributes to calmer digestive rhythms and improved stress tolerance. These effects are cumulative and subtle, but they often precede or accompany improvements in behavioural steadiness, cognitive engagement and emotional resilience.

In animals receiving chronic medication–especially non-steroidal anti-inflammatory drugs, corticosteroids or long-term analgesics–the gastrointestinal tract often bears secondary strain from oxidative load and reduced mucosal defence. Lion's Mane's antioxidant compounds help protect epithelial cells from medication-induced stress and may contribute to more predictable digestive tolerance in these patients. Integrative practitioners commonly report smoother appetite patterns, reduced sensitivity to dietary change and fewer episodes of stress-related gastrointestinal upset when Lion's Mane is included as part of a broader Mycotherapy strategy.

Taken together, Lion's Mane provides a multi-level regulatory influence on the gastrointestinal system, microbiome ecology and the neurochemical pathways that link gut and brain. Its benefits develop gradually, typically emerging over two to six weeks of consistent administration, and align closely with its broader role as a modulator of physiological stability rather than a rapid symptomatic agent. For animals with chronic enteropathy, intermittent digestive sensitivity, stress-amplified gastrointestinal disturbance or combined gastrointestinal–neurological presentations, Lion's Mane represents a valuable, evidence-aligned therapeutic tool within integrative veterinary practice.

3.6 Hepatic and Renal Considerations

Lion's Mane exerts a meaningful influence on gastrointestinal and microbiome physiology, reflecting its long history of use in traditional medicine for digestive complaints and its modern recognition as a mushroom that interacts across the gut–brain axis. Much of its gastrointestinal relevance arises from the combined actions of its polysaccharides, fibre-bound compounds, antioxidant constituents and neurotrophic molecules, which together create a regulatory environment that supports epithelial integrity, microbial composition and mucosal immune balance.

Preclinical research demonstrates that Lion's Mane can help attenuate gastrointestinal inflammation by modulating nuclear factor kappa B activity and reducing the expression of pro-inflammatory cytokines, including interleukin 6, tumour necrosis factor alpha and interleukin 1 beta. These downstream effects correspond with reduced oxidative load, smoother mucosal signalling and less tissue irritation in models of gastritis and chemically induced colitis. Although veterinary-specific trials remain limited, these mechanistic findings align closely with clinical observations that animals experiencing intermittent gastrointestinal discomfort, stress-responsive digestive changes or chronic inflammatory bowel patterns may benefit from the mushroom's regulatory action when used consistently.

Lion's Mane also supports the structural integrity of the gastrointestinal barrier. Its polysaccharides and proteoglucans have been shown to enhance tight-junction stability and reduce oxidative injury to the epithelial lining, helping to maintain appropriate permeability and protect against microbial translocation. This is particularly relevant to dogs and cats with chronic enteropathy, stress-related gastrointestinal sensitivity or dysbiosis-associated hepatic strain, where subtle improvements in barrier stability can translate into broader systemic benefits.

The mushroom's prebiotic effects contribute further to its gastrointestinal utility. Fibre retained within full-spectrum extracts, especially those produced by Sub-critical water extraction, provides substrate for beneficial microbial taxa and promotes short-chain fatty acid production. These metabolites, particularly butyrate, are essential for epithelial energy supply, immune modulation and local anti-inflammatory function. Canine nutrition studies on mushroom supplementation have consistently shown improvements in microbial richness and shifts towards more favourable taxa, suggesting that Lion's Mane may play a supportive role in restoring gastrointestinal ecological balance.

The gut–brain axis represents another domain where Lion's Mane exerts influence. By modulating inflammation in the gut and supporting microbial stability, the mushroom may help regulate vagal signalling and stress-related digestive patterns, contributing to improved behavioural steadiness in animals with concurrent gastrointestinal and emotional sensitivity. These effects are supported by translational research showing that Lion's Mane can reduce microglial activation and attenuate neuroinflammatory pathways, forming a link between digestive health and behavioural resilience.

Overall, Lion's Mane's gastrointestinal actions are cumulative, regulatory and best suited to long-term management of chronic or stress-associated digestive disturbance. Its value lies not in rapid symptomatic relief but in supporting the gradual restoration of mucosal stability, microbial diversity and inflammatory equilibrium. Veterinary clinicians integrating Lion's Mane into gastrointestinal protocols typically observe improvements in stool consistency, appetite stability and digestive comfort over several weeks, particularly when combined with dietary management and additional Mycotherapy species such as Reishi or Turkey Tail in more complex cases.

3.7 Cardiovascular and Respiratory Physiology

Although Lion's Mane is most strongly associated with neurological and gastrointestinal benefits, emerging preclinical evidence suggests that it may also exert modest yet clinically relevant effects on cardiovascular and respiratory physiology. These actions stem primarily from its antioxidant constituents, its influence on systemic inflammation and its capacity to support metabolic efficiency, rather than from direct vascular or bronchodilatory mechanisms. As such, Lion's Mane is not considered a cardiovascular or respiratory mushroom in the same sense as Reishi, yet it contributes meaningfully to overall physiological stability in animals experiencing chronic inflammatory strain, age-related metabolic decline or environmental respiratory sensitivity.

Oxidative stress plays a central role in age-related cardiovascular decline, diminished endothelial responsiveness and increased susceptibility to inflammatory airway patterns. Lion's Mane's antioxidant peptides, polyphenols and fibre-bound compounds help reduce lipid peroxidation and protect mitochondrial integrity within metabolically demanding tissues. Preclinical studies demonstrate improved antioxidant enzyme activity, enhanced mitochondrial stability and attenuation of inflammatory mediators, effects that may indirectly support vascular resilience and circulatory efficiency. In clinical settings, integrative practitioners occasionally observe subtle improvements in stamina, recovery and general vitality in older animals receiving Lion's Mane, although these reports remain anecdotal and should not be interpreted as evidence of direct cardiac modulation.

Lion's Mane may also exert influence on lipid handling and metabolic pathways that intersect with cardiovascular physiology. Translational studies have shown reduced cholesterol and triglyceride accumulation alongside improved lipid metabolism, suggesting potential supportive value for overweight, senior or endocrine-compromised animals. While dogs and cats are less prone to atherosclerotic disease than humans, improved lipid regulation can still contribute to healthier energy utilisation and reduced metabolic strain.

Respiratory effects have also been noted in preclinical work, where Lion's Mane extracts reduced airway inflammation and modulated cytokine activity within lung tissue. These actions appear related to the mushroom's broad anti-inflammatory profile, including reduced levels of cyclo-oxygenase 2 and other inflammatory mediators. Although these findings are early and not yet validated in controlled veterinary trials, they offer a theoretical basis for Lion's Mane's use as a gentle background support in animals experiencing respiratory irritation, inflammatory airway patterns or reduced respiratory resilience associated with age or chronic illness.

In veterinary practice, Lion's Mane should not be used as a primary therapeutic agent for cardiovascular or respiratory disease, but may offer supportive benefits as part of a comprehensive Mycotherapy strategy aimed at reducing systemic inflammation, improving oxidative defence and stabilising metabolic function. Any improvements are subtle, cumulative and dependent on consistent administration, reflecting the mushroom's broader role as a systemic regulatory agent rather than a targeted organ-specific intervention.

3.8 Oncology and Adjunctive Cancer Support

Lion's Mane plays a more indirect yet clinically meaningful role in integrative oncology, offering support not through cytotoxic or tumour-suppressing effects but through its broader influence on inflammation, neurobiology, gastrointestinal integrity and mitochondrial stability. Although it lacks the polysaccharopeptide-driven immune-enhancing profile of Turkey Tail or the triterpene-mediated anti-inflammatory potency of Reishi, Lion's Mane provides a stabilising foundation for animals undergoing cancer treatment by helping preserve cognitive function, digestive comfort and overall physiological resilience. Much of the evidence is preclinical or based on translational models, but the convergence of mechanistic research and clinical experience suggests that Lion's Mane may help mitigate secondary effects of chronic oncological disease.

Cancer alters systemic physiology through chronic inflammation, metabolic strain, immune fatigue and neuroendocrine disruption. Lion's Mane's β-glucans interact with immune receptors such as Dectin-1 and complement receptor 3, supporting improved macrophage and dendritic cell function without provoking excessive stimulation. This regulatory influence may help soften the inflammatory terrain that contributes to fatigue, malaise and reduced appetite in many oncology patients. Preclinical findings demonstrating reduced activity of nuclear factor kappa B and down-regulation of pro-inflammatory cytokines, including interleukin-6, tumour necrosis factor alpha and interleukin-1 beta, provide a scientific rationale for its inclusion in long-term terrain-supportive protocols.

Cancer and its treatments also influence behaviour, cognition and emotional regulation. Animals frequently experience altered sleep patterns, reduced engagement, agitation or increased stress reactivity during the course of their illness. Lion's Mane's well-documented ability to reduce neuroinflammation, stabilise microglial activity and support mitochondrial function within neuronal tissue may contribute to improved steadiness and cognitive comfort. These effects align with the mushroom's recognised role in promoting nerve growth factor activity and supporting neuronal resilience, and while clinical trials in veterinary oncology are lacking, many integrative clinicians report calmer demeanour, steadier sleep and improved daily engagement in senior or medically fragile patients receiving Lion's Mane persistently.

Gastrointestinal integrity is a critical determinant of quality of life in animals with cancer, as both disease and treatment can disrupt mucosal stability and appetite. Lion's Mane has demonstrated protective effects in preclinical gastric and colitis models, where it supports epithelial repair, reduces inflammatory signalling and enhances tight-junction integrity. Through its fibre-rich matrix and prebiotic polysaccharides, Lion's Mane can also contribute to improved microbiome composition and short-chain fatty acid production, offering additional support for appetite consistency and digestive comfort. These effects do not constitute direct anticancer activity but remain highly relevant in maintaining patient stability during therapy.

Mitochondrial protection represents another pathway through which Lion's Mane may benefit oncology patients. Cancer and chemotherapy place considerable oxidative and metabolic demand on tissues with high energetic requirements. By reducing lipid peroxidation and supporting mitochondrial membrane stability, Lion's Mane's antioxidant compounds may help preserve stamina and recovery capacity, although evidence in animals is currently limited to translational studies and anecdotal reports.

Lion's Mane should not be misconstrued as a tumour-regressing agent. It does not demonstrate the angiogenesis inhibition or apoptosis-inducing properties characteristic of Reishi, nor the immune-priming potency associated with Turkey Tail. Its value lies instead in the subtle, cumulative support it provides to the broader physiological environment, helping to maintain comfort, cognitive steadiness and digestive resilience in animals undergoing conventional oncology care. Caution remains appropriate when combining Lion's Mane with immunosuppressive oncology drugs, but experience suggests that its regulatory action rarely conflicts with pharmacological protocols when introduced gradually and monitored appropriately.

Overall, Lion's Mane offers a gentle but meaningful contribution to terrain-based oncology support. Its primary strengths involve stabilising the neuroimmune environment, protecting gastrointestinal integrity, modulating chronic inflammation and supporting mitochondrial efficiency. These benefits unfold gradually and should always be integrated within evidence-informed oncology plans centred on diagnostic clarity, pharmacological necessity and individualised care.

3.9 Veterinary Pharmacology and Drug Interaction Considerations

Lion's Mane has a distinctive pharmacological profile shaped by its neurotrophic compounds, polysaccharides, antioxidant molecules and fibre-bound constituents. For veterinary clinicians, its pharmacokinetics and potential drug interactions must be understood through a combination of preclinical studies, nutritional trials in dogs and accumulated integrative practice. While Lion's Mane is generally well tolerated, its neuroactive and metabolic effects necessitate thoughtful integration, especially in fragile, medicated or neurologically compromised patients.

Absorption and bioavailability

The bioactive compounds in Lion's Mane follow different physiological routes. Its polysaccharides exhibit minimal systemic absorption, exerting most of their activity through engagement with gut-associated lymphoid tissue, modulation of mucosal immunity and prebiotic effects on the microbiome. In contrast, the erinacines and hericenones, particularly the diterpenoid erinacines found in the mycelial mass used in some research extracts, demonstrate neurotrophic activity after systemic absorption in preclinical models. These compounds appear to cross the blood–brain barrier in rodent studies, influencing nerve growth factor signalling and neuronal resilience. Although pharmacokinetic studies in dogs or cats are lacking, the cumulative behavioural and cognitive effects observed clinically suggest that absorbed fractions do reach the central nervous system.

Hepatic handling and detoxification pathways

Lion's Mane interacts with hepatic enzyme systems in a mild and largely supportive manner. Preclinical findings indicate that the mushroom may modulate phase II detoxification pathways, particularly glutathione-dependent processes, and exert antioxidant protection within hepatic tissue. These actions are beneficial in older animals or those on long-term medication. However, the influence of Lion's Mane on cytochrome P450 enzymes remains incompletely characterised, and although adverse interactions have not been reported, conservative introduction is sensible in patients receiving narrow-therapeutic-index drugs such as anticonvulsants, chemotherapeutics or certain cardiac medications. Full-spectrum SCWE extracts provide additional predictability by reducing solvent artefacts and maintaining a coherent biochemical matrix.

Central nervous system - active medications

Given Lion's Mane's influence on nerve growth factor activity, neuroinflammation and neurochemical balance, theoretical interactions with CNS-active pharmaceuticals warrant consideration. Animals receiving anxiolytics, antidepressants, gabapentin or anti-seizure drugs may exhibit enhanced steadiness, calmer demeanour or improved recovery from stress when Lion's Mane is introduced, but these effects derive from regulatory neurobiology rather than direct pharmacological potentiation. No evidence suggests that Lion's Mane interferes negatively with behavioural medications, although caution and incremental dosing are recommended in patients with seizure disorders or those undergoing behavioural medication adjustments.

Endocrine and metabolic medications

Lion's Mane's reported effects on glucose regulation, lipid metabolism and insulin sensitivity remain primarily preclinical, yet they introduce a theoretical consideration for diabetic animals receiving insulin or oral hypoglycaemics. A low-and-slow titration approach, paired with closer glucose monitoring during the initial weeks, ensures safe integration. Animals with hypothyroidism, Cushing's syndrome or metabolic syndrome may benefit from Lion's Mane's broader anti-inflammatory and antioxidant effects, but these benefits are supportive and should never replace primary endocrine therapy.

Gastrointestinal medication interactions

Lion's Mane's fibre content and prebiotic activity may influence the absorption of oral medications in a small subset of patients, particularly drugs requiring empty-stomach administration or narrow absorption windows. Administering Lion's Mane separately from oral antibiotics, thyroxine or specific cardiac drugs can minimise theoretical interference. SCWE extracts, which maintain native fibre architecture while avoiding excessive bulk, improve overall predictability in this domain.

Platelet function and coagulation

Unlike Reishi, Lion's Mane shows no strong evidence of clinically relevant antiplatelet effects. Some preclinical studies suggest mild influence on oxidative stress within platelets, but this has not translated into bleeding concerns in veterinary practice. Nevertheless, for animals undergoing surgical procedures or those with known coagulopathies, a cautious approach and clear treatment timelines are advisable.

General pharmacological summary

Overall, Lion's Mane's pharmacology is best described as mild, regulatory and supportive, with low likelihood of significant pharmacokinetic conflict when introduced appropriately. Most considerations involve neurological conditions, metabolic disease, polypharmacy or fragile hepatic physiology. With gradual titration and clinical monitoring, Lion's Mane integrates safely with most veterinary medications, contributing to a cumulative improvement in resilience rather than exerting strong pharmacodynamic shifts.

3.10 Clinical Application in Veterinary Practice

Overview and therapeutic positioning

Lion's Mane occupies a distinctive place within veterinary Mycotherapy because of its multi-system actions across the nervous, immune and gastrointestinal networks. Beyond its well-recognised neurotrophic effects, it demonstrates meaningful influence on gut–brain axis physiology through prebiotic polysaccharides, polyphenols and ergothioneine-rich antioxidant components. Emerging canine research now shows that Lion's Mane can modulate the gut microbiota in aged dogs, promoting a shift toward more balanced, anti-inflammatory microbial communities. These findings reinforce its relevance not only for neurological health but for broader systemic wellness where gastrointestinal, metabolic and behavioural pathways overlap.

In clinical settings, Lion's Mane is seldom used as a stand-alone intervention. Its strength lies in functioning as a long-term terrain-supportive agent that harmonises with integrative treatment plans. It is particularly valuable in animals presenting with cognitive decline, chronic gastrointestinal sensitivity, neuroimmune dysregulation, stress-related behaviours or age-related functional slowing. By supporting neuronal stability, gut barrier integrity, microbial diversity and oxidative balance, Lion's Mane contributes to a more resilient physiological baseline.

Its therapeutic role therefore aligns with the principles of functional and integrative veterinary practice: enhancing adaptability, restoring communication between systems, and supporting the animal's inherent capacity for repair and healthy ageing. As evidence grows, particularly in senior dogs, it reinforces the position of Lion's Mane as a foundational mushroom for maintaining long-term neurocognitive and gastrointestinal vitality.

Lion's Mane and the aged canine microbiome

Recent canine data provide some of the strongest species-specific support for Lion's Mane in veterinary practice. In a 16-week controlled trial, Cho et al. (2022) demonstrated that *Hericium erinaceus* fruiting-body powder produced a dose-dependent restructuring of the gut microbiota in aged dogs, significantly reducing the Firmicutes/Bacteroidetes ratio — a biomarker associated with obesity and metabolic dysregulation in dogs. The high-dose group showed marked reductions in pro-inflammatory taxa, including *Streptococcus*, *Campylobacter* and *Tyzzerella*, alongside increases in fibre-associated *Bacteroidetes* and *Prevotella*. Importantly, microbial richness and evenness remained stable, suggesting that Lion's Mane modulates composition without destabilising the gut ecosystem. These findings align with known prebiotic actions of Lion's Mane polysaccharides and polyphenols, supporting its role in aged animals where immune resilience, gut barrier integrity and metabolic balance are priority concerns.

Neurological and cognitive support

In senior animals, Lion's Mane is frequently integrated into care plans for cognitive ageing, disorientation, disrupted sleep cycles and behavioural slowing. Improvements typically emerge gradually over several weeks, reflecting the mushroom's influence on nerve growth factor signalling, synaptic resilience and the reduction of neuroinflammatory mediators such as interleukin-6 and tumour necrosis factor-alpha. When paired with Reishi, practitioners often report enhanced emotional steadiness, more predictable circadian rhythms and improved engagement with daily routines.

Lion's Mane may also support animals recovering from neurological trauma or chronic neuroinflammation. While these applications are grounded primarily in preclinical data and practitioner experience, the mushroom's neurotrophic influence and effects on neuronal mitochondrial stability appear to be particularly relevant during convalescence.

Stress physiology, behaviour and emotional regulation

Lion's Mane plays a meaningful role in supporting animals with chronic stress reactivity, noise sensitivity, environmental anxiety or post-traumatic behavioural patterns. While not a sedative, its modulation of the hypothalamic–pituitary–adrenal axis, combined with its antioxidant and mitochondrial-stabilising effects within neuronal tissue, may contribute to a calmer behavioural threshold. Practitioners often note subtle improvements in resilience, adaptability and overall affect when Lion's Mane is used consistently within multimodal behavioural plans.

Gastrointestinal and gut–brain axis applications

Digestive health represents another core domain for Lion's Mane in veterinary practice. Animals with gastritis, intermittent nausea, stress-responsive gastrointestinal upset or chronic inflammatory enteropathies may experience improved mucosal stability, appetite consistency and stool quality over time. Lion's Mane's fibre-rich matrix and prebiotic influence support microbial diversity and reinforce short-chain fatty acid production, complementing dietary adjustments and other Mycotherapy species such as Turkey Tail or Chaga. Its effects on the enteric nervous system also make it valuable in cases where gastrointestinal symptoms intersect with stress or neurological imbalance.

Metabolic and performance support

Performance and working animals may benefit from Lion's Mane's subtle metabolic and mitochondrial effects, particularly when fatigue, mild coordination changes or reduced recovery capacity are observed. By supporting mitochondrial redox stability and antioxidant defence, Lion's Mane can contribute to improved cellular resilience under physical or metabolic strain.

Multimodal integration and long-term use

Across species, Lion's Mane is best utilised as part of a multimodal plan that may include behavioural therapy, environmental modification, nutritional strategies and additional complementary mushrooms. Its effects are cumulative rather than acute, making consistent daily administration essential. When used with SCWE full-spectrum extracts, the combination of neurotrophic compounds, prebiotic fibre and small-molecule antioxidants is preserved, supporting long-term nervous system and gastrointestinal harmony.

Integration with other functional mushrooms

Lion's Mane is a highly adaptable mushroom that pairs effectively with a wide range of functional mushrooms due to its unique neurotrophic compounds (erinacines, hericenones), gut–brain axis modulation and influence on neuronal regeneration. Its actions are complemented by species that support immunity, mitochondrial health, stress physiology and metabolic steadiness. The following pairings reflect the most clinically relevant combinations for veterinary patients.

- **With Reishi** - Lion's Mane and Reishi offer a powerful combination for animals experiencing stress-linked neurological, behavioural or gastrointestinal concerns. Reishi stabilises the HPA axis and modulates inflammatory pathways, creating a calmer physiological environment in which Lion's Mane's neurotrophic actions can be more effective. Together they support cognitive ageing, anxiety-related digestive fragility, autonomic dysregulation and nervous system recovery after illness or stress. This pairing is especially valuable in senior animals, reactive temperaments, chronic stress states and gut–brain axis dysfunction.

- **With Turkey Tail** - Lion's Mane adds neuroprotective and neuroregenerative support to Turkey Tail's immune-priming and microbiome-modulating profile. This combination is relevant in oncology care, where nervous system stability, appetite, behaviour and quality of life may be affected by disease processes or treatment burden. Turkey Tail helps stimulate balanced immune activity, while Lion's Mane supports neural resilience and reduces gut–brain axis disruption. Together they reinforce systemic resilience in animals facing chronic immune challenges or cancer-related frailty.

- **With Chaga** - Chaga's potent antioxidant and gastrointestinal-supportive properties amplify Lion's Mane's effects on gut–brain communication, mucosal repair and oxidative stress management. This pairing benefits animals with chronic digestive issues, dysbiosis, inflammatory bowel tendencies or stress-related gastrointestinal upset. Chaga buffers oxidative load and supports mucosal immunity, while Lion's Mane promotes nerve regeneration within the enteric nervous system. Together they offer integrated support for digestion, cognition and stress physiology.

- **With Cordyceps** - Cordyceps contributes respiratory efficiency, endurance and mitochondrial energy support, complementing Lion's Mane's neural recovery and neurotrophic influence. This pairing is especially useful for working and performance animals, senior animals with fatigue or mobility decline, and those recovering from chronic illness or neurological injury. Cordyceps enhances oxygen utilisation and cellular ATP production, while Lion's Mane supports neural healing, proprioception and neuromuscular resilience. The synergy strengthens stamina and neurological steadiness simultaneously.

- **With Golden Oyster** - Lion's Mane and Golden Oyster create one of the most compelling neuroprotective combinations available in functional mushroom practice. Lion's Mane stimulates nerve growth factor pathways and regenerative activity, while Golden Oyster provides ergothioneine-driven mitochondrial protection, redox stability and cellular longevity support. This pairing is particularly relevant for cognitive ageing, neurodegenerative patterns, chronic inflammatory neurological conditions, and behavioural fragility linked to oxidative burden. Together they reinforce long-term brain vitality, mitochondrial resilience and nervous system performance across life stages.

> Synergistic pairings or triads of mushrooms can act across multiple physiological pathways, broadening the supportive effect and contributing to a full-spectrum, terrain-based Mycotherapy strategy.

3.11 Safety, Contraindications and Monitoring

Lion's Mane is regarded as one of the safest medicinal mushrooms across companion species, supported by nutritional trials in aged dogs, extensive preclinical toxicology work and a long record of use in traditional medicine. Nevertheless, thoughtful clinical oversight is essential, particularly in neurologically compromised animals, those receiving CNS-active medications or individuals with complex metabolic disease.

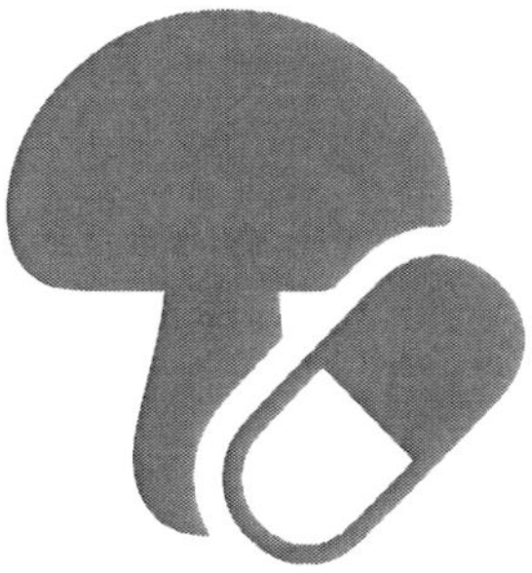

General tolerability

Most animals tolerate Lion's Mane without difficulty. Mild digestive changes such as soft stools or temporary appetite fluctuation may occur during the first few days, particularly at higher doses or in sensitive gastrointestinal patients. Introducing the mushroom gradually over five to seven days reduces these effects significantly. SCWE full-spectrum extracts tend to exhibit superior tolerability due to maintained fibre architecture and absence of solvent residues.

Neurological considerations

Because Lion's Mane influences nerve growth factor signalling and neuroinflammatory pathways, caution is appropriate in animals with seizure disorders or those undergoing changes to behavioural or anti-seizure medication. Although no data suggest that Lion's Mane provokes seizures, any neuroactive substance introduced into an unstable neurological environment requires incremental dosing and close observation.

Metabolic and endocrine disease

In diabetic animals, Lion's Mane's mild glucose-regulatory effects suggest that blood glucose should be monitored more closely during the initial integration period. Hypoglycaemia is unlikely but theoretically possible in animals receiving insulin or oral hypoglycaemics. Animals with thyroid or adrenal disorders generally tolerate Lion's Mane well, and may benefit from its systemic antioxidant effects, but the mushroom should never replace primary endocrine therapy.

Hepatic and renal considerations

Lion's Mane provides antioxidant support to hepatic tissue, but animals with advanced liver disease or markedly reduced metabolic reserve should begin at reduced doses with regular monitoring. Renal considerations are limited, as Lion's Mane is not associated with high oxalate content, yet fragile geriatric cats with low hydration status benefit from conservative titration.

Drug interactions

The most relevant interaction domains include CNS-active medications, endocrine therapies and drugs requiring narrow absorption timing. Spacing administration appropriately and monitoring clinical response reduce the likelihood of interference. SCWE extracts provide predictable pharmacological behaviour and minimise interaction risk by avoiding dual-extraction alcohols and starch-heavy mycelial substrates.

Monitoring

Veterinary monitoring should include assessment of digestive tolerability, behavioural changes, appetite stability and neurological status during the first month. Animals with metabolic, endocrine or hepatic disease warrant periodic laboratory evaluation. Documentation of cognitive, behavioural or gastrointestinal changes contributes to growing clinical insight within veterinary Mycotherapy and helps refine individualised dosing strategies.

3.12 Evidence Quality Commentary

The evidence base for Lion's Mane spans neurobiology, gastrointestinal physiology, microbiome science and metabolic regulation, but remains weighted toward preclinical and translational research rather than species-specific veterinary trials. Mechanistic clarity is strongest in the domains of nerve growth factor signalling, microglial modulation, oxidative stress reduction and mucosal protection, with multiple independent laboratories corroborating these findings. These data provide a compelling scientific rationale for Lion's Mane's integration into neurological, behavioural and gastrointestinal care, despite the absence of large-scale veterinary clinical trials.

Canine nutrition studies contribute an important translational bridge, demonstrating improved serum biomarkers of tissue repair, enhanced antioxidant status and beneficial shifts in microbiome composition in older dogs receiving Lion's Mane supplementation. While these studies do not assess cognitive function directly, they reinforce the mushroom's safety, tolerability and physiological relevance across species.

Anecdotal veterinary evidence, while not equivalent to controlled data, remains valuable given the mushroom's consistent behavioural and cognitive effects across senior pets, anxious animals and neurologically compromised patients. These clinical impressions align closely with Lion's Mane's mechanistic foundation, increasing confidence in its practical relevance.

As with all mushrooms, extract fidelity remains central to evidence interpretation. Many published studies utilise laboratory isolates or alcohol-based extracts that do not reflect the composition of real-world supplements. SCWE full-spectrum extracts, which retain both hydrophilic and lipophilic compounds along with native prebiotic fibre, most closely approximate the whole-mushroom profile used in traditional practice. This alignment strengthens translational relevance and supports the use of SCWE in clinical settings.

Overall, evidence quality for Lion's Mane can be characterised as high in mechanistic domains, moderate in translational relevance and emerging in species-specific veterinary research. Its regulatory, cumulative nature makes it a low-risk adjunct in multimodal care when applied with clinical judgement.

LION'S MANE (HERICIUM ERINACEUS) – Evidence Quality Commentary Table

This spectrum of evidence is summarised in the following table:

Domain	Evidence Strength	Primary Evidence Type
Neurotrophic and neuroregenerative activity	High	Preclinical rodent models, in vitro neurite–outgrowth studies, mechanistic
Cognitive support and ageing–related decline	Moderate to high	Preclinical, translational human data, early animal cognition models
Gut–brain axis modulation	Moderate	Preclinical GI–neural pathway studies, microbiome–modulating mechanisms
Gastrointestinal support and mucosal repair	Moderate	Preclinical anti–ulcer models, GI anti–inflammatory studies

Domain	Evidence Strength	Primary Evidence Type
Immunomodulation	Moderate	Preclinical immune-signalling studies, β-glucan mechanisms
Anti-inflammatory and antioxidant effects	Moderate	Preclinical antioxidant and cytokine-modulation studies
Behavioural and stress resilience	Emerging to moderate	Preclinical anxiolytic models, translational human evidence
Neuropathy and nerve-injury recovery	Emerging	Preclinical nerve-injury models, mechanistic pathways
Metabolic regulation	Emerging	Preclinical glucose and lipid-modulation studies
Oncology adjunct use	Emerging	Limited preclinical studies; practitioner interest growing
Clinical veterinary trials	Limited	No formal veterinary trials; extrapolated translational data

Lion's Mane is distinguished by its unique neurotrophic profile. Compounds such as the **erinacines** (mycelial origin) and **hericenones** (fruiting-body origin) stimulate nerve growth factor (NGF) pathways, promote neurite extension and support neuronal plasticity. These mechanisms form the basis of its value in animals experiencing cognitive decline, neurological stress, sensory processing changes or gut-brain dysregulation. Although formal veterinary trials are limited, the mechanistic evidence is robust and supported by translational human studies demonstrating improvements in cognition, mood and neuroinflammatory markers.

Beyond neurological applications, Lion's Mane provides gastrointestinal benefits through modulation of mucosal inflammation, enhancement of epithelial integrity and shifts in microbiome composition. This connection to the gut-brain axis is particularly relevant in animals with chronic anxiety, stress-related digestive issues or ageing-associated behavioural changes. Its immunomodulatory and antioxidant actions further contribute to multi-system steadiness, though these effects are secondary to its primary neurotrophic profile.

Within Mycotherapy, extract fidelity is critical. Fruiting-body SCWE preparations retain the full complement of β-glucans, phenolics and hydrophilic bioactive molecules essential for immune and gastrointestinal activity, while also preserving heat-sensitive compounds relevant to neurological support. Grain-grown mycelium provides erinacines but lacks the broader fruiting-body matrix, and alcohol tinctures fail to capture key β-glucans and polysaccharides. SCWE full-spectrum extracts therefore offer the most balanced and clinically dependable option for veterinary practice.

Lion's Mane is best positioned as a long-term, terrain-supportive neurotrophic agent – ideal for cognitive ageing, neurological steadiness, gastrointestinal-neurological interplay and behavioural dysregulation. Its actions are gradual, cumulative and regulatory rather than rapid, aligning with the foundational principles of terrain-based Mycotherapy.

3.13 Conclusion – Integrative Significance and Extraction Considerations

Lion's Mane provides a distinctive contribution to integrative veterinary medicine through its combined influence on neuronal resilience, gut–brain communication, gastrointestinal integrity and systemic inflammatory balance. Its neurotrophic compounds support nerve growth factor activity and neuronal recovery, while its polysaccharides and fibre-bound constituents help stabilise the gastrointestinal environment and foster microbial diversity. Recent canine research reinforces these actions, demonstrating that Lion's Mane can beneficially influence the gut microbiota in aged dogs, reducing dysbiosis-associated taxa and supporting a more balanced microbial profile. These effects make Lion's Mane particularly relevant to senior animals, those recovering from neurological stress or injury and individuals experiencing chronic gastrointestinal sensitivity or stress-associated behavioural change.

The mushroom's systemic benefits develop gradually, requiring consistent administration and thoughtful integration within broader veterinary care plans. When used alongside Reishi for stress modulation, Turkey Tail for immune intelligence or Golden Oyster for mitochondrial protection, Lion's Mane contributes to a synergistic Mycotherapy strategy that supports long-term resilience and vitality.

Extract fidelity remains essential for expressing Lion's Mane's full therapeutic value. SCWE whole-food extracts preserve both hydrophilic and lipophilic compounds, as well as the natural prebiotic fibre that underpins many of its gut–brain and immunological benefits. This method avoids the biochemical fragmentation associated with alcohol-based tinctures and the dilution inherent in grain-grown mycelium products, providing a physiologically coherent preparation that reflects the mechanisms described throughout this monograph.

Used judiciously and monitored with clinical insight, Lion's Mane offers a safe, predictable and scientifically grounded contribution to integrative veterinary care. Its long-term use supports cognitive clarity, emotional stability and gastrointestinal resilience, helping animals maintain functional vitality throughout the course of their lives.

> Lion's Mane provides a distinctive contribution to integrative veterinary medicine through its combined influence on neuronal resilience, gut-brain communication, gastrointestinal integrity and systemic inflammatory balance.

Key sources (summary)

Cho et al., 2022; Friedman, 2015; Kawagishi & Zhuang, 2008; Mori et al., 2009; Zhang et al., 2016; Wong et al., 2020; Nagano et al., 2010; Satou et al., 2019; Ma et al., 2023; Lin et al., 2017; Lull et al., 2005; Memorial Sloan Kettering Cancer Center, 2024; Bosch et al., 2015. **Full professional reference list available in the Master References section.**

> "The natural world is the greatest source of excitement, the greatest source of visual beauty, the greatest source of intellectual interest. *Sir David Attenborough (b. 1926)*"

4 CHAGA (Inonotus obliquus)

4.1 Introduction to Chaga – *The Brain Booster and Gut Warrior*

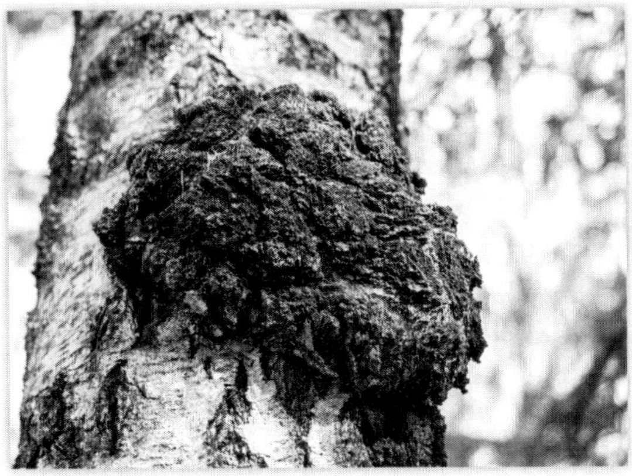

Chaga (Inonotus obliquus) occupies a unique position within medicinal Mycotherapy due to its exceptionally dense profile of antioxidant, immune-regulating and tissue-protective compounds. Historically revered across Siberian, Scandinavian and northern Asian medical traditions, Chaga has been described for centuries as a tonic for vitality, resilience and recovery from chronic illness. Modern analytical research confirms much of this empirical knowledge, identifying Chaga as one of nature's richest sources of polyphenols, melanins, betulinic acid, antioxidant peptides and complex polysaccharides that collectively influence oxidative balance, immune modulation and metabolic stability.

For veterinary medicine, Chaga's relevance arises from its capacity to buffer oxidative stress, calm excessive inflammatory responses, support detoxification pathways and contribute to mucosal and hepatic resilience. These domains underpin many chronic conditions seen in companion animals, including gastrointestinal sensitivity, dermatological reactivity, immune dysregulation, environmental toxin exposure and age-related decline. Although species-specific clinical trials remain limited, translational evidence from human studies, rodent research, in vitro investigations and emerging veterinary applications collectively provide a strong mechanistic rationale for its inclusion in integrative care.

Within the broader framework of veterinary Mycotherapy, Chaga is best understood as a terrain-supporting mushroom rather than a rapid symptomatic agent. Its benefits develop gradually through the cumulative restoration of antioxidant capacity, mitochondrial stability, immune equilibrium and gut–liver axis function. These mechanisms are particularly valuable for animals living with chronic inflammatory burden, environmental pollutants, metabolic imbalance or systemic oxidative stress. When used consistently and integrated within comprehensive treatment plans, Chaga contributes meaningfully to long-term physiological balance and improved resilience across multiple interconnected systems.

> Chaga occupies a unique position within medicinal Mycotherapy due to its exceptionally dense profile of antioxidant, immune-regulating and tissue-protective compounds.

4.2 Taxonomy, Morphology and Extract Science

Chaga's biological identity differs from many other medicinal mushrooms commonly used in veterinary practice. It is not the fruiting body that is traditionally harvested, but rather a hardened, melanised sterile conk (sclerotium) formed on birch trees (Betula species). This sclerotium contains exceptionally high concentrations of melanin pigments, phenolic compounds, triterpenes and polysaccharides that accumulate through the fungus–birch interaction. The presence of betulin and betulinic acid, derived from birch bark, is a distinguishing feature of Chaga and contributes significantly to its antioxidant and cytoprotective profile.

Microscopically, the sclerotium is composed of dense, melanised hyphal masses with embedded polyphenolic complexes. These structural features explain both its unusually high oxidative stability and its intense free-radical scavenging capacity. Chaga's polysaccharides include β-glucans and heteroglucans that interact with immune receptors and gut-associated lymphoid tissue, while its melanins provide broad-spectrum antioxidant effects and contribute to tissue repair and barrier protection.

Extract Science and the Role of SCWE

Due to its dense structure and the insolubility of many of its compounds, extraction quality is essential in determining Chaga's therapeutic value. Sub-critical water extraction (SCWE) provides a controlled, solvent-free method capable of liberating both hydrophilic and lipophilic constituents from the sclerotium, including polysaccharides, phenolic antioxidants, triterpenes, betulinic acid and natural fibre. This produces a full-spectrum extract that maintains the biochemical ecology of the whole organism.

By contrast, alcohol tinctures capture triterpenes but leave behind the substantial polyphenol–melanin complex and much of the indigestible prebiotic fibre, while hot-water extractions may under-represent lipophilic compounds. Myceliated grain products introduce unnecessary starch, dilute active compounds and lack the birch-derived triterpenes central to Chaga's pharmacology.

For veterinary application, SCWE extracts provide the most predictable, physiologically coherent preparation, particularly for gastrointestinal, hepatic, oxidative and immune-focused protocols. Extract fidelity is critical, as Chaga's wide-ranging effects depend on the synergy between polysaccharides, triterpenes, melanins, antioxidant enzymes and fibre-bound complexes functioning as a natural matrix.

4.3 Bioactive Constituents and Mechanistic Overview

Chaga's therapeutic profile is defined by a dense and unusually complex matrix of bioactive compounds that work collectively to moderate inflammation, buffer oxidative stress, support cellular repair and maintain immune equilibrium. Unlike many mushrooms where individual compound groups dominate the pharmacology, Chaga's effects emerge from the interplay of polysaccharides, phenolic antioxidants, melanins, triterpenes and betulinic derivatives that accumulate through its specialised ecological relationship with birch trees. This biochemical diversity underpins its broad relevance within veterinary Mycotherapy, particularly for animals living with chronic inflammation, oxidative burden, immune imbalance or environmental toxin exposure.

The polysaccharide fraction is composed of β-glucans and heteroglucans that interact with pattern-recognition receptors along the gut–immune axis. These compounds influence macrophage surveillance, support balanced cytokine expression and contribute to the stability of mucosal immunity. Although veterinary-specific studies remain limited, preclinical evidence demonstrates improved phagocytic capacity, modulation of interleukin 6, tumour necrosis factor alpha and immunoglobulin responses, and normalisation of T-helper activity. These findings provide a mechanistic foundation for Chaga's gradual, regulatory immune influence rather than a strongly stimulatory effect.

Chaga's phenolic antioxidants and melanin complexes are central to its reputation as one of nature's most powerful antioxidant sources. The melanin fraction alone exhibits unusually high free-radical scavenging potential and offers extensive protection against lipid peroxidation, DNA damage and mitochondrial injury. These antioxidant systems are particularly relevant to senior animals, those exposed to environmental pollutants, high-intensity working animals and individuals undergoing chronic inflammatory stress. Chaga's ability to reinforce endogenous antioxidant enzymes such as superoxide dismutase, catalase and glutathione peroxidase provides broad cellular defence, with downstream implications for systemic resilience.

The triterpene profile, including betulin, betulinic acid and lupeol derivatives, contributes additional layers of cytoprotective and anti-inflammatory activity. Betulinic acid is of particular interest due to its extensive documentation in preclinical models of inflammation, oxidative injury and tumour biology. These compounds influence pathways such as nuclear factor kappa B, cyclo-oxygenase 2 and inducible nitric oxide synthase, helping to mitigate inflammatory escalation in gastrointestinal, hepatic, dermatological and respiratory tissues. Although many findings arise from translational or rodent studies, the underlying mechanisms align closely with clinical presentations encountered in veterinary practice.

Chaga's fibre-bound bioactive complexes are another defining feature. The structural matrix of the sclerotium contains indigestible polysaccharides tightly associated with phenolic and melanin compounds, providing slow-release interaction with the gut mucosa and sustained modulation of the gut–immune interface. These retained fibre structures also function as prebiotic substrates, supporting microbial diversity and short-chain fatty acid production. This activity carries relevance for animals with stress-responsive gastrointestinal sensitivity, chronic enteropathies or microbiome instability. Extracts that remove or degrade this structural fibre lose a significant portion of Chaga's physiological coherence.

Finally, Chaga contains a range of minor constituents including antioxidant peptides, sterols and trace minerals that contribute to its overall adaptogenic profile. These compounds support mitochondrial efficiency, stabilise cellular membranes and reinforce tissue repair mechanisms under conditions of chronic physiological challenge. Taken together, Chaga's biochemical assembly offers a multi-layered defence system particularly suited to companion animals experiencing oxidative stress, immune fatigue, toxin exposure or age-related decline.

Sub-critical water extraction plays a critical role in preserving this complexity. SCWE allows both hydrophilic and lipophilic constituents to be recovered in physiologically relevant ratios, maintaining the polyphenol–melanin structure, the betulinic triterpenes and the natural fibre-based matrix. This ensures that veterinary patients receive an extract that reflects the therapeutic integrity of the whole organism rather than a fractionated or solvent-biased preparation. The result is a more predictable, whole-system regulatory influence consistent with the mechanistic pathways described above.

4.4 Immune Modulation and Inflammatory Regulation

Chaga exerts a distinctive regulatory influence on the immune system that is neither suppressive nor excessively stimulatory. Instead, its actions unfold gradually through modulation of key immune pathways, correction of dysregulated cytokine patterns and reinforcement of mucosal and systemic defence mechanisms. This regulatory profile aligns well with clinical situations in which chronic inflammation, immune imbalance or environmental stress play a central role in disease progression.

The mushroom's polysaccharides, particularly its β-glucans and heteroglucans, interact with pattern-recognition receptors such as Dectin-1, complement receptor 3 and Toll-like receptor 2. Engagement of these receptors activates balanced macrophage and dendritic cell responses, enhancing immune vigilance without provoking the hyperreactive patterns commonly associated with allergic, dysbiotic or stressed animals. Preclinical evidence demonstrates improvement in phagocytic efficiency, enhanced antigen presentation and restoration of more appropriate T-helper cell ratios, particularly where Th1–Th2 imbalance underpins chronic inflammatory cycles.

Chaga's phenolic and melanin complexes add another dimension to immune regulation by moderating oxidative drivers of inflammation. Oxidative stress amplifies inflammatory signalling in many tissues, including the gastrointestinal tract, skin, liver and respiratory system. Chaga's antioxidants attenuate this amplification by reducing reactive oxygen species and stabilising endogenous antioxidant enzymes. This dual antioxidant–immunoregulatory action is particularly relevant to senior animals and individuals living with chronic metabolic strain, chronic enteropathies or low-grade allergic patterns.

Inflammatory cascades driven by nuclear factor kappa B, interleukin 6 and tumour necrosis factor alpha are consistently down-regulated in preclinical models when Chaga extracts are used. These pathways are central to a wide range of veterinary conditions, from dermatitis and atopy to chronic gastrointestinal inflammation and environmentally induced respiratory sensitivity. Chaga's ability to reduce inducible nitric oxide synthase and cyclo-oxygenase 2 activity further contributes to tissue-level stability by diminishing inflammatory mediator production, helping to restore equilibrium in tissues subjected to persistent inflammatory load.

Although direct veterinary clinical trials remain limited, practitioner observations support Chaga's usefulness in cases marked by immune fragmentation, flare-prone inflammation or inadequate immune recovery following illness or stress. In such contexts, Chaga functions as a slow, stabilising influence on immune tone. Its actions rarely produce immediate symptomatic shifts but instead provide the foundation upon which longer-term improvement in resilience, comfort and inflammatory balance can occur.

Chaga's immune-modulating profile can be especially valuable when used alongside other mushrooms whose actions complement its antioxidant and regulatory effects. For example, pairing Chaga with Reishi in chronic inflammatory conditions or with Turkey Tail in cases requiring gut–immune support can create a more comprehensive immunological environment. These combinations, however, must be implemented with attention to each animal's clinical context, medication regimen and sensitivity to immune-modifying interventions.

Overall, Chaga's influence on inflammatory and immune pathways is best understood as a cumulative recalibration of regulatory systems rather than a direct pharmacological suppression of symptoms. This orientation makes it particularly well suited to chronic and multi-systemic cases where stability, resilience and long-term modulation are primary therapeutic goals.

4.5 Antioxidant, Oxidative Stress and Cellular Defence Mechanisms

Chaga is distinguished within functional mushrooms by its exceptional antioxidant density and its ability to modulate oxidative pathways that influence cellular health, mitochondrial efficiency and tissue resilience. Its antioxidant profile is generated from multiple compound classes, including melanins, polyphenols, triterpenes and antioxidant peptides. The synergy of these constituents produces a breadth of antioxidant activity rarely seen in botanical or fungal therapeutics, positioning Chaga as a uniquely valuable tool in conditions where oxidative stress drives or exacerbates disease.

The melanin fraction, which defines Chaga's characteristic deep pigmentation, is one of the most potent naturally occurring free-radical scavenging complexes identified in medicinal fungi. This melanin matrix binds and neutralises reactive oxygen species with high efficiency, while also protecting DNA from oxidative injury. Preclinical studies demonstrate reduced lipid peroxidation, improved mitochondrial membrane integrity and increased resistance to oxidative damage under environmental or chemical stress. These findings align with clinical observations in senior animals, working dogs, convalescent patients and individuals exposed to environmental toxins or chronic inflammatory load.

Chaga's polyphenolic compounds complement the melanin fraction by reinforcing endogenous antioxidant enzymes. Studies report increased activity of superoxide dismutase, catalase and glutathione peroxidase following Chaga administration, indicating a strengthening of intrinsic cellular defence systems. These enzymes are essential for neutralising reactive oxygen species generated during chronic inflammation, metabolic stress, strenuous activity or exposure to pollutants. By enhancing these endogenous antioxidant pathways, Chaga extends its influence beyond simple radical scavenging toward long-term cellular protection and tissue resilience.

The triterpenes, particularly betulin and betulinic acid, contribute further to Chaga's cytoprotective mechanisms. These compounds demonstrate the ability to reduce mitochondrial oxidative burden, modulate nuclear factor kappa B activity and influence apoptotic signalling in damaged or stressed cells. Preclinical research highlights betulinic acid's capacity to help stabilise cellular membranes, reduce DNA fragmentation and support orderly cellular repair. Although these findings derive primarily from rodent and in vitro studies, the mechanistic relevance to veterinary physiology is strong, particularly in cases of chronic hepatic strain, metabolic disease, environmental toxicity or degenerative conditions.

Chaga also provides protection to tissues with high oxidative turnover, such as the liver, gastrointestinal mucosa, skin and respiratory epithelium. Its antioxidant peptides and phenolic–melanin complexes help mitigate the secondary oxidative consequences of inflammation, infection, allergen exposure and chronic medication. In gastrointestinal tissues, this influence contributes to stabilised mucosal integrity and reduced permeability. In hepatic tissue, the combined antioxidant and anti-inflammatory effects may help reduce hepatocellular stress associated with medication, environmental toxins or metabolic load.

The relevance of oxidative stress in modern veterinary medicine cannot be overstated. Many chronic conditions, including dermatitis, inflammatory bowel disease, hepatic dysfunction, chronic respiratory irritation, cognitive decline and neoplastic processes, involve a significant oxidative component. Chaga's unparalleled antioxidant matrix therefore provides a foundational defence system that can support healing and resilience across numerous clinical contexts.

Sub-critical water extraction enhances these benefits by preserving the integrity of the melanin–polyphenol complex and ensuring retention of antioxidant peptides and triterpenes. Solvent-based extractions or unprocessed raw Chaga often degrade or fail to capture the full antioxidant assembly, resulting in extracts that lack the depth of cellular defence described in preclinical literature. SCWE full-spectrum extracts more faithfully reflect the natural biochemical order of the sclerotium, delivering predictable antioxidant influence suited to veterinary practice.

In summary, Chaga's antioxidant capacity is not defined by a single compound but by the synergistic cooperation of its phenolics, melanins, peptides and triterpenes. This multi-layered defence system contributes to cellular protection, improved metabolic resilience and enhanced physiological integrity across a wide range of veterinary presentations. Its role in oxidative stress modulation is among the strongest mechanistic foundations for its inclusion in integrative care, particularly for senior animals, chronically medicated patients, environmentally exposed individuals and those recovering from illness or systemic inflammation.

> Chaga is distinguished within functional mushrooms by its exceptional antioxidant density and its ability to modulate oxidative pathways that influence cellular health, mitochondrial efficiency and tissue resilience.

4.6 Gastrointestinal, Microbiome and Mucosal Integrity

Chaga has a long ethnomedical history as a gastrointestinal restorative, particularly in the context of gastric discomfort, mucosal sensitivity and inflammatory or stress-related digestive disturbance. Modern research supports many aspects of this traditional use, indicating that Chaga influences gastrointestinal physiology at multiple levels, including modulation of inflammation, protection of epithelial integrity, support of microbial balance and reduction of oxidative injury within the digestive tract. These combined actions give Chaga a distinctive role in cases where gastrointestinal and systemic inflammation coexist or where the gut forms a central component of chronic disease patterns.

One of Chaga's primary contributions lies in its ability to regulate inflammatory pathways within the gastrointestinal mucosa. Its polyphenolic compounds and triterpenes, including betulinic acid, help down-regulate nuclear factor kappa B activation, reducing expression of pro-inflammatory cytokines such as interleukin 6 and tumour necrosis factor alpha. In preclinical models of chemically induced gastritis and enteritis, Chaga extracts reduce inflammatory infiltration, limit mucosal damage and support more rapid recovery of epithelial tissue. These findings offer mechanistic insight into why many practitioners observe improvements in stool quality, reduced gastrointestinal reactivity and enhanced comfort in animals with chronic enteropathies, stress-sensitive digestion or diet-associated inflammatory patterns.

Chaga also contributes meaningfully to mucosal defence. The gastrointestinal barrier is constantly challenged by dietary antigens, microbial products and oxidative stress. Increased permeability is a central driver of chronic inflammation in many animals, feeding into systemic immune imbalance, hepatic load and behavioural vulnerability through the gut–brain axis. Chaga's antioxidant constituents, including its melanin–polyphenol complexes and antioxidant peptides, help protect epithelial cells from oxidative injury and lipid peroxidation. This stabilisation of the mucosal barrier may reduce susceptibility to flare cycles in animals with mixed gastrointestinal and allergic presentations, where oxidative stress and inflammation perpetuate permeability.

The mushroom's polysaccharides and fibre-rich matrix further reinforce gastrointestinal resilience by supporting the microbiome. Chaga provides indigestible polysaccharides that act as prebiotic substrates, selectively nourishing beneficial microbial populations. Preclinical studies demonstrate increased microbial richness and shifts toward anti-inflammatory taxa following Chaga supplementation. These microbial changes support the production of short-chain fatty acids, including butyrate, which promote epithelial repair, help regulate intestinal immune function and contribute to improved metabolic balance. In veterinary contexts, these mechanisms align with practitioner reports of steadier gastrointestinal patterns, improved appetite regularity and reduced sensitivity to dietary transitions.

The gut–liver axis is particularly relevant in the context of Chaga's effects. Increased intestinal permeability and dysbiosis can elevate hepatic stress through the portal circulation. By strengthening mucosal integrity, reducing endothelial oxidative load and modulating inflammatory pathways, Chaga helps reduce hepatic burden indirectly. This is especially valuable in animals receiving chronic medication, recovering from toxin exposure or experiencing multi-system inflammatory patterns that involve both gastrointestinal and hepatic systems.

Chaga's influence on the gut–brain axis provides further relevance for animals with stress-responsive gastrointestinal symptoms. Chronic stress disrupts gastrointestinal motility, alters microbial composition and destabilises mucosal immune activity. Chaga's antioxidant and mucosal-calming properties, combined with its influence on systemic inflammatory and oxidative pathways, contribute to more stable digestive patterns in animals whose gastrointestinal symptoms are closely linked to environmental, emotional or physiological stressors.

Sub-critical water extraction preserves the structural and biochemical components upon which Chaga's gastrointestinal benefits depend. Preparations produced via SCWE retain the natural fibre, polysaccharides, polyphenols and melanin complexes that interact directly with the gut–immune axis. In contrast, solvent-based extracts often lose fibre and structural compounds essential for prebiotic and mucosal-supportive effects, while raw or unprocessed Chaga poses risks due to inconsistent compound extraction and elevated oxalate content. SCWE full-spectrum extracts therefore offer the most predictable and physiologically coherent gastrointestinal benefits.

When the anti-inflammatory, antioxidant, prebiotic and mucosal-stabilising mechanisms described above are considered collectively, it becomes clear that Chaga offers a multi-layered regulatory influence across the gastrointestinal system. Its benefits emerge gradually, reflecting cumulative modulation of gut–immune signalling, oxidative stability, epithelial resilience and the gut–liver axis. These properties make Chaga particularly well suited to long-term strategies for chronic enteropathies, stress-responsive digestive disturbances, metabolic–inflammatory overlap and cases involving combined gut and hepatic strain. For many animals, Chaga provides a gentle yet meaningful stabilising effect on the gastrointestinal terrain that underpins wider systemic health.

4.7 Metabolic and Endocrine Regulation

Chaga's influence on metabolic and endocrine physiology arises from its combined effects on oxidative balance, inflammatory tone, mitochondrial function and gut–liver axis regulation. Although veterinary-specific studies are still limited, a growing body of preclinical research highlights Chaga's capacity to improve glucose handling, modulate lipid metabolism and support metabolic stability in the face of chronic physiological strain. These actions position Chaga as a valuable adjunct for animals exhibiting metabolic imbalance, age-related endocrine fragility or chronic inflammatory states that overlap with metabolic dysfunction.

> Chaga offers a valuable foundation-building tool within integrative metabolic care.

One of the most consistently documented metabolic effects of Chaga involves its ability to improve insulin sensitivity and support glucose regulation. In rodent models of metabolic syndrome, Chaga extracts reduce fasting glucose, improve glucose tolerance and enhance insulin receptor signalling. These outcomes arise from reductions in systemic inflammation, decreases in oxidative stress and improvements in mitochondrial efficiency. For veterinary patients, these mechanisms carry relevance for animals with inflammatory-driven metabolic tendencies, including overweight senior dogs, cats with early insulin resistance or animals experiencing metabolic instability due to chronic stress, endocrine disease or long-term medication.

Chaga's antioxidant activity also contributes to more efficient mitochondrial function, which plays a central role in metabolic health. By protecting mitochondrial membranes from oxidative injury and reinforcing endogenous antioxidant defences, Chaga supports more stable energy metabolism. This may explain why practitioners often observe improved stamina, fewer fatigue episodes and steadier energy patterns in older or convalescent animals receiving Chaga consistently. These observations remain anecdotal but align closely with mechanistic pathways described in preclinical models.

Lipid regulation is another domain where Chaga shows meaningful influence. Triterpenes such as betulin and betulinic acid help modulate lipid metabolism by influencing sterol-regulatory element binding proteins, reducing lipid accumulation and improving hepatic lipid handling. Although companion animals have different lipid profiles compared with humans, these mechanisms may still contribute to improved metabolic resilience, particularly in overweight animals, those with endocrine disorders or senior animals with chronic inflammatory load. These effects are modest rather than dramatic, reflecting Chaga's role as a regulator rather than a corrective agent.

Chaga may also play a supportive role in endocrine health due to its capacity to reduce inflammatory signalling and oxidative stress that disrupt endocrine rhythms. Chronic inflammation contributes to altered cortisol secretion, impaired thyroid hormone conversion and increased metabolic variability. Chaga's broad anti-inflammatory and antioxidant activity helps buffer these disruptions at a systemic level. While Chaga does not mimic or replace endocrine hormones, its ability to reduce oxidative and inflammatory burden may help stabilise endocrine physiology indirectly.

The gut–liver axis is another essential part of Chaga's metabolic relevance. Dysbiosis, intestinal permeability and microbial endotoxin exposure contribute to hepatic inflammation and metabolic strain. By strengthening epithelial integrity, modulating microbial composition and reducing oxidative load within the gut and liver, Chaga helps maintain metabolic stability. This indirect hepatic support is particularly relevant for animals on chronic medication, individuals with combined gastrointestinal and metabolic presentations and senior animals exhibiting low-grade metabolic fragility.

Taken together, Chaga's metabolic and endocrine effects are best understood as cumulative, gentle and multi-layered rather than corrective or rapid. Its regulatory influence emerges gradually over weeks, contributing to improved metabolic steadiness, better energy utilisation and a more resilient physiological baseline. For animals with metabolic–inflammatory overlap, age-related metabolic drift or chronic stress-associated endocrine dysregulation, Chaga offers a valuable foundation-building tool within integrative metabolic care.

4.8 Dermatological and Oxidative Skin Support

Skin and coat health are intimately tied to systemic inflammation, oxidative balance, immune activity and metabolic stability. Chaga's dense antioxidant matrix, combined with its anti-inflammatory and immune-regulatory properties, provides a compelling rationale for its use in veterinary dermatology. While direct clinical trials in animals remain limited, preclinical data and practitioner experience suggest that Chaga may benefit animals with chronic inflammatory skin conditions, environmental sensitivities or oxidative-stress driven dermal changes.

Chaga's melanin and polyphenol complexes contribute significantly to its dermatological relevance. These compounds exhibit strong ultraviolet-absorbing and free-radical-scavenging activity, helping protect skin cells and keratinocytes from oxidative and photodamage. This may be particularly relevant for light-coated animals, those recovering from inflammatory skin flare cycles and senior animals with reduced dermal antioxidant capacity. Although most evidence derives from cell and rodent models, the underlying mechanisms align with patterns observed in veterinary practice, where improvements in coat gloss, skin tone and overall dermal resilience are often reported after several weeks of consistent supplementation.

The mushroom's influence on inflammatory pathways also contributes to improved dermatological stability. Chronic inflammatory skin disease involves dysregulated cytokine expression, mast-cell activation and persistent oxidative burden. Chaga's triterpenes, including betulinic acid, help down-regulate nuclear factor kappa B and associated cytokines such as interleukin 6 and tumour necrosis factor alpha. By reducing these inflammatory mediators, Chaga may help decrease the severity and frequency of dermatological flare-ups, particularly in animals with combined inflammatory and oxidative components to their skin disease.

> Chaga's dense antioxidant matrix, combined with its anti-inflammatory and immune-regulatory properties, provides a compelling rationale for its use in veterinary dermatology

Chaga's capacity to modulate immune responses extends to mucosal and dermal immunity. Its polysaccharides support more balanced T-helper activity and promote appropriate innate immune surveillance, which may help reduce excessive or misdirected inflammatory reactions. Practitioners often note improvements in animals with environmental sensitivities or mixed inflammatory–allergic dermatitis, although such observations remain anecdotal and should be interpreted alongside standard dermatological care.

Oxidative stress plays a central role in chronic skin conditions, contributing to impaired barrier function, delayed healing and increased sensitivity. Chaga's ability to reinforce endogenous antioxidant enzymes, such as superoxide dismutase and glutathione peroxidase, may help restore dermal resilience in animals experiencing chronic skin irritation, coat deterioration or slow recovery after inflammatory episodes. These mechanisms are especially relevant in senior animals, where oxidative stress accumulates across multiple organ systems, including the skin.

Chaga also contributes indirectly to dermatological health through its effects on gastrointestinal and hepatic function. The gut–skin axis is well established, with dysbiosis and increased intestinal permeability contributing to skin inflammation in many animals. By supporting microbial balance, reducing mucosal inflammation and improving hepatic clearance of inflammatory mediators, Chaga may help stabilise dermatological patterns that involve gastrointestinal and hepatic overlap.

Sub-critical water extraction is particularly relevant to dermatological applications because it preserves the melanin–polyphenol complexes that form the backbone of Chaga's antioxidant and tissue-protective effects. These structures are partially lost or degraded in solvent-based extracts or unprocessed preparations. SCWE therefore provides a structurally faithful extract that retains the molecular components responsible for Chaga's broad dermatological and oxidative benefits.

Overall, Chaga offers a gentle but cumulative influence on skin and coat health. Its effects emerge gradually, reflecting improvements in oxidative balance, immune stability, mucosal and hepatic support and overall metabolic resilience. For animals with chronic inflammatory skin conditions, environmental sensitivities or age-related dermal decline, Chaga provides a versatile and well-tolerated supportive agent when integrated thoughtfully within a comprehensive dermatological care plan.

4.9 Cardiovascular and Vascular Health

The cardiovascular relevance of Chaga in veterinary medicine arises primarily from its capacity to modulate oxidative stress, support vascular integrity and influence lipid and glucose handling through interconnected metabolic pathways. Although direct veterinary cardiovascular trials are limited, the mechanistic and translational evidence offers a coherent rationale for its cautious and supportive use, particularly in ageing animals, performance dogs, endocrine-related metabolic dysfunction and individuals with chronic inflammatory burden.

Oxidative stress plays a central role in the deterioration of vascular health across species, contributing to endothelial dysfunction, impaired nitric oxide signalling and reduced vascular elasticity. Chaga's dense profile of antioxidant compounds, including polyphenols, melanin complexes and antioxidant peptides, helps buffer oxidative injury within vascular tissues. Preclinical studies indicate that these compounds reduce lipid peroxidation, stabilise endothelial cells and support mitochondrial function in cardiomyocytes. This antioxidant reinforcement is especially relevant in senior animals, where cumulative oxidative load contributes to reduced stamina, slower recovery, altered circulation and diminished resilience under stress.

In addition to antioxidant support, Chaga exhibits several metabolic effects with cardiovascular implications. Rodent and translational studies demonstrate improvements in lipid handling, including reductions in total cholesterol and low-density lipoprotein, alongside enhanced glucose regulation and insulin sensitivity. While companion animals have species-specific metabolic profiles that do not mirror human lipid physiology, improvements in metabolic balance can still reduce inflammatory pressure on the cardiovascular system. In overweight animals, or those with endocrine disorders such as hypothyroidism or Cushing's syndrome, this broader metabolic support may contribute indirectly to improved vascular stability and energy metabolism.

Chaga's anti-inflammatory properties further influence cardiovascular health by modulating inflammatory pathways that contribute to endothelial irritation and systemic vascular stress. Its triterpenes and polyphenols down-regulate nuclear factor kappa B activation and reduce production of inflammatory cytokines such as interleukin 6 and tumour necrosis factor alpha. By decreasing inflammatory load, Chaga may help reduce background cardiovascular strain, particularly in animals with chronic inflammatory diseases, long-term medication exposure or mixed allergic–vascular presentations.

Although Chaga is not a cardiac botanical in the traditional sense, its metabolic, antioxidant and anti-inflammatory profile provides a meaningful supportive matrix for animals with early cardiovascular vulnerability or subclinical decline. Senior dogs with reduced circulatory efficiency, working dogs under high oxidative load and animals recovering from illness or surgery may benefit from this systemic stabilisation. In these contexts, practitioners sometimes observe subtle improvements in stamina, post-exercise recovery and general vitality, although such findings remain anecdotal and should not be interpreted as direct cardiac treatment effects.

Caution is advised when Chaga is used alongside antihypertensive medications or agents that influence vascular tone. Preclinical work suggests that Chaga may contribute to mild reductions in blood pressure through improved endothelial responsiveness and reduced inflammatory signalling. While the effect is modest, additive actions are possible in animals already receiving pharmaceuticals for cardiac or vascular conditions. As with all supportive Mycotherapy interventions, individual clinical judgement and careful monitoring are essential.

Sub-critical water extraction enhances Chaga's cardiovascular applicability by preserving the full spectrum of bioactive compounds that underpin these interconnected mechanisms. SCWE extracts retain the natural fibre, polyphenols, triterpenes and melanin complexes essential for modulating oxidative and inflammatory pathways. This contrasts with solvent-based tinctures and raw preparations, which may lose structural compounds, introduce ethanol residues or present inconsistent oxalate concentrations. For animals with metabolic or cardiovascular sensitivity, the biochemical stability and predictability of SCWE preparations provide additional reassurance.

Chaga's cardiovascular relevance arises not from direct effects on cardiac contractility or vascular tone but from its broader influence on metabolic, oxidative and inflammatory pathways. By reducing oxidative burden, moderating cytokine activity and supporting lipid balance, Chaga contributes indirectly to vascular resilience and long-term physiological stability. Its effects are cumulative and supportive rather than acute, making it most appropriate as part of comprehensive care plans targeting healthy ageing, metabolic balance and whole-body vitality.

4.10 Veterinary Pharmacology and Drug Interaction Considerations

Chaga's pharmacological profile is defined by its concentration of polyphenols, melanins, triterpenes (including betulinic acid), antioxidant peptides and polysaccharides. These compounds exert significant influence on oxidative pathways, inflammatory signalling, hepatic detoxification and metabolic regulation. While broadly supportive and generally low risk, Chaga's potency warrants careful consideration when administered alongside pharmaceuticals or in animals with complex internal-medicine needs. The following domains outline the clinically relevant interactions and pharmacological behaviours observed in current translational research.

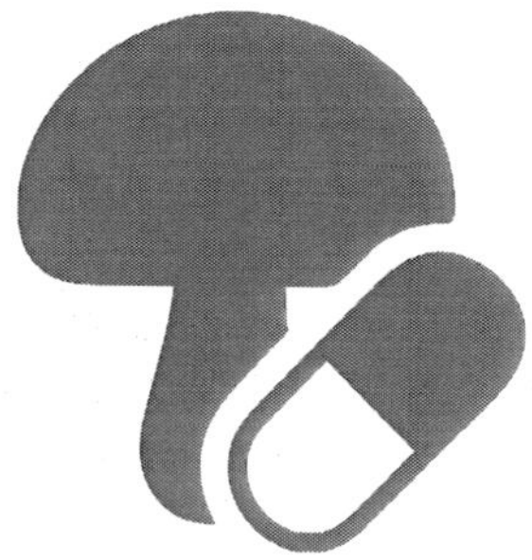

Chaga's pharmacological profile is defined by its concentration of polyphenols, melanins, triter penes (including betulinic acid), antioxidant peptides and polysaccharides.

Influence on hepatic detoxification and drug metabolism

Chaga modulates hepatic detoxification pathways, particularly phase I and phase II enzyme systems associated with oxidative defence and metabolic clearance. Preclinical data suggest effects on glutathione-dependent pathways and selected cytochrome P450 mechanisms, although species-specific veterinary data remain limited. This influence may theoretically alter the metabolism of medications reliant on hepatic transformation, such as phenobarbital, certain chemotherapeutics and long-term corticosteroids.

Clinicians should monitor hepatic trends when Chaga is introduced in animals with pre-existing liver compromise or those receiving medications with narrow therapeutic indices. Although Chaga's effects are modulatory rather than disruptive, prudent oversight improves predictability in medically fragile animals.

Effects on glucose regulation and interaction with hypoglycaemic medications

Rodent and cell-based studies demonstrate that Chaga can influence glucose metabolism through enhanced insulin sensitivity, modulation of hepatic glucose production and improved glucose uptake. These effects stem from its polyphenols and triterpenes, which reduce oxidative stress in pancreatic and hepatic tissues.

While clinical hypoglycaemia is unlikely, cautious titration is warranted in diabetic animals receiving insulin or oral hypoglycaemics. Subtle reductions in blood glucose have been reported anecdotally in veterinary practice, making early monitoring advisable in the first two to three weeks of use.

Interaction with gastrointestinal and hepatic medications

Chaga's mucosal-protective and anti-inflammatory properties can help buffer gastrointestinal irritation associated with non-steroidal anti-inflammatory drugs, corticosteroids and long-term analgesic therapy. These interactions are generally supportive, but clinicians should remain observant for changes in stool quality or appetite during concurrent use.

In animals receiving hepatically metabolised drugs, Chaga's influence on detoxification enzymes may alter the rate of metabolic clearance. Although predictable pharmacokinetic interactions are not established, geriatric patients and individuals on polypharmacy protocols benefit from periodic reassessment of hepatic parameters during the introductory phase.

Interaction with immunomodulatory and chemotherapeutic agents

Chaga regulates innate and adaptive immune pathways through modulation of macrophage activity, natural killer cell function and cytokine balance. While these effects are typically harmonising rather than stimulating, they intersect with pharmaceutical immune-modification strategies.

Animals receiving ciclosporin, corticosteroids, oclacitinib or targeted chemotherapeutics require individualised assessment to ensure that Chaga's immune effects do not counteract the therapeutic intent. In oncology cases, Chaga's antioxidant and apoptotic-modulating properties may enhance physiological resilience and treatment response. Collaboration between treating veterinarians and Mycotherapy practitioners is recommended to ensure coherence across modalities.

Oxalate considerations and renal pharmacology

Chaga contains naturally high levels of oxalates, making renal considerations a central aspect of its pharmacological profile. Although SCWE extracts significantly reduce soluble oxalate fractions compared with raw or powdered Chaga, they do not eliminate them entirely.

Animals with a history of calcium-oxalate urolithiasis, chronic kidney disease or metabolic predisposition to crystal formation should be approached with caution. Concurrent use with diuretics, angiotensin-converting enzyme inhibitors or medications affecting calcium balance warrants additional monitoring of hydration status, renal parameters and urinary comfort.

Anticoagulant and antiplatelet considerations

Chaga's triterpenes and antioxidant compounds exhibit mild antiplatelet activity in preclinical models. While clinically significant bleeding tendencies are extremely rare, animals receiving antiplatelet or anticoagulant therapies such as aspirin analogues or heparins require conservative monitoring. Temporary withholding before surgical or dental procedures may be appropriate depending on the individual.

Advantages of SCWE extracts in pharmacological predictability

Extraction fidelity plays a major role in Chaga's pharmacological reliability. SCWE preserves both hydrophilic and lipophilic compounds, maintains fibre-bound polysaccharides and removes solvent residues. This whole-food biochemical coherence supports more predictable interactions, particularly in elderly or polypharmacy patients.

In contrast, alcohol tinctures can distort the triterpene–polysaccharide balance, and myceliated grain products introduce starch and lack the bioactive constituents central to Chaga's therapeutic mechanisms. For animals receiving medications with narrow therapeutic windows, SCWE extracts deliver a more stable and physiologically aligned profile.

Summary of pharmacological and interaction considerations

Chaga's pharmacological actions are predominantly supportive, but its potency as an antioxidant, hepatic modulator and metabolic regulator requires thoughtful integration. Key considerations include oxalate load, theoretical glucose-lowering synergy, mild antiplatelet activity and the need for monitoring in animals receiving immunomodulators or hepatically cleared pharmaceuticals. When used within a structured Mycotherapy framework and accompanied by appropriate clinical oversight, SCWE Chaga can be incorporated safely into treatment plans for animals experiencing oxidative stress, chronic inflammation, hepatic strain, metabolic challenges or environmental toxin exposure.

4.11 Clinical Application in Veterinary Practice

Chaga's clinical relevance in veterinary medicine is grounded in its exceptional antioxidant capacity, broad immunological influence and its supportive effects on hepatic, gastrointestinal and metabolic stability. Unlike mushrooms whose primary domain is neurological (Lion's Mane) or immunological (Turkey Tail), Chaga acts as a systemic regulator that reduces underlying physiological strain. Its greatest value emerges in conditions characterised by oxidative load, chronic inflammatory activity, environmental toxin burden and impaired cellular recovery. These patterns are increasingly recognised in modern veterinary practice, particularly in ageing animals, individuals exposed to chronic stress or those receiving long-term pharmaceutical intervention.

CHAGA (INONOTUS OBLIQUUS) – Evidence Quality Commentary Table

This spectrum of evidence is summarised in the following table:

Domain	Evidence Strength	Primary Evidence Type
Antioxidant capacity and oxidative defence	High	Preclinical, biochemical assays, in vivo antioxidant models
Anti-inflammatory activity	Moderate to high	Preclinical, mechanistic animal studies
Immune modulation	Moderate	Preclinical, rodent and cell-based studies
Gastrointestinal and mucosal support	Moderate	Preclinical, anti-ulcer and mucosal-protective models
Hepatic support and detoxification pathways	Moderate	Preclinical, hepatoprotective animal models
Metabolic and glycaemic regulation	Emerging to moderate	Preclinical metabolic-syndrome models
Behavioural and stress resilience	Emerging	Preclinical neuroinflammatory models
Antimicrobial properties	Emerging	In vitro and limited in vivo research
Oncology adjunct use	Emerging	Preclinical anti-proliferative studies; strong practitioner interest

Domain	Evidence Strength	Primary Evidence Type
Clinical veterinary trials	Limited	No formal veterinary trials; translational rationale only

Chaga's evidence base is dominated by strong antioxidant and anti-inflammatory findings, reflecting its unusually high concentration of polyphenols, melanin complexes and triterpenes such as inotodiol. These constituents consistently demonstrate potent free-radical buffering capacity, modulation of inflammatory signalling and protection of cellular structures under oxidative load. Although direct veterinary studies remain limited, comparative physiology and mechanistic data provide a solid rationale for its use in animals experiencing chronic inflammatory conditions, metabolic strain, environmental toxicity or gastrointestinal mucosal vulnerability.

Within a Mycotherapy context, Chaga contributes to terrain stability by supporting mitochondrial protection, moderating oxidative injury and assisting hepatic detoxification pathways. SCWE full-spectrum extracts retain the full complement of phenolics, melanin-bound antioxidants, polysaccharides and sterol derivatives without denaturing heat-sensitive compounds. This contrasts with high-heat or alcohol-based preparations, which may lose key antioxidant fractions or over-represent lipophilic triterpenes at the expense of the native whole-mushroom matrix.

For veterinarians, Chaga functions best as a complementary, long-term supportive agent – particularly in chronic inflammatory states, oxidative stress syndromes, gastrointestinal fragility and metabolic imbalance – rather than as a rapid or stand-alone intervention.

Support in chronic inflammatory and oxidative conditions

Animals living with chronic inflammatory disease often experience ongoing oxidative stress, mitochondrial fatigue and impaired tissue recovery. Chaga's melanin complexes, polyphenols and triterpenes exert antioxidant effects that reduce cellular damage and stabilise inflammatory pathways. Clinicians frequently incorporate Chaga into protocols for animals with long-standing dermatitis, joint inflammation, recurrent infections or multi-system inflammatory tendencies. Its effects are gradual, reflecting deeper changes in redox balance rather than rapid symptomatic shifts. Over several weeks, practitioners often report improved stamina, brighter demeanour, reduced inflammatory volatility and enhanced resilience to environmental triggers.

Gastrointestinal and hepatic applications

Chaga's historical use for gastric discomfort aligns with its contemporary value in animals experiencing gastrointestinal sensitivity or stress-responsive digestive disturbance. Its polysaccharides, mucosal-supportive fibre and antioxidant compounds help stabilise epithelial integrity, which may contribute to improved stool quality and reduced reactivity to dietary fluctuations. In animals with low-grade inflammatory bowel tendencies or chronic enteropathies, Chaga may support greater comfort and digestive consistency.

Its influence on hepatic pathways is also clinically meaningful. Animals exposed to chronic medication, environmental pollutants or metabolic strain often benefit from Chaga's hepatoprotective properties. Although not a replacement for targeted hepatic therapies, its ability to support glutathione-related processes and protect hepatocytes from oxidative injury can enhance overall hepatic resilience. Senior animals, or those receiving anticonvulsants, corticosteroids or long-term analgesics, may exhibit improved tolerance and steadier enzyme trends when Chaga is incorporated carefully into care plans.

Metabolic and endocrine relevance

Chaga's influence on glucose and lipid metabolism, although primarily supported by preclinical models, provides a rationale for its use in animals with metabolic–inflammatory overlap. Senior animals with weight fluctuations, reduced vitality or impaired metabolic flexibility may benefit from its regulatory effects on insulin sensitivity and oxidative pathways. In overweight pets or those with mild endocrine imbalance, Chaga supports a steadier metabolic baseline that complements dietary and lifestyle interventions. Any use alongside hypoglycaemic medications should be monitored, but the mushroom's activity is generally moderate and regulatory rather than pharmacologically forceful.

Adjunctive role in oncology and immune support

Chaga's relevance in oncology is grounded in both its antioxidant defence and its influence on apoptosis pathways. While not an anticancer treatment, its cellular-protective and immune-stabilising mechanisms can be valuable during chemotherapy or chronic tumour management. Chaga may help reduce treatment-associated oxidative burden and support tissue resilience, contributing to steadier energy levels and improved comfort. Its role is supportive and terrain-focused, strengthening cellular integrity and immune surveillance rather than exerting direct tumouricidal activity.

Dermatological and skin–coat health applications

Because oxidative stress and inflammatory activity often contribute to dermatological conditions, Chaga's antioxidant and cytokine-balancing mechanisms can indirectly support skin recovery. Animals with chronic itch, inflamed skin or environmentally driven sensitivities may show improved dermal comfort when Chaga is incorporated as part of an integrative plan. Improved coat sheen and general vitality are also frequently noted by practitioners in ageing animals.

Suitability across life stages and species

Chaga is generally well suited to dogs, cats and selected small mammals when administered as a SCWE full-spectrum extract. Mature and senior animals tend to experience the greatest benefit because oxidative load, metabolic inefficiency and cumulative inflammatory strain are more pronounced in later life. Environmentally sensitive breeds, animals undergoing rehabilitation and individuals with chronic gastrointestinal or hepatic vulnerability also represent suitable candidates. As with all Mycotherapy, Chaga performs best when integrated into a comprehensive care plan that includes diagnostic assessment, nutritional guidance and targeted pharmaceutical or nutraceutical support where required.

Clinical summary

Chaga's role in veterinary practice is defined not by dramatic short-term effects but by gradual restoration of physiological balance. Its actions build over weeks, helping animals cope more effectively with chronic inflammation, environmental stressors and metabolic strain. Practitioners often value Chaga for the stronger baseline of resilience and vitality it cultivates, particularly in ageing or medically complex patients. As long as its oxalate considerations are respected and its use is monitored in animals receiving specific medications, Chaga offers a stable, predictable and scientifically coherent contribution to long-term integrative care.

Integration with other functional mushrooms

Chaga offers a unique combination of antioxidant strength, hepatic support, immune modulation and gastrointestinal stability, making it a versatile integrative partner for many functional mushrooms. Its melanin complexes, polyphenols, betulinic compounds and SOD-like activity complement species that support immunity, neurotrophic pathways, mitochondrial resilience and metabolic balance. The following pairings represent the most clinically relevant combinations in veterinary practice.

- **With Reishi** - Chaga and Reishi form a deeply harmonising combination for animals requiring balanced immune modulation, hepatic steadiness and allergy support. Reishi's triterpenoids influence mast-cell behaviour, autonomic tone and inflammatory cascades, while Chaga contributes potent antioxidant buffering and mucosal stability. Together, they support chronic dermatitis, seasonal allergies, hepatic workload due to medication or age, and immune dysregulation driven by stress or environmental triggers. This pairing is especially useful for animals with mixed inflammatory–allergic presentations or chronic hepatic strain.

- **With Turkey Tail** - Turkey Tail amplifies Chaga's actions by contributing broad-spectrum β-glucans and PSP/PSK-associated immune support. This pairing is notable in integrative oncology settings, where Chaga's antioxidant defence and DNA-protective influence help buffer oxidative stress, while Turkey Tail strengthens immune surveillance and cellular resilience.

Animals experiencing chronic illness, treatment-related oxidative burden or immune compromise may benefit from the combination's synergistic effects across the redox–immune interface.

- **With Lion's Mane** - Lion's Mane adds a neurotrophic and enteric-nervous-system dimension to Chaga's gastrointestinal and antioxidant profile. Together, they support animals with chronic digestive vulnerability, stress-linked gastrointestinal upset, inflammatory bowel tendencies or gut–brain axis fragility. Chaga's polyphenols and fibre-rich matrix assist mucosal repair and oxidative balance, while Lion's Mane enhances neuronal integration within the gut and stabilises stress physiology. This pairing is particularly valuable in animals displaying concurrent digestive and behavioural or cognitive symptoms.

- **With Cordyceps** - Cordyceps builds upon Chaga's tissue-protective influence by improving mitochondrial efficiency, oxygen utilisation and metabolic resilience. Chaga stabilises oxidative load and supports hepatic and gastrointestinal tissues, while Cordyceps enhances endurance, stamina and post-exertional recovery. This combination benefits working dogs, performance animals and those recovering from chronic metabolic or inflammatory stress. In senior animals, the pairing can help support energy steadiness, mobility and oxidative repair capacity.

- **With Golden Oyster** - Chaga and Golden Oyster create a formidable antioxidant and cytoprotective combination. Golden Oyster's ergothioneine-rich profile protects mitochondrial membranes, modulates redox status and enhances cellular longevity, while Chaga delivers strong polyphenolic and melanin-based antioxidant influence. This pairing supports animals exposed to environmental toxins, chronic oxidative stress, age-related tissue degeneration or inflammatory cycles driven by metabolic strain. It is particularly relevant for senior animals and those undergoing prolonged medical treatment or rehabilitation.

> Synergistic pairings or triads of mushrooms can act across multiple physiological pathways, broadening the supportive effect and contributing to a full-spectrum, terrain-based Mycotherapy strategy.

4.12 Safety, Contraindications and Monitoring

Chaga is generally well tolerated across species when used in full-spectrum, fruiting-body extracts produced via Sub-critical water extraction. Its high antioxidant capacity and broad regulatory influence make it suitable for long-term support in chronic inflammatory, metabolic and oxidative conditions. Nonetheless, Chaga's unique biochemical profile, particularly its naturally elevated oxalate content, necessitates thoughtful clinical application. Safety in veterinary Mycotherapy always depends upon dose, extract quality, the physiological resilience of the patient and the surrounding pharmaceutical context.

Digestive tolerance and gastrointestinal sensitivity

Most animals tolerate Chaga without difficulty when it is introduced gradually. Mild digestive adjustments, such as soft stools or changes in appetite during the first week, are occasionally reported, especially in animals with highly sensitive gastrointestinal tracts. These effects reflect the mushroom's rich fibre matrix and polysaccharide profile and usually stabilise with careful titration. For animals with chronic enteropathies, slow onboarding and concurrent dietary stability are recommended to avoid misinterpretation of benign digestive transitions as adverse reactions.

Oxalate content and renal considerations

Chaga's natural oxalate concentration constitutes its most clinically significant safety consideration. Although SCWE extraction reduces the proportion of soluble oxalates compared with raw or ground Chaga, a measurable oxalate load remains. Animals with a history of calcium-oxalate uroliths, chronic kidney disease or metabolic conditions that predispose to crystallisation require conservative dosing and closer monitoring. Veterinary oversight is strongly recommended in cats, where renal sensitivity is more common.

Animals receiving medications that influence renal perfusion or electrolyte handling, such as diuretics or angiotensin-converting enzyme inhibitors, should be assessed with particular care. Monitoring hydration, urinalysis and renal parameters at baseline and periodically during supplementation helps ensure ongoing physiological safety.

Hepatic and metabolic caution in medically fragile animals

Chaga's influence on hepatic detoxification pathways, while beneficial in many contexts, requires careful interpretation in animals with severely compromised hepatobiliary function. Although preclinical evidence supports hepatoprotective properties, fragile animals may be less equipped to metabolise additional nutraceutical inputs. In such cases, lower doses, extended titration periods and routine biochemical monitoring are recommended. Similarly, animals with advanced metabolic disease, including those with tightly regulated diabetes mellitus, should be observed for changes in glycaemic control during the introduction period.

Interactions with pharmaceutical agents

Chaga's pharmacological actions are broadly supportive, yet several theoretical interactions warrant clinical attention. Its capacity to influence insulin sensitivity and glucose uptake suggests a potential additive effect when used alongside insulin or oral hypoglycaemic agents. Careful monitoring of glycaemic trends during the first two to three weeks is appropriate, particularly for animals with brittle diabetes or variable insulin responses.

Its mild antiplatelet properties have been described in preclinical models, although clinically significant effects are rare. Animals receiving anticoagulant or antiplatelet medications such as heparins or aspirin analogues should be monitored with additional caution, especially before procedures involving anaesthesia or tissue manipulation.

Chaga's immune-modulating actions, including enhancement of macrophage and natural killer cell activity, require prudence when combined with immunosuppressive therapies such as ciclosporin or corticosteroids. The mushroom tends to normalise rather than stimulate immune responses, yet individual responses may vary. Oncology patients receiving complex chemotherapy protocols may benefit from coordinated communication between clinicians to ensure supportive Mycotherapy aligns with pharmacological goals.

Pregnancy, lactation and paediatric use

Formal evidence regarding Chaga's safety in pregnancy or lactation is extremely limited. Although no concerning signals have emerged from traditional use or modern clinical observation, conservative practice recommends avoiding Chaga in pregnant or nursing animals unless the expected benefit clearly outweighs theoretical risks. Young animals generally tolerate Chaga well but should begin at lower doses to respect developmental variability in metabolic capacity.

Extraction quality and safety fidelity

Extraction method is a central determinant of Chaga's safety profile. Sub-critical water extraction preserves the mushroom's natural biochemical matrix while reducing oxalate concentration and eliminating solvent residues. Alcohol tinctures may concentrate undesirable compounds and introduce ethanol exposure, while myceliated grain products significantly dilute therapeutic constituents with starch. For medically fragile, elderly or polypharmacy patients, SCWE extracts provide the most predictable and physiologically aligned option.

Monitoring recommendations

Monitoring should be tailored to the patient's medical context and the intended therapeutic goal rather than applied uniformly. Clinicians may consider:

- assessment of stool quality, appetite and demeanour during the first week
- urinalysis and renal parameters in animals with renal sensitivity or oxalate history
- hepatic enzyme trends in patients receiving hepatically metabolised medications
- blood glucose review in diabetic animals
- evaluation of bruising or bleeding tendencies in those on anticoagulant or antiplatelet therapy
- documentation of vitality, coat condition and inflammatory indicators in senior animals

Thoughtful monitoring ensures that Chaga's supportive effects are realised safely and predictably, particularly in complex internal medicine or oncology cases.

4.13 Evidence Quality Commentary

Chaga occupies a distinctive position among medicinal mushrooms due to its exceptionally rich antioxidant profile and long historical use as a restorative agent. The contemporary evidence base is shaped by preclinical studies, translational research, in vitro oncology work and a growing body of practitioner observations in veterinary contexts. While formal clinical trials in companion animals remain limited, the consistency of mechanistic findings provides a strong rationale for its inclusion in integrative care.

Strength of mechanistic evidence

Mechanistic studies support Chaga's influence across multiple biological systems. Its polyphenols, melanin complexes, triterpenes and polysaccharides demonstrate antioxidant, anti-inflammatory, immunomodulatory and hepatoprotective effects in a range of experimental models. These findings are coherent and reproducible, emphasising regulation of nuclear factor kappa B signalling, attenuation of oxidative DNA damage, enhancement of glutathione-related pathways and stabilisation of cytokine activity. Such mechanistic alignment underpins Chaga's value in chronic inflammation, oxidative stress and metabolic dysregulation.

Translational and veterinary relevance

The translational step from preclinical research to veterinary application is supported by emerging evidence in canine and feline models, including studies exploring Chaga's influence on tumour biology, broad-spectrum antiviral activity and gastrointestinal–immune interactions. Although early, these studies align closely with the mechanistic signals described in rodent and cell-culture work. Practitioner experience further supports improvement in stamina, coat quality, digestive regularity and general resilience in senior or chronically inflamed animals. While anecdotal, such observations carry weight when they consistently mirror mechanistic expectations.

Limitations in species-specific clinical trials

As with most medicinal mushrooms, controlled clinical trials in companion animals remain sparse. This limitation is not unique to Chaga but reflects broader constraints in veterinary nutritional research. Consequently, Chaga's evidence profile relies heavily on mechanistic, preclinical and translational signals rather than robust randomised controlled trials. This does not diminish its therapeutic potential but highlights the need for careful interpretation and integration within evidence-informed practice. Its role should be understood as supportive and regulatory rather than curative or disease-specific.

Importance of extract fidelity in evidence translation

The majority of research supporting Chaga's actions is based on fruiting-body material or purified compounds, not myceliated grain products. Extracts lacking fibre, phenolic compounds or triterpene-rich fractions do not reflect the biochemical complexity underpinning published findings. SCWE preparations most closely align with the research base, particularly in their ability to retain polysaccharides, triterpenes, melanins, polyphenols and the native fibre matrix. This fidelity is essential if clinicians intend to rely on research-driven or mechanistic expectations.

Clinical interpretation

In clinical practice, Chaga should be regarded as a terrain-building agent. Its value lies in supporting antioxidant status, reducing inflammatory load, enhancing mucosal and hepatic resilience and improving recovery capacity. These benefits develop gradually and are most meaningful when incorporated into long-term integrative protocols. Chaga's evidence profile supports its use in senior vitality, chronic inflammatory disease, toxin exposure, gastrointestinal fragility and supportive oncology care, provided dosing is individualised and monitoring remains attentive.

4.14 Conclusion – Integrative Significance and Extraction Considerations

Chaga stands out within veterinary Mycotherapy as a uniquely potent source of antioxidant, anti-inflammatory and regulatory support. Its rich matrix of melanins, polyphenols, triterpenes, antioxidant peptides and polysaccharides gives rise to a broad spectrum of physiological effects that influence oxidative load, mucosal stability, immune balance, hepatic resilience and metabolic integrity. These actions develop gradually and contribute to a strengthened physiological terrain that better withstands chronic disease, environmental stressors and age-related decline.

The mushroom's value in veterinary medicine is not defined by acute symptomatic change but by cumulative stabilisation. Chaga supports systems that struggle under chronic inflammatory pressure, metabolic imbalance or environmental toxicity, making it particularly appropriate for senior animals, those with chronic dermatitis or gastrointestinal fragility, and patients undergoing long-term pharmaceutical therapy. In oncology contexts, its antioxidant and immunological actions complement conventional treatment without attempting to replace it. In metabolic and hepatic conditions, it provides reinforcement for tissues vulnerable to oxidative injury and impaired detoxification.

Extract fidelity is central to Chaga's therapeutic predictability. The biochemical complexity described throughout this monograph is preserved only when extraction methods retain both hydrophilic and lipophilic fractions as well as the structural fibre matrix that shapes gastrointestinal and immunological interactions. Sub-critical water extraction achieves this by producing a solvent-free, grain-free, whole-food extract with consistent constituent ratios. This fidelity is particularly important for veterinary patients with increased sensitivity, such as elderly animals, those with multi-systemic disease or individuals receiving polypharmacy. Products based on raw powder, alcohol tincture or grain-grown mycelium do not represent the same research-valid profile and may introduce oxalate or solvent-related concerns absent from SCWE preparations.

Used within a multimodal framework that includes nutritional management, pharmaceutical treatment when necessary and attentive monitoring, Chaga provides a stable, predictable and physiologically coherent contribution to veterinary care. Its enduring relevance arises from its capacity to reduce oxidative burden, restore mucosal and hepatic resilience, support immune balance and contribute meaningfully to long-term vitality. When applied judiciously, with appropriate patient selection and extract quality, Chaga remains one of the most valuable antioxidant-focused mushrooms in modern integrative veterinary practice.

> Chaga stands out within veterinary Mycotherapy as a uniquely potent source of antioxidant, anti-inflammatory and regulatory support.

Key sources (summary)

Babitskaya et al., 2002; Shashkina et al., 2006; Lee & Yun, 2011; Kim et al., 2005; Song & Park, 2013; Zhao et al., 2018; Park et al., 2004; Ma et al., 2013; Lu et al., 2011; Kim & Choi, 2016; Alhallaf et al., 2024; Choi & Kim, 2016; Jeong & Cho, 2010; Yoon & Kim, 2018; Memorial Sloan Kettering Cancer Center, 2024; Rizzo & Moore, 2022. **Full professional reference list available in the Master References section.**

> “Herbal medicine works by engaging the body's own intelligence – not replacing it.”
>
> *Dr Rob Silver, DVM, MS*

5

CORDYCEPS (Cordyceps militaris)

5.1 Introduction to Cordyceps – *The Vitality and Endurance Enhancer*

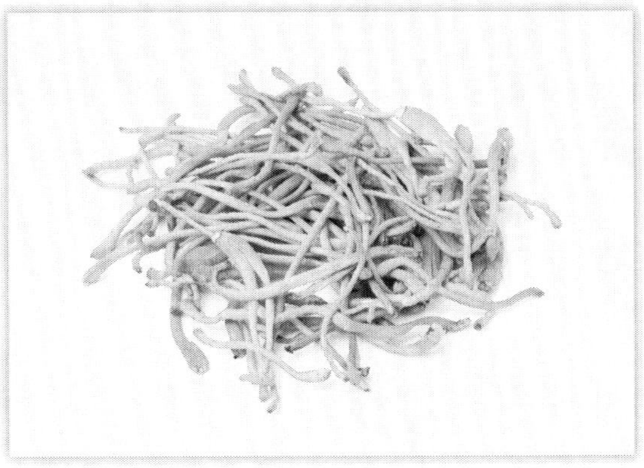

Cordyceps militaris occupies a distinctive place in veterinary Mycotherapy as a mushroom associated with stamina, recovery and adaptive resilience. Traditional East Asian medicine regarded Cordyceps as a restorative tonic for fatigue, respiratory weakness, sexual vitality and age-related decline. While the wild caterpillar fungus Ophiocordyceps sinensis was historically reserved for elite or royal use due to its scarcity, modern cultivation of C. militaris on plant-based substrates has made a consistent, standardisable fruiting-body source available for clinical and nutritional purposes.

In a veterinary context, Cordyceps is primarily considered when there is a need to reinforce cellular energy, improve recovery from exertion or chronic illness, and support respiratory and metabolic stability. Preclinical and translational research suggests that its nucleoside analogues and polysaccharides can influence adenosine triphosphate (ATP) production, mitochondrial efficiency, oxygen utilisation and antioxidant defence. These properties align with clinical goals in working dogs, performance animals, senior patients with fatigue, and animals recovering from systemic disease, oncology treatment or chronic inflammatory burden.

Cordyceps is also increasingly discussed in relation to immune modulation, respiratory function, hepatic and renal support, and metabolic balance. The mushroom's actions are not simply stimulating; rather, they fit the profile of a gentle adaptogen that helps normalise physiological responses to stress, demand and disease. As with other medicinal mushrooms, the bulk of research is preclinical or derived from human and rodent models, and direct veterinary trials remain limited. For this reason, Cordyceps is best positioned as an adjunctive, terrain-strengthening intervention within integrative veterinary practice rather than as a stand-alone therapeutic.

> Cordyceps militaris occupies a distinctive place in veterinary Mycotherapy as a mushroom associated with stamina, recovery and adaptive resilience.

5.2 Taxonomy, Cultivation and Extract Science

Cordyceps militaris is an ascomycete fungus within the family Cordycipitaceae. In nature it parasitises insect pupae and larvae, forming characteristic bright orange club-shaped fruiting bodies. For ethical, safety and standardisation reasons, modern medicinal use relies on controlled cultivation of C. militaris on plant-based substrates rather than wild insect hosts. This approach allows precise control of species identity, substrate composition and contamination risk, and it tends to yield higher and more reproducible levels of cordycepin than are typically seen in wild Ophiocordyceps sinensis.

From an extraction perspective, several important distinctions influence clinical relevance. Many commercial Cordyceps products are based on mycelium grown on grain, producing powders that contain a high proportion of substrate starch and relatively low levels of characteristic nucleosides, triterpenes and polysaccharides. Others use simple hot-water extraction, which captures water-soluble polysaccharides but may underrepresent more lipophilic constituents and does not preserve the original fibre matrix. Alcohol-based dual extracts introduce solvent residues and can skew the ratio of nucleosides to polysaccharides in ways that do not fully reflect the whole fruiting body.

Sub-critical water extraction (SCWE) offers a more comprehensive approach for veterinary use. By using pressurised water at controlled temperatures, SCWE is able to solubilise both hydrophilic and moderately lipophilic compounds without synthetic solvents. This process yields a full-spectrum extract that preserves beta-glucans, cordycepin, adenosine and related nucleosides, fungal sterols, polyphenols and the natural fibre that shapes gut–immune and metabolic interactions. For animals, especially those that are elderly, medically fragile or highly active, this whole-food profile provides a more physiologically coherent representation of Cordyceps than grain-grown mycelium or solvent-focused extracts.

In veterinary Mycotherapy, the choice of extract is therefore central to pharmacological predictability. Fruiting-body only, SCWE-derived preparations align more closely with the traditional and preclinical evidence base, avoid dilution with cereal starch and provide a stable, reproducible platform for long-term use in performance, senior-care and recovery protocols.

5.3 Bioactive Constituents and Mechanistic Relevance

The therapeutic profile of Cordyceps militaris arises from the interaction of several key classes of compounds, each of which contributes distinct but overlapping actions relevant to veterinary physiology.

Cordycepin (3′-deoxyadenosine) is the signature nucleoside analogue of Cordyceps. It structurally resembles adenosine but lacks a hydroxyl group on the ribose moiety, enabling it to interfere selectively with nucleic acid synthesis, cell-signalling pathways and inflammatory cascades. Preclinical research attributes to cordycepin a range of actions including modulation of adenosine receptors, inhibition of abnormal cell proliferation, induction of apoptosis in malignant cells, and down-regulation of inflammatory mediators such as nuclear factor kappa B (NF-kappa B), interleukin 6 (IL-6) and tumour necrosis factor alpha (TNF-alpha). These mechanisms underpin many of the proposed oncology, anti-inflammatory and anti-fatigue uses of Cordyceps.

Adenosine and related nucleosides support cardiovascular and respiratory physiology by influencing vasodilation, platelet function and oxygen utilisation. Through adenosine receptor interactions, these compounds can promote improved blood flow, modulate vascular tone and support myocardial and skeletal muscle oxygen delivery. In the context of performance and recovery, this contributes to smoother circulation, better tissue perfusion and reduced perception of fatigue.

Polysaccharides, including beta-glucans and heteropolysaccharides, exert classical mushroom-derived immunomodulatory effects. They interact with pattern-recognition receptors such as Dectin-1 and Toll-like receptors on macrophages and dendritic cells, enhancing immune surveillance while promoting regulatory cytokine patterns rather than indiscriminate immune stimulation. These polysaccharides also have prebiotic potential in the gut, supporting microbial diversity and short-chain fatty acid production.

Additional bioactive components include **ergosterol and other sterols**, small peptides, trace minerals and antioxidant compounds that collectively support endogenous antioxidant enzyme systems such as superoxide dismutase, catalase and glutathione peroxidase. These pathways are especially relevant in animals exposed to sustained exercise, chronic inflammatory conditions or age-related oxidative accumulation.

The overall clinical relevance of these constituents lies not in any single molecule but in their combined impact on energy metabolism, immune competence, inflammatory balance and organ resilience. In veterinary practice this translates into potential benefits for animals requiring enhanced endurance, improved recovery, immune support, respiratory steadiness or longer-term metabolic stability.

5.4 Energy Metabolism, Mitochondrial Function and Performance Physiology

> Cordyceps is most widely recognised for its influence on energy metabolism and physical performance.

Cordyceps is most widely recognised for its influence on energy metabolism and physical performance. This reputation is supported by preclinical and human data showing improvements in exercise capacity, delayed onset of fatigue and more efficient utilisation of oxygen during exertion. For veterinary patients, these mechanisms are of particular interest in working dogs, sporting animals, agility dogs, performance horses and companion animals that experience chronic fatigue or reduced vitality.

At the cellular level, cordycepin and adenosine appear to enhance mitochondrial ATP generation by supporting oxidative phosphorylation and improving electron transport chain efficiency. This improved mitochondrial function reduces reliance on anaerobic glycolysis during exertion, which in turn moderates lactic-acid accumulation and associated muscle fatigue. Animal models have demonstrated extended swimming and running times, reduced markers of exercise-induced oxidative damage, and faster restoration of baseline energy parameters following exertion when Cordyceps is administered.

In addition to mitochondrial support, Cordyceps influences oxygen delivery by promoting mild vasodilation and improving microcirculatory flow. This ensures that oxygen and nutrients are more effectively transported to active muscle, cardiac tissue and vital organs during activity or recovery. For working and performance animals, this combination of improved energy production and enhanced circulatory efficiency may manifest clinically as greater stamina, more rapid post-exercise recovery, and a smoother, less laboured pattern of exertion.

Senior animals and those recovering from illness or prolonged convalescence also stand to benefit from these mechanisms. In such cases, Cordyceps is less about pushing performance and more about helping restore baseline vitality and tolerance for normal daily activity. Improvements are typically gradual and unfold over several weeks, aligning with the cumulative nature of Mycotherapy. In veterinary practice, it is important to introduce Cordyceps as part of a comprehensive approach that also addresses nutrition, conditioning, pain management and any underlying disease processes.

5.5 Immune and Inflammatory Modulation

Although Cordyceps is best known for its impact on stamina and energy, its immunological profile is equally relevant to veterinary medicine. Polysaccharides and cordycepin together shape immune function across both innate and adaptive arms, with a tendency towards regulatory balance rather than simple stimulation.

Cordyceps polysaccharides engage pattern-recognition receptors on macrophages, neutrophils and dendritic cells, promoting enhanced phagocytic activity, improved antigen presentation and more efficient coordination between innate and adaptive immunity. Experimental models show increased natural killer cell activity and modulation of T-helper cell function, with evidence of more balanced Th1 and Th2 responses and support for regulatory T-cell stability. For animals experiencing recurrent infections, immune exhaustion or age-related decline in immune vigilance, these actions provide a plausible mechanism for improved immune resilience.

> Although Cordyceps is best known for its impact on stamina and energy, its immunological profile is equally relevant to veterinary medicine.

Cordycepin contributes a distinct anti-inflammatory dimension. By inhibiting NF-kappa B activation and reducing transcription of pro-inflammatory cytokines such as IL-6 and TNF-alpha, cordycepin helps dampen chronic inflammatory signalling across multiple tissues. Preclinical studies have demonstrated reductions in airway inflammation, attenuation of inflammatory markers in joint and soft-tissue models, and protection of tissues from oxidative–inflammatory injury. These effects are of potential value in animals with chronic respiratory sensitivities, low-grade musculoskeletal inflammation or systemic inflammatory burden secondary to metabolic or neoplastic disease.

From a clinical standpoint, this combination of immune support and inflammatory modulation suggests a role for Cordyceps in animals recovering from infection, undergoing vaccination, living with chronic inflammatory conditions or experiencing immune compromise due to age or oncology treatment. At the same time, caution is warranted in animals with autoimmune disease or those receiving targeted immunosuppressive therapy, as any agent that shapes immune tone must be integrated with clear therapeutic intent and monitoring. In most cases, Cordyceps is best employed at moderate doses as a background regulator rather than as an aggressive immunological intervention.

5.6 Respiratory and Cardiovascular Support

The traditional association of Cordyceps with lung and 'Kidney' support in East Asian medicine translates in modern terms to a combined influence on respiratory and cardiovascular physiology. For veterinary patients, this is particularly relevant in animals with reduced exercise tolerance, mild chronic bronchial irritation, age-related cardiopulmonary stiffness or high oxygen demand due to performance work.

Respiratorily, Cordyceps appears to exert both anti-inflammatory and functional effects. Experimental models indicate that cordycepin and related compounds can reduce inflammatory cell infiltration in airway tissue, suppress production of pro-inflammatory cytokines within the respiratory mucosa, and support a less reactive bronchial environment. Some studies suggest mild bronchodilatory influence, likely mediated through adenosine receptor interactions and modulation of smooth-muscle tone. These mechanisms provide a rationale for considering Cordyceps as part of integrative support for animals with low-grade chronic bronchitis, exercise-associated airway sensitivity or environmental irritant exposure, always alongside appropriate diagnostics and conventional care.

Cardiovascularly, adenosine and other nucleosides in Cordyceps support vasodilation and improved endothelial responsiveness, which can help optimise tissue perfusion and oxygen delivery. Preclinical work has reported modest improvements in lipid handling and endothelial function, suggesting potential benefit for animals with emerging metabolic strain or early vascular compromise. For geriatric patients, these circulatory effects may contribute to a more even distribution of blood flow, reduced sensation of exertional fatigue and better tolerance of moderate exercise.

In theory, Cordyceps may also influence platelet function and blood pressure through its adenosine-related actions, although clinically significant hypotension or bleeding effects are rarely reported at typical nutritional doses. Nonetheless, animals receiving antihypertensive medication, anticoagulants or antiplatelet drugs should be monitored carefully when Cordyceps is introduced, particularly in the perioperative period or where cardiac function is already fragile.

Overall, Cordyceps offers gentle yet meaningful cardiopulmonary support by improving oxygen uptake, circulation and inflammatory stability across the heart–lung axis. For veterinarians, its role is best conceived as a long-term adjunct that enhances physiological reserve and exercise tolerance rather than as a direct substitute for bronchodilators, cardiac medication or disease-specific interventions.

5.7 Gastrointestinal, Microbiome and Gut–Liver Axis Support

Cordyceps exerts a stabilising influence on gastrointestinal health through a combination of metabolic, immunological and antioxidant mechanisms that collectively support the digestive terrain. Although traditionally associated with vitality and respiratory resilience, emerging research highlights its relevance to gastrointestinal and gut–liver dynamics due to its polysaccharides, nucleosides and antioxidant compounds that act on mucosal integrity, immune tone and microbial ecology. Preclinical studies, including zebrafish colitis models and rodent models of gastrointestinal inflammation, demonstrate that Cordyceps polysaccharides can reduce mucosal ulceration, normalise inflammatory signalling and promote epithelial repair. These findings offer translational relevance for animals with chronic enteropathy, stress-sensitive digestion or gastrointestinal irritation associated with chronic medication use.

Within the gut–immune interface, Cordyceps appears to modulate both innate and adaptive responses by influencing macrophage activity and cytokine expression. This regulatory activity may help reduce inappropriate inflammatory escalation while maintaining adequate immune vigilance. It also contributes to microbial balance by providing prebiotic substrates that favour beneficial bacterial species while moderating dysbiosis. Senior animals and individuals recovering from prolonged illness often show improved stool quality, steadier appetite and enhanced digestive resilience when Cordyceps is integrated gradually into their care. In animals with combined gastrointestinal and hepatic strain, the mushroom's antioxidant compounds help reduce hepatic oxidative load, supporting more predictable detoxification and reducing the physiological stress imposed by chronic inflammation or long-term pharmaceutical use.

Cordyceps therefore contributes to gastrointestinal stability not through strong symptomatic shifts but through the gradual recalibration of mucosal integrity, immune behaviour and microbial balance. Its actions are cumulative rather than immediate, and its value is most clearly seen when used consistently as part of broader gastrointestinal and metabolic support strategies in veterinary practice.

5.8 Liver, Kidney and Detoxification Support

Cordyceps has long been regarded as a restorative mushroom for liver and kidney function, a perspective now supported by growing translational research demonstrating protective effects on hepatocytes, renal tubules and metabolic detoxification pathways. Its nucleosides, polysaccharides and antioxidant compounds contribute to reduced oxidative stress within hepatic and renal tissues, improved enzymatic defence mechanisms and enhanced resilience against metabolic or medication-induced injury. Human studies involving chronic hepatitis B and renal insufficiency provide evidence for reductions in hepatic inflammation, improvements in liver enzyme profiles and stabilisation of renal biomarkers following Cordyceps supplementation. Although species-specific veterinary trials are limited, these observations offer plausible relevance to dogs and cats experiencing hepatocellular strain, chemotherapy-associated toxicity or chronic metabolic burden.

> Cordyceps has long been regarded as a restorative mushroom for liver and kidney function.

Within hepatic physiology, Cordyceps appears to influence both mitochondrial integrity and phase II detoxification pathways, supporting glutathione turnover and reducing lipid peroxidation. This may be particularly meaningful in animals on long-term pharmaceuticals or those recovering from toxin exposure or metabolic illness. In the kidney, Cordyceps may help enhance renal perfusion, reduce oxidative injury and support filtration efficiency through actions that include modulation of inflammatory mediators and stabilisation of tubular function. These mechanisms provide a rationale for its adjunctive use in early chronic kidney disease, medication-associated renal stress or convalescence after systemic illness, provided that dosing is conservative and monitoring is maintained.

The interconnectedness of hepatic and renal systems means that Cordyceps often exerts its strongest influence when integrated into multimodal plans aimed at reducing metabolic strain, improving oxidative defence and supporting tissue recovery. Its actions unfold steadily over weeks and complement dietary and pharmaceutical strategies rather than competing with them. While not a primary treatment for organ-specific disease, Cordyceps provides a meaningful regulatory foundation that helps maintain physiological stability, particularly in senior or medically complex animals.

5.9 Oncology and Adjunctive Cancer Support

Cordyceps has become increasingly relevant in integrative oncology due to its combined influence on immune surveillance, mitochondrial function, cellular metabolism and treatment tolerance. Much of the research underpinning its oncology relevance is preclinical, yet consistent mechanistic patterns provide a legitimate rationale for supportive use in veterinary cancer care when applied under professional oversight. Cordycepin and related nucleoside analogues have demonstrated the capacity to induce apoptosis, inhibit tumour cell proliferation and modulate signalling pathways involved in cancer progression, including nuclear factor kappa B, PI3K–AKT and MAPK pathways. Polysaccharides contribute complementary activity by enhancing macrophage and natural killer cell function and supporting T-cell responsiveness, thereby strengthening immune recognition of abnormal cells.

In oncology settings, Cordyceps may help counteract treatment-related fatigue by improving mitochondrial ATP production and supporting more efficient oxygen utilisation. This effect is often reported anecdotally by veterinarians and pet owners as improved stamina, brighter demeanour and better recovery between chemotherapy sessions. Preclinical studies suggest that Cordyceps may also help maintain white blood cell counts during chemotherapeutic protocols, though this evidence is not yet sufficiently mature to guide specific dosing recommendations. Its antioxidant activity further contributes to tissue resilience by reducing oxidative stress associated with chronic malignancy and pharmaceutical intervention.

Clinical caution is warranted, particularly in hormone-sensitive cancers or haematological malignancies, where immune or metabolic modulation could theoretically aggravate disease behaviour. For solid tumours managed with chemotherapy or radiation, Cordyceps is generally used as an adjunct to improve vitality, appetite and immune stability rather than as a direct anti-cancer agent. Its most meaningful role lies in enhancing quality of life, supporting immune competence and providing metabolic reinforcement during prolonged cancer management. When integrated thoughtfully alongside veterinary supervision, Cordyceps offers a supportive, low-risk contribution to broader oncology protocols, strengthening the physiological terrain in which conventional therapies operate.

5.10 Veterinary Pharmacology and Drug Interactions

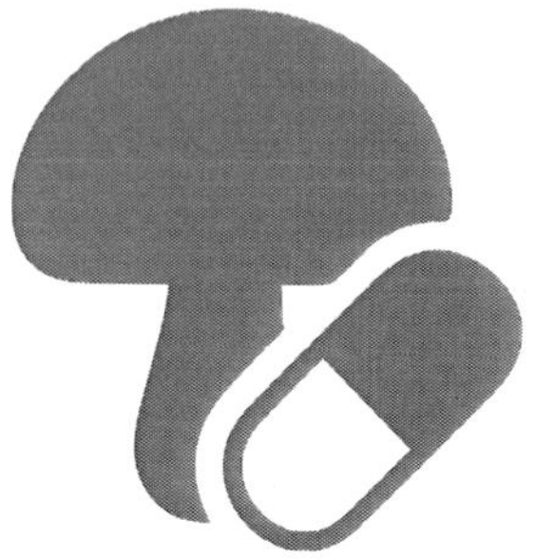

Cordyceps exhibits a pharmacological profile that is both broad in its physiological reach and generally predictable in its clinical behaviour when high-quality fruiting-body preparations are used. Its primary bioactive compounds, including cordycepin, adenosine, polysaccharides, sterols and antioxidant constituents, influence mitochondrial activity, immune regulation, inflammatory signalling, vascular tone and metabolic stability. These actions contribute to its therapeutic versatility, but they also introduce considerations when animals are receiving pharmaceuticals with narrow therapeutic indices or significant immunological or metabolic effects. The following domains outline the areas most relevant to veterinary practice, with emphasis on mechanisms that carry clinically meaningful implications.

Influence on hepatic and renal drug metabolism

Cordyceps affects several metabolic pathways that are relevant to the clearance and distribution of pharmaceuticals. Cordycepin and related nucleosides interact with enzymes involved in oxidative metabolism, and Cordyceps polysaccharides may modulate pathways associated with hepatic detoxification, including aspects of the cytochrome P450 system. Although veterinary-specific pharmacokinetic trials are limited, these mechanisms suggest a theoretical potential for altered metabolism of drugs processed heavily through hepatic pathways, particularly phenobarbital, certain chemotherapeutics and long-term corticosteroids. In most cases the effect appears to be stabilising rather than disruptive, but animals with pre-existing hepatic compromise should undergo periodic monitoring during the first weeks of supplementation.

Renal considerations are generally favourable. Some human and preclinical studies suggest that Cordyceps may support renal perfusion and reduce oxidative injury within the kidneys. This may benefit animals receiving nephrotoxic medication, yet it also requires cautious integration in those with reduced renal reserve, particularly if diuretics, angiotensin-modulating drugs or renal-protective nutraceuticals are being used concurrently. Slow titration and monitoring of hydration status and renal parameters are recommended in such cases.

Interaction with glucose regulation and endocrine medications

Cordyceps has demonstrated mild but measurable effects on glucose metabolism in preclinical models, including improvements in insulin sensitivity and modulation of hepatic glucose handling. While these actions are generally regulatory, they raise theoretical considerations when used alongside insulin or oral hypoglycaemic drugs in diabetic animals. Close observation during the initial two to three weeks of supplementation helps identify any additive glucose-lowering effects, although such interactions appear uncommon and typically subtle. Cordyceps' broader influence on adrenal balance and metabolic stress may also intersect with endocrine medications, yet these effects tend to reflect systemic support rather than direct hormonal modulation.

Interaction with immunomodulatory and chemotherapeutic agents

Cordyceps exerts a bidirectional regulatory influence on innate and adaptive immune pathways, enhancing macrophage, T-cell and natural killer cell activity while moderating excessive pro-inflammatory signalling. This dual behaviour can complement recovery from infection or chronic illness but requires thoughtful application when animals are receiving immunosuppressive drugs such as ciclosporin, corticosteroids or oclacitinib. In most cases Cordyceps' influence does not oppose pharmaceutical immunosuppression but may narrow the margin between intended therapeutic effects and immune-activation thresholds in sensitive individuals. Case-by-case assessment and gradual introduction are therefore recommended.

In oncology contexts, Cordyceps may provide metabolic and immune reinforcement that supports tolerance to chemotherapy or radiation. Preclinical research suggests potential synergistic benefits when cordycepin is combined with certain chemotherapeutic agents, particularly via modulation of apoptosis pathways and reduced oxidative stress. While promising, these findings require careful clinical interpretation and should always be coordinated with the attending oncologist to ensure alignment with treatment goals.

Cardiovascular and anticoagulant considerations

Cordyceps nucleosides contribute to mild vasodilatory activity, which may enhance circulation and tissue oxygenation. This action is usually advantageous but may interact with antihypertensive or vasodilatory medications, particularly in senior animals with cardiovascular instability. Preclinical data also indicate that Cordyceps may exhibit modest antiplatelet properties by reducing platelet aggregation, although clinically significant bleeding events have not been documented in veterinary practice. Nonetheless, animals receiving anticoagulants such as aspirin analogues, heparins or other antiplatelet agents should be monitored conservatively, particularly before surgical or dental procedures.

Advantages of SCWE extracts for predictable pharmacology

Extraction fidelity plays a critical role in the pharmacological reliability of Cordyceps. SCWE extracts retain the full spectrum of bioactive nucleosides, polysaccharides, peptides and antioxidant compounds in their natural ratios, providing predictable clinical behaviour and avoiding the variability associated with alcohol tinctures or myceliated grain powders. Alcohol-based extracts may concentrate certain fractions while excluding fibre-bound constituents, creating inconsistent pharmacokinetics. Myceliated grain products lack meaningful levels of cordycepin, contain a high proportion of starch and do not reflect the biochemical profile used in much of the scientific literature. For veterinary patients receiving pharmaceuticals with narrow therapeutic indices, the consistency of SCWE full-spectrum extracts offers a significantly safer and more predictable option.

Summary of pharmacological interaction considerations

Cordyceps possesses a broad but generally favourable interaction profile when integrated thoughtfully into veterinary treatment plans. Its influence on hepatic and renal pathways, immune responsiveness, vascular tone and endocrine resilience introduces considerations in animals receiving complex medication regimes, yet most interactions are regulatory rather than disruptive. With gradual dosage escalation, appropriate monitoring and preference for SCWE fruiting-body extracts, Cordyceps can be incorporated safely alongside conventional therapies to support energy metabolism, tissue resilience, immune competence and overall recovery in companion animals.

5.11 Clinical Application in Veterinary Practice

Cordyceps occupies a distinctive therapeutic niche within veterinary Mycotherapy because it influences several foundational systems simultaneously: mitochondrial energy metabolism, respiratory and circulatory efficiency, immune balance, metabolic stability and recovery from physiological stress. Its benefits develop gradually and depend on consistent administration, reflecting its role as a regulator rather than an acute symptomatic agent. For clinicians, its value lies in its capacity to restore physiological resilience in animals experiencing fatigue, chronic inflammation, metabolic dysregulation or long-term convalescence.

> Cordyceps occupies a distinctive therapeutic niche within veterinary Mycotherapy

Application in active, working and performance animals

Cordyceps is particularly suited to animals with sustained activity demands. Its nucleosides support ATP synthesis, oxygen utilisation and mitochondrial efficiency, creating a stable metabolic foundation for exertion and recovery. Dogs engaged in agility, sporting or working roles may display improvements in stamina, reduced post-exertional fatigue and quicker recovery trajectories. Although veterinary trials are limited, these observations align with preclinical findings in mammalian models and longstanding traditional use. Its cumulative effects are most evident when used continuously during training cycles or long-term conditioning plans.

Support in convalescence and chronic fatigue

Animals recovering from illness, surgery or chronic inflammatory disease often experience reduced vitality, impaired metabolic stability and diminished resilience. Cordyceps may help restore energy balance by supporting mitochondrial function and moderating the inflammatory burden that contributes to fatigue. Clinicians frequently report that animals appear more engaged, brighter and physically steadier after several weeks of supplementation. These outcomes are particularly relevant in senior animals whose metabolic reserves are diminished or whose recovery is hindered by low-grade systemic inflammation.

Respiratory and cardio-respiratory applications

Cordyceps has a long traditional association with respiratory support, and modern preclinical data suggest mild bronchodilatory, anti-inflammatory and circulation-enhancing effects. These properties may provide adjunctive benefit in animals with chronic cough, mild bronchial irritation, reduced exercise tolerance or age-related respiratory decline. In cardio-respiratory overlap cases, such as senior dogs with sluggish circulation and intermittent respiratory stiffness, Cordyceps may contribute to improved tissue oxygenation and comfort. It should not replace pharmacological management for significant respiratory disease but acts as a supportive background therapy.

Immune modulation in chronic illness

Cordyceps' immune effects are regulatory rather than stimulatory, supporting both innate and adaptive pathways without provoking excessive immune activation. This makes it suitable for animals with chronic infections, immunosenescence, post-viral recovery or chronic inflammatory disease. In these contexts, immune balance is often disrupted by prolonged stress, oxidative burden and metabolic strain. Cordyceps may help re-establish a more stable immunological environment, improving resilience while reducing the inflammatory noise that contributes to systemic deterioration. Clinical improvements are gradual, reflecting the time required for immune recalibration.

Adjunctive support in oncology care

Cordyceps is frequently integrated into supportive oncology plans due to its potential to bolster mitochondrial efficiency, improve stamina, enhance immune surveillance and moderate inflammation. Preclinical evidence suggests cordycepin may influence apoptosis pathways, reduce oxidative DNA damage and support treatment tolerance during chemotherapy or radiation. In clinical practice, improved appetite, energy and comfort are among the most consistently observed effects. These benefits complement, rather than replace, conventional oncology interventions and should always be coordinated with veterinary oversight to ensure alignment with therapeutic goals.

Role in senior wellness and healthy ageing

Ageing animals commonly experience reduced energy, impaired endurance, diminished immune function and fluctuating metabolic stability. Cordyceps addresses several of these domains simultaneously through its effects on mitochondrial health, circulation, oxidative stress and immune balance. Senior dogs and cats may show subtle but meaningful improvements in vitality, mobility, coat quality and day-to-day engagement. As with other mushrooms, benefits unfold progressively and are dependent on consistent long-term administration.

Integration with other functional mushrooms

Cordyceps is a highly complementary species in veterinary Mycotherapy due to its influence on mitochondrial energy production, oxygen utilisation, adrenal steadiness and metabolic recovery. It integrates well with mushrooms that modulate immune patterns, support neurotrophic health, buffer oxidative stress or stabilise inflammatory cascades. The following pairings represent the most relevant clinical synergies in companion and performance animals.

- **With Reishi** - Cordyceps and Reishi form a balanced adaptogenic pairing that supports adrenal resilience, hepatic steadiness and allergy modulation. Reishi's triterpenoids influence mast-cell behaviour, autonomic tone and inflammatory responses, while Cordyceps enhances mitochondrial ATP production and oxygen utilisation. This combination is particularly helpful for animals with chronic fatigue, mild hepatic compromise, stress-exacerbated allergies or HPA-axis dysregulation. In working and performance animals, the duo supports steady energy output without overstimulation.
- **With Turkey Tail** - Turkey Tail enhances Cordyceps' capacity to support immune resilience, especially in chronic disease or oncology settings. Cordyceps contributes metabolic stability and improved oxygenation, helping maintain stamina and recovery during periods of systemic strain, while Turkey Tail strengthens immune surveillance and balanced β-glucan-driven activity. This pairing is useful for animals undergoing integrative cancer care, chronic infections or age-related immune decline, where both stamina and immune modulation are required.
- **With Chaga** - Chaga adds a potent antioxidant and hepatic-protective dimension to Cordyceps' mitochondrial and metabolic influence. While Cordyceps improves respiratory efficiency and endurance, Chaga buffers oxidative stress and supports gastrointestinal and

hepatic tissues. Together, they benefit performance animals, senior animals with reduced stamina, and those recovering from chronic inflammatory or metabolic challenges. The combination also stabilises oxidative burden in animals exposed to environmental toxins or high physical workload.

- **With Maitake** - Cordyceps and Maitake complement each other in cases involving metabolic fragility, chronic inflammation or oncology support. Maitake's influence on insulin signalling, lipid regulation and NK-cell activity integrates well with Cordyceps' role in enhancing oxygenation, mitochondrial performance and recovery capacity. This synergy supports overweight animals, endocrine-vulnerable individuals, and those undergoing long-term immune or metabolic stress. It is also relevant for chronic inflammatory presentations where metabolic and immune pathways intersect.
- **With Lion's Mane** - This pairing merges Cordyceps' metabolic and mitochondrial stability with Lion's Mane's neurotrophic and neuroprotective effects. The combination supports neural recovery, proprioceptive steadiness, stamina and cognitive vitality, particularly in older animals or those recovering from neurological challenges. Lion's Mane enhances gut–brain axis function and nerve regeneration, while Cordyceps improves cellular energy availability, enabling more efficient repair and functional recovery.
- **With Golden Oyster** - Cordyceps and Golden Oyster create a high-value mitochondrial and metabolic synergy. Golden Oyster's ergothioneine-rich profile protects mitochondrial membranes, stabilises redox processes and supports long-term cellular resilience. Cordyceps contributes ATP generation, oxygen utilisation and metabolic output. Together, they support endurance, exercise recovery, healthy ageing and resilience during chronic disease or environmental stress. This pairing is particularly relevant for performance animals, senior animals and those requiring long-term cytoprotective and metabolic support.

> Synergistic pairings or triads of mushrooms can act across multiple physiological pathways, broadening the supportive effect and contributing to a full-spectrum, terrain-based Mycotherapy strategy.

5.12 Safety, Contraindications and Monitoring

Cordyceps is widely recognised for its favourable safety profile across species, particularly when high-quality fruiting-body SCWE extracts are used. It is generally well tolerated, even in senior or medically compromised animals, yet its broad physiological activity requires thoughtful integration, dose individualisation and periodic monitoring in certain clinical contexts.

General tolerability and digestive sensitivity

Most animals tolerate Cordyceps without difficulty when introduced gradually. The most common transient response is mild gastrointestinal sensitivity, particularly soft stools or temporary appetite fluctuation during the initial titration period. These effects typically resolve within a few days and are uncommon with SCWE extracts, which preserve natural fibre and polysaccharide ratios without the irritant potential associated with alcohol tinctures or grain-grown mycelium powders.

Considerations in immune-mediated disease

Cordyceps modulates immune function through a balanced influence on macrophage activity, T-cell signalling and cytokine pathways. Although its effects are regulatory, caution is appropriate in animals with active autoimmune disease or those requiring strict pharmacological immunosuppression. In such cases, Cordyceps should be introduced conservatively and only under veterinary supervision, with clear monitoring for shifts in clinical status. Most well-controlled immune-mediated cases tolerate Cordyceps without issue, but individual responses vary and require case-specific evaluation.

Endocrine and metabolic considerations

Preclinical studies demonstrate mild improvements in glucose regulation, insulin sensitivity and lipid metabolism. For diabetic animals receiving insulin or oral hypoglycaemic agents, the possibility of additive glucose-lowering effects warrants early monitoring during the first two to three weeks of introduction. In animals with endocrine instability, particularly adrenal or thyroid dysregulation, Cordyceps' adaptogenic effects may support systemic balance, yet should not replace conventional management.

Hepatic, renal and detoxification considerations

Cordyceps offers hepatoprotective and reno-protective benefits in several preclinical and human studies, yet medically fragile animals require conservative integration. Those with advanced hepatic insufficiency, chronic kidney disease or concurrent nephrotoxic medication use should be monitored periodically for changes in liver and renal parameters. SCWE extracts provide a safer profile than raw powders or tinctures due to predictable constituent ratios and fibre retention, but careful titration remains appropriate in animals with reduced metabolic reserve.

Cardiovascular and anticoagulant considerations

Cordyceps' mild vasodilatory and antiplatelet activities, while generally advantageous, require attention in animals receiving antihypertensives or anticoagulants. Although clinically significant bleeding events are exceedingly rare, planned surgical or dental procedures may warrant a temporary dose reduction or short withdrawal period. Cardiovascularly fragile animals may also benefit from slower dose escalation to avoid excessive circulatory shifts.

Hormone-sensitive neoplasia

Due to its influence on metabolic and immunological pathways, cautious use is advised in hormone-sensitive cancers or cases where immune suppression is therapeutically essential. No direct pro-hormonal action has been demonstrated for Cordyceps, yet theoretical concerns remain due to limited species-specific research. Oncology oversight is recommended when integrating Cordyceps into complex cancer cases.

Extraction quality and safety implications

Extraction methodology strongly influences safety and clinical predictability. SCWE fruiting-body extracts retain cordycepin, adenosine, β-glucans, peptides and fibre in ratios consistent with published research, offering superior tolerability compared to tinctures or myceliated-grain powders. Alcohol tinctures may pose metabolic strain and exclude key fibre-bound compounds, while grain-grown mycelium products dilute active constituents with starch and lack therapeutic nucleosides.

Monitoring recommendations

The following monitoring principles apply during Cordyceps integration, particularly in chronic disease or polypharmacy scenarios:

- review stool quality, appetite and behaviour during the first 7–10 days
- monitor glucose levels closely in diabetic animals for 2–3 weeks
- assess renal and hepatic markers periodically in senior or metabolically fragile animals
- evaluate stamina, recovery, respiratory comfort and quality-of-life indicators in performance or convalescent animals
- maintain communication between practitioners when used alongside oncology or internal medicine protocols

Cordyceps' safety profile is excellent when applied with appropriate clinical judgement. With careful titration, high-quality SCWE extracts and meaningful monitoring, it can be integrated smoothly into a wide range of veterinary care plans, supporting energy metabolism, immune resilience and recovery with a low risk of adverse effects.

> From the evidence presented, Cordyceps contains bioactive compounds linked to mitochondrial and antioxidant pathways, and when paired with natural honey – rich in polyphenols and prebiotic sugars – the combination may help support cellular resilience, energy steadiness and digestive health in animals.

5.13 Evidence Quality Commentary

The evidence base for Cordyceps militaris aligns closely with the pattern observed in other functional mushrooms used in veterinary Mycotherapy: strong mechanistic grounding, moderate translational relevance and still-emerging species-specific clinical validation. Its physiological actions have been repeatedly demonstrated across laboratory, rodent and human studies, particularly in relation to mitochondrial efficiency, ATP production, oxygen utilisation, immune modulation and reductions in inflammatory signalling. These domains show high internal consistency, with cordycepin, adenosine analogues, β-glucans and sterols identified as the principal drivers of these effects. Such mechanistic reproducibility across multiple research platforms provides a compelling foundation for application in companion animals, even in the absence of extensive canine or feline clinical trials.

Translational evidence suggests meaningful potential in performance enhancement, fatigue reduction, recovery from exertion and metabolic stability. Improvements in VO2 max, lactic-acid handling and mitochondrial enzyme activity observed in controlled human and animal models resonate with the anecdotal improvements reported by integrative veterinarians working with working dogs, senior pets and convalescent animals. Immune-modulating activity is similarly well supported, with consistent documentation of enhanced macrophage function, improved T-cell responsiveness and increased natural killer cell activity. The reduction of key inflammatory mediators such as interleukin 6, tumour necrosis factor alpha and cyclo-oxygenase 2 reinforces Cordyceps' relevance in chronic inflammatory conditions, metabolic-inflammatory overlap and tissue recovery following stress or illness.

Limitations in the evidence arise primarily from heterogeneity in extract types and the predominance of studies using isolated compounds or mycelial products rather than whole fruiting-body preparations. This variability underscores the importance of extraction fidelity in veterinary practice, as differences in constituent balance directly influence potency, tolerability and clinical predictability. SCWE full-spectrum extracts provide a closer match to the biochemical complexity described in the scientific literature, retaining both nucleosides and fibre-bound polysaccharides essential to Cordyceps' regulatory profile.

Taken as a whole, the available evidence positions Cordyceps militaris as a scientifically grounded and low-risk adjunct with particular relevance to metabolic resilience, performance support, chronic inflammation and recovery from illness or physiological strain. While further veterinary-specific research is needed, the convergence of mechanistic data, translational studies and growing practitioner experience provides a reliable foundation for its use within integrative veterinary care.

> Cordyceps has been shown in animal studies to enhance mitochondrial function and improve cellular oxygen handling – mechanisms that may help support stamina, recovery and overall physiological resilience in animals.

* * *

CORDYCEPS (CORDYCEPS MILITARIS) – Evidence Quality Commentary Table

This spectrum of evidence is summarised in the following table:

Domain	Evidence Strength	Primary Evidence Type
Mitochondrial support and cellular energetics	Moderate to high	Preclinical metabolic and endurance models; mechanistic pathways
Exercise tolerance and fatigue resistance	Moderate	Preclinical and translational human studies
Respiratory and oxygen–utilisation support	Moderate	Preclinical respiratory models; extrapolated human endurance data
Immunomodulation	Moderate	Preclinical immune–signalling studies; β–glucan and cordycepin pathways
Anti–inflammatory and antioxidant activity	Moderate	Preclinical cytokine–modulation and oxidative–stress studies
Endocrine and stress–response regulation	Emerging to moderate	Preclinical adrenal–axis and stress–response models
Metabolic regulation (lipids and glucose)	Emerging	Preclinical metabolic–syndrome and glycaemic–control models
Hepatic and renal support	Emerging	Preclinical organ–protective studies
Reproductive and libido effects	Emerging	Preclinical hormonal and reproductive studies
Antimicrobial and antiparasitic activity	Emerging	In vitro studies; limited in vivo findings
Oncology adjunct use	Emerging	Mechanistic insights; early preclinical evidence; practitioner interest
Clinical veterinary trials	Limited	Minimal formal veterinary trials; translational rationale only

Cordyceps is defined by its influence on cellular energetics, mitochondrial resilience and oxygen utilisation. Compounds such as **cordycepin**, **adenosine derivatives** and **polysaccharides** support ATP dynamics, enhance mitochondrial efficiency and modulate respiratory pathways involved in endurance and fatigue resistance. These properties make Cordyceps of particular interest in animals experiencing reduced stamina, convalescence, age–related metabolic decline or chronic conditions characterised by low vitality.

Its immunomodulatory and anti–inflammatory properties add broader utility, with preclinical studies demonstrating modulation of cytokine profiles, enhancement of macrophage and NK–cell activity and attenuation of oxidative stress. These effects contribute to steadier immune performance and may assist animals recovering from chronic infections or immune imbalance. Although early, there is emerging interest in its potential adjunctive role in oncology, where mitochondrial support, improved energy utilisation and moderated inflammatory signalling may influence quality of life and treatment tolerance.

Cordyceps also shows emerging effects on endocrine balance and stress–response pathways, particularly through influences on adrenal signalling and metabolic homeostasis. These findings, while preliminary, offer a rationale for its use in animals with chronic stress, metabolic irregularities or age–related endocrine shift.

From a Mycotherapy perspective, extract fidelity is essential. **Cordyceps militaris fruiting–body SCWE extracts** provide the richest concentration of cordycepin, β–glucans and phenolics while avoiding the starch dilution seen in grain–based mycelium products. SCWE extraction preserves thermolabile nucleoside analogues and hydrophilic immune–active constituents critical to its physiological effects.

In integrative veterinary practice, Cordyceps is best positioned as a **multi–system vitality and resilience agent** – supporting mitochondrial steadiness, immune competence and physiological recovery in both acute depletion and chronic disease contexts. Its actions are gradual, cumulative and regulatory, consistent with the principles of terrain–based Mycotherapy.

> Cordyceps militaris offers a distinctive contribution to integrative veterinary care by supporting physiological resilience across energy metabolism, oxygen utilisation, immune stability and stress regulation.

5.14 Conclusion – Integrative Significance and Extraction Considerations

Cordyceps militaris offers a distinctive contribution to integrative veterinary care by supporting physiological resilience across energy metabolism, oxygen utilisation, immune stability and stress regulation. Its influence on mitochondrial ATP generation and oxygen delivery distinguishes it from other functional mushrooms, making it particularly useful for animals experiencing reduced stamina, post-exertional fatigue, chronic illness, respiratory vulnerability or age-related declines in vitality. Rather than functioning as a stimulant, Cordyceps acts as a metabolic regulator that gradually restores efficiency and endurance, supporting sustained well-being in both companion and performance animals.

Its capacity to modulate inflammatory pathways, enhance antioxidant defences and stabilise immune responses further broadens its applications. These actions align with clinical observations of improved recovery after illness, more consistent energy patterns in senior animals and enhanced coping capacity during physiological stress. In oncology or chronic-disease settings, Cordyceps may contribute to quality-of-life improvements through its regulatory effects on immune tone, mitochondrial function and tissue resilience, although such applications must be approached with case-specific judgement.

Extract quality remains central to achieving predictable and clinically relevant outcomes. SCWE full-spectrum extracts preserve the structural and biochemical matrix of the fruiting body, including nucleosides, β-glucans, sterols, peptides and prebiotic fibre. This contrasts sharply with alcohol tinctures, which skew constituent ratios, and myceliated-grain preparations, which dilute active compounds with starch. The whole-food integrity of SCWE extracts provides a physiologically coherent preparation that aligns with the pathways described across Cordyceps' evidence base, improving reliability in animals with chronic disease, metabolic fragility or complex medication regimens.

When introduced gradually, monitored appropriately and integrated into broader multimodal care plans, Cordyceps militaris offers a steady, cumulative and clinically meaningful contribution to health. Its value lies not in rapid, dramatic shifts but in the incremental restoration of metabolic balance, respiratory efficiency, immune harmony and cellular vitality. Applied with thoughtful veterinary oversight, it stands as a versatile and well-tolerated adjunct within modern Mycotherapy.

> Cordyceps offers a distinctive contribution to integrative veterinary care.

Key sources (summary)

Tuli et al., 2013; Zhou et al., 2009; Wasser, 2011–2023; Jin & Zhong, 2016; Das, 2010; Kuo et al., journal of Ethnopharmacology; Park et al., Journal of Agricultural and Food Chemistry; Li et al., Journal of Clinical Gastroenterology; Hsu et al., Phytomedicine; Liu et al., Molecular Carcinogenesis; Veterinary Mycotherapy School (MykoTroph), 2023; Chinese Pharmacopoeia Committee (multiple editions). **Full professional reference list available in the Master References section.**

> "The body has an incredible power to heal itself if given the right tools. *Source: The Nature of Animal Healing (1999) Dr Marty Goldstein, DVM*"

6

MAITAKE (Grifola frondosa)

6.1 Introduction to Maitake – *The Metabolic Harmoniser*

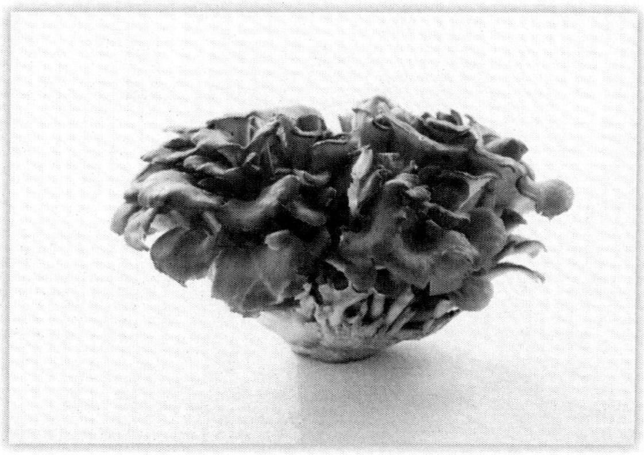

Maitake (*Grifola frondosa*) occupies a distinct place within Mycotherapy as a mushroom that harmonises metabolic, immune and inflammatory functions in a coordinated manner. It is often described as a 'metabolic harmoniser' because its actions extend across glucose regulation, lipid balance, innate and adaptive immune function, and terrain-level inflammatory tone. This breadth originates from the mushroom's highly structured β-glucans, glycoproteins and secondary metabolites, which interact with physiological networks rather than isolated sites of action.

In veterinary practice, Maitake is especially relevant for animals in which metabolic strain, chronic inflammation and immune dysregulation intersect. Ageing dogs, overweight or insulin-resistant animals, chronically stressed patients and those with recurrent infections frequently exhibit these overlapping patterns. Preclinical research demonstrates that Maitake influences insulin receptor sensitivity, modulates hepatic lipid metabolism, enhances mitochondrial efficiency and improves innate immune responsiveness. Although formal veterinary clinical trials are limited, these mechanistic pathways are shared across mammalian species and align closely with clinical patterns observed in dogs and cats with chronic or degenerative health challenges.

A defining part of Maitake's clinical relevance lies in the accessibility of its bioactive compounds. The fruiting body contains a dense, chitin-rich cell-wall structure, which naturally restricts the release of β-glucans and polysaccharide–protein complexes during digestion. Traditional decoctions often failed to fully liberate these compounds. Modern extraction methods, particularly Sub-critical water extraction (SCWE), provide a more precise means of releasing the mushroom's bioactive matrix without degrading thermolabile constituents. SCWE allows water to remain in a semi-compressed state, improving the solubilisation of high-molecular-weight β-glucans, glycoproteins and phenolic compounds while preserving nutritional co-factors. This results in extracts that more accurately reflect the mushroom's full therapeutic potential.

> In veterinary practice, Maitake is especially relevant for animals in which metabolic strain, chronic inflammation and immune dysregulation intersect.

From a clinical perspective, the value of SCWE lies not in marketing, but in pharmacotechnical relevance. Soluble β-glucans must be adequately released to interact with intestinal immune receptors such as Dectin-1, complement receptor 3 and toll-like receptors within the gut-associated lymphoid tissue. By enhancing cell-wall breakdown and polysaccharide accessibility, SCWE supports clearer physiological recognition of Maitake's compounds. When applied to whole fruiting bodies rather than isolated fractions, SCWE also retains the mushroom's synergistic fibre, sterols, phenolics and micronutrients, allowing it to contribute to metabolic steadiness, immune balance and gastrointestinal terrain health.

Clinically, Maitake's effects are gradual, cumulative and terrain-modifying. Animals may exhibit improvements in vitality, steadier appetite, enhanced resilience to infections, better metabolic indicators and reduced inflammatory burden over time. Maitake is rarely used in isolation; it integrates naturally with other medicinal mushrooms such as Turkey Tail (immune modulation), Reishi (homeostatic calm and inflammatory regulation) and Lion's Mane (gut–brain–metabolic synchrony). Its long culinary history, favourable safety profile and multi-pathway influence make it a valuable component of integrative veterinary strategies, particularly for animals experiencing chronic or age-related physiological decline.

6.2 Taxonomy, Morphology and Extract Science

Maitake (*Grifola frondosa*) belongs to the Basidiomycota division, class Agaricomycetes, and family Meripilaceae. Its taxonomic consistency across diverse growing regions ensures a relatively stable biochemical profile, particularly regarding its hallmark 1,3- and 1,6-β-glucans. For Mycotherapy, this stability is advantageous, as variations in β-glucan branching patterns can significantly influence immunological recognition and metabolic modulation. *G. frondosa* is therefore considered one of the more predictable species in terms of therapeutic composition.

Morphologically, Maitake forms a large, perennial, polyporoid fruiting body characterised by its multi-branched, layered fronds which resemble overlapping feathers. This extensive architecture provides substantial surface area for environmental nutrient exchange and supports dense development of fungal tissue. The fronded structure contributes directly to Maitake's high polysaccharide content, particularly within its robust fungal cell wall. This wall is composed of chitin, β-glucans, mannans, glycoproteins and structural proteins, creating a rigid and relatively impermeable matrix that protects the mushroom in nature but also influences extraction requirements for therapeutic use.

For veterinarians, understanding Maitake's morphological and structural features is important because they govern the accessibility of bioactive compounds. Raw Maitake powder retains the integrity of the chitinous cell wall, meaning that only partial breakdown occurs within the gastrointestinal tract. While the non-solubilised fraction offers pre-biotic fibre that can support beneficial microbiota, the immunologically active β-glucans and polysaccharide–protein complexes remain largely inaccessible when the cell wall is not adequately disrupted. This is particularly relevant in dogs and cats, whose digestive capacities differ from humans and who often exhibit diminished enzymatic digestion in chronic disease states.

Extraction science therefore plays a crucial role in translating Maitake's biochemical potential into clinically effective preparations. Traditional extraction approaches, including hot-water decoction or alcohol precipitation, have historically yielded isolated fractions such as the well-known 'D-fraction' and related polysaccharide complexes. These extracts demonstrate potent immunomodulatory effects in preclinical research but may exclude secondary metabolites, fibres, and redox-active compounds that contribute to the mushroom's full therapeutic footprint.

Sub-critical water extraction (SCWE) offers a more integrative approach that aligns with the principles of Mycotherapy. SCWE uses water under precisely controlled temperature and pressure, maintaining it in a semi-compressed state that enhances its solvating power. This allows for deeper penetration of the chitinous cell wall and improved solubilisation of high-molecular-weight β-glucans, glycoproteins, phenolic compounds, sterols and trace elements while preserving thermolabile constituents. The result is an extract that maintains the biochemical context of the whole mushroom and provides a more complete representation of its natural therapeutic synergy.

For companion animals, SCWE has practical value because the resulting extracts present β-glucans in a more bioavailable, physiologically recognisable form. Enhanced solubility facilitates interaction with key pattern-recognition receptors in the gut-associated lymphoid tissue, such as Dectin-1 and complement receptor 3, while the preserved whole-mushroom matrix continues to support gastrointestinal terrain, redox balance and metabolic steadiness. This synergy is central to Mycotherapy's systems-based philosophy, which values the coordinated modulation of physiological networks rather than isolated pharmacological effects.

From a veterinary perspective, Maitake's taxonomic reliability, structural complexity and responsiveness to advanced extraction techniques underpin its clinical utility. These features ensure that the mushroom's principal bioactive compounds can be delivered in forms that are physiologically intelligible, therapeutically meaningful and suited to integration within metabolic, immune and inflammatory protocols for companion animals.

6.3 Bioactive Constituents – Mechanistic Relevance

Maitake's therapeutic profile arises from a diverse matrix of bioactive constituents that operate across multiple physiological systems. Although the mushroom is most widely recognised for its β-glucans, its clinical effects result from the synergistic activity of polysaccharides, glycoproteins, sterols, phenolic compounds, enzymes, micronutrients and pre-biotic fibres that together influence metabolic regulation, immune responsiveness and inflammatory tone.

The predominant bioactive molecules are highly branched 1,3-β-glucans with 1,6-linked side chains. These complex architectures allow Maitake β-glucans to bind effectively to innate immune receptors such as Dectin-1, complement receptor 3 and various toll-like receptors located within the gut-associated lymphoid tissue. Engagement of these receptors triggers downstream signalling cascades that modulate macrophage activation, support dendritic cell maturation, enhance natural killer cell function and influence T-helper cell differentiation. Importantly, Maitake's β-glucans demonstrate regulatory rather than purely stimulatory activity. They enhance deficient immune responses but do not indiscriminately amplify inflammation, a key reason why Maitake is well suited to chronic, low-grade inflammatory states common in ageing animals.

Beyond β-glucans, Maitake contains a structurally varied group of α-glucans, mannans and chitin–glucan complexes which contribute to its pre-biotic, immunological and metabolic effects. Certain α-glucans exhibit antioxidant and cytokine-modulating actions in preclinical studies, attenuating pro-inflammatory pathways and supporting redox homeostasis. This is particularly relevant in animals with chronic inflammatory burden, metabolic dysfunction or age-related oxidative stress.

Polysaccharide–protein complexes add an additional layer of mechanistic nuance. The best known of these, the 'D-fraction', has demonstrated potent effects on antigen presentation, innate immune priming and cytokine modulation in preclinical cancer models. These complexes act at lower doses than isolated β-glucans and illustrate the importance of retaining the mushroom's broader molecular context in extraction processes. Glycoproteins and lectin-like molecules within Maitake may also influence cellular communication and signalling within the immune system.

Maitake's secondary metabolites contribute to its relevance in metabolic and oxidative pathways. Ergosterol and its derivatives support membrane stability and exhibit antioxidant behaviour. Phenolic compounds and organic acids provide additional redox-modulating activity, assisting in the reduction of oxidative stress which often accompanies chronic disease. Trace minerals and enzyme cofactors offer further metabolic support and may influence mitochondrial resilience, energy utilisation and tissue repair.

Of particular importance for veterinary integrative practice is Maitake's influence on metabolic signalling. Well-characterised polysaccharide fractions such as GF5000 and F2 improve insulin receptor sensitivity, modulate hepatic lipid metabolism and influence adipokine patterns in preclinical models of metabolic syndrome and pre-diabetes. These actions can translate conceptually to overweight dogs, insulin-resistant cats and animals exhibiting chronic metabolic strain. Improved gut microbiota composition has also been documented in association with Maitake polysaccharides, reinforcing the mushroom's role in supporting gastrointestinal and metabolic health.

Collectively, these constituents form a biochemical ecosystem rather than a single active agent. The interplay between β-glucans, polysaccharide–protein complexes, sterols, phenolics, micronutrients and fibres underpins Maitake's systems-level effects. This integrated activity is central to Mycotherapy, where the aim is not to isolate or amplify individual compounds, but to provide a coordinated, physiologically coherent stimulus that supports the terrain across immune, metabolic and inflammatory axes.

> Maitake exerts a broad and regulatory influence on the immune system, an effect that aligns well with the terrain-based principles of Mycotherapy.

6.4 Immune System Modulation

Maitake exerts a broad and regulatory influence on the immune system, an effect that aligns well with the terrain-based principles of Mycotherapy. Rather than functioning as a simple immune stimulant, Maitake supports immune recalibration. It enhances deficient or suppressed immune activity while maintaining appropriate checks on inflammatory or dysregulated responses. This dual-action pattern is particularly relevant in animals experiencing immune fatigue, chronic inflammation or age-related immunosenescence.

The primary mechanisms begin in the gastrointestinal tract, where orally administered β-glucans interact with receptors within the gut-associated lymphoid tissue. Maitake's highly branched 1,3-/1,6-β-glucans bind to Dectin-1 on macrophages and dendritic cells, complement receptor 3 on neutrophils and natural killer cells, and specific toll-like receptors that coordinate innate immune engagement. Activation of these receptors influences antigen uptake, promotes dendritic cell maturation and primes macrophages to perform more efficient phagocytosis. These early events shape downstream adaptive responses, including improved T-helper cell balance and enhanced cytotoxic potential.

Preclinical research has demonstrated that Maitake supports healthy Th1-weighted immunity, which is crucial for antiviral defence and tumour surveillance. At the same time, it can attenuate overactive Th2 patterns by modulating cytokine expression and improving regulatory T cell behaviour within certain inflammatory contexts. This immunological balancing effect explains why Maitake is suitable for animals with chronic low-grade immune stress rather than for conditions requiring aggressive immunostimulation.

Polysaccharide–protein complexes such as the 'D-fraction' add further depth to Maitake's immune properties. These complexes have shown the capacity to increase production of interleukin-2, interleukin-12 and interferon-γ in preclinical models. The result is enhanced innate immune vigour without premature or excessive activation. This is a clinically meaningful distinction for veterinarians working with geriatric animals or patients receiving chemotherapy, where preserving immune competence without provoking inflammatory toxicity is a central concern.

> Maitake exerts a broad and regulatory influence on the immune system, an effect that aligns well with the terrain-based principles of Mycotherapy.

Although controlled veterinary trials are still emerging, practitioner observations frequently report improved resilience, steadier convalescence after infections and enhanced general vitality when Maitake is used within a broader integrative plan. Caution remains appropriate in animals with unstable immune-mediated disease, where immune modulation must be introduced slowly and with clear monitoring parameters.

Overall, Maitake functions as a physiological signal that helps restore immune clarity and responsiveness. Its regulatory nature makes it especially suited to chronic and terrain-based cases where the aim is to strengthen host defence without destabilising immune balance.

6.5 Inflammation and Oxidative Stress Pathways

Chronic inflammation and oxidative stress underpin many of the clinical presentations in which Maitake becomes relevant within integrative veterinary medicine. These include ageing-related decline, metabolic dysfunction, gastrointestinal disorders, osteoarthritis and tumour micro-environment dysregulation. Maitake influences inflammatory pathways through a combination of polysaccharide signalling, antioxidant activity and metabolic normalisation.

At the cellular level, Maitake's β-glucans modulate key inflammatory intermediaries by influencing receptor-mediated signalling. Engagement of Dectin-1 and toll-like receptors can lead to downregulation of nuclear factor kappa B, one of the major transcription factors responsible for amplifying inflammatory responses. This modulation has been demonstrated in preclinical models of metabolic syndrome and hepatic inflammation, where Maitake administration reduced circulating concentrations of interleukin-6 and tumour necrosis factor-α. Although these studies were not conducted in veterinary species, the underlying pathways are conserved across mammals and align with clinical patterns observed in dogs and cats presenting with chronic inflammatory burden.

Maitake's α-glucan fractions contribute further antioxidant and cytokine-modulating effects. These smaller polysaccharides have shown the ability to enhance endogenous antioxidant enzymes such as superoxide dismutase and glutathione peroxidase in preclinical systems. By improving redox homeostasis, these compounds may help reduce oxidative damage to tissues that are particularly vulnerable in chronic diseases, including hepatic tissue, neural tissue and the gastrointestinal mucosa.

Secondary metabolites, including ergosterol derivatives, phenolic compounds and organic acids, add additional layers to Maitake's redox and anti-inflammatory profile. Ergosterol and its oxidation products possess mild antioxidant capacity, while phenolic constituents can neutralise reactive oxygen species. These actions are subtle but meaningful within a terrain-based approach, especially for animals experiencing long-term inflammation where mitochondrial strain and oxidative load exacerbate fatigue, degenerative processes and immune dysregulation.

An additional aspect of Maitake's influence on inflammation arises indirectly through metabolic regulation. By supporting healthier insulin responsiveness and reducing lipotoxic inflammatory signalling, Maitake helps reduce some of the upstream metabolic drivers of chronic inflammation. This metabolic–inflammatory synchrony is particularly beneficial for overweight dogs, pre-diabetic cats and older animals with inflammatory tendencies linked to diminished metabolic resilience.

Clinically, Maitake is best used as a background modulator rather than a fast-acting anti-inflammatory agent. Its role is to shift inflammatory tone gradually, support tissue resilience and contribute to a more stable redox environment. For animals with chronic disease, this may translate into improved comfort, steadier energy levels, reduced inflammatory markers and better tolerance of other therapies. When integrated with dietary strategies, omega-3 fatty acids, joint support or mitochondrial cofactors, Maitake's benefits can align naturally with broader integrative goals.

Chronic inflammation and oxidative stress underpin many of the clinical presentations in which Maitake becomes relevant within integrative veterinary medicine.

6.6 Gastrointestinal, Microbiome and Metabolic Health

The gastrointestinal system plays a central role in Maitake's therapeutic profile. Because β-glucans and polysaccharide–protein complexes exert their primary effects through interaction with the gut-associated lymphoid tissue, Maitake functions partly as a gastrointestinal immune modulator. However, its actions extend beyond immune signalling into microbial composition, epithelial integrity and systemic metabolic pathways.

Maitake polysaccharides act as selective substrates for beneficial gut bacteria, particularly those responsible for producing short-chain fatty acids. This pre-biotic activity promotes a healthier microbial community, favouring species associated with anti-inflammatory and metabolic benefits. P reclinical models have demonstrated increases in butyrate-producing bacteria following Maitake supplementation, which is significant because butyrate supports intestinal barrier integrity, mucosal healing and anti-inflammatory signalling throughout the body reclinical models have demonstrated increases in butyrate-producing bacteria following Maitake supplementation, which is significant because butyrate supports intestinal barrier integrity, mucosal healing and anti-inflammatory signalling throughout the body.

Maitake's influence on the microbiome also connects directly to metabolic regulation. Key polysaccharide fractions, such as GF5000 and F2, have been shown to improve insulin receptor sensitivity, modulate hepatic lipid metabolism and reduce hepatic inflammation in rodent models of metabolic syndrome. Improved gut microbial diversity and reductions in endotoxin-associated inflammation appear to contribute to these benefits. These findings are relevant for animals exhibiting metabolic fragility, including overweight dogs, insulin-resistant cats and older animals with gastrointestinal irregularities linked to dysbiosis.

The mushroom's fibre-rich matrix supports stool quality and gastrointestinal motility, providing a stabilising effect in animals prone to loose stools or gut sensitivity. In dogs and cats with chronic gastrointestinal dysregulation, Maitake may contribute to improved digestive consistency and reduced inflammatory burden in the intestinal mucosa. The preserved fibre and micronutrient context within SCWE whole-mushroom extracts is particularly suited to this terrain-supportive role.

Maitake's systemic metabolic effects stem from its combined actions on gut health, immune signalling and hepatic pathways. By improving insulin responsiveness, reducing lipotoxicity and modulating inflammatory drivers, Maitake facilitates a more coherent metabolic environment. This makes it valuable in early-stage metabolic dysfunction, pre-diabetes, hepatic steatosis tendencies and chronic inflammatory conditions associated with metabolic strain.

From a clinical perspective, Maitake fits naturally into integrative protocols for dogs or cats with gastrointestinal fragility, metabolic risk profiles, weight challenges or chronic inflammatory tendencies. It complements dietary modifications, pre-biotic fibres, probiotics, hepatoprotective measures and anti-inflammatory strategies. Its benefits emerge progressively, reflecting the gradual recalibration of the gut–immune–metabolic axis rather than immediate symptomatic changes.

> Maitake's systemic metabolic effects stem from its combined actions on gut health, immune signalling and hepatic pathways.

6.7 Neurological and Behavioural Health

Maitake's direct neurotrophic effects are less pronounced than those of Lion's Mane, yet its systemic actions across metabolism, immunity and inflammation indirectly influence neurological and behavioural wellbeing in animals. The brain is highly responsive to metabolic efficiency, oxidative balance and inflammatory tone, and Maitake's capacity to modulate these systems provides secondary neuroprotective value. This is particularly relevant for ageing dogs and cats, animals with chronic inflammatory burden and those experiencing stress-related behavioural changes.

Insulin signalling plays a central role in brain health. Preclinical studies indicate that Maitake polysaccharides improve insulin receptor sensitivity and modulate glucose metabolism in peripheral tissues. Although not studied directly in canine or feline neurons, improved systemic insulin regulation can reduce neuroinflammatory signalling and support mitochondrial stability within the central nervous system. This may benefit animals with early cognitive decline or metabolic fragility that manifests behaviourally as disorientation, reduced engagement or altered sleep–wake patterns.

Chronic inflammation is another key driver of neurological dysfunction in animals. Maitake's influence on inflammatory mediators, including reductions in interleukin-6 and tumour necrosis factor-α in preclinical systems, may indirectly support microglial tempering and protect neural tissues from inflammatory injury. Phenolic compounds, ergosterol derivatives and antioxidant cofactors further contribute to redox balance, which is crucial for maintaining neuronal integrity in geriatric animals. These effects should not be interpreted as direct neuroregenerative actions, but rather as contributors to a healthier internal terrain that supports cognitive resilience.

The gut–brain axis provides an additional pathway through which Maitake may influence behaviour and neurological health. By supporting a more diverse, short-chain-fatty-acid-producing microbiome, Maitake indirectly modulates vagal signalling, intestinal barrier function and systemic inflammatory tone. These interactions are increasingly recognised as influential in behavioural stability, stress resilience and emotional regulation in companion animals. Dogs experiencing stress-linked gastrointestinal disturbance, for example, may benefit from improved microbial composition and reduced inflammatory signalling.

Clinically, Maitake is best positioned as part of a broader integrative strategy for neurological and behavioural support, often alongside Lion's Mane, Reishi, omega-3 fatty acids, mitochondrial cofactors, environmental enrichment and, where appropriate, conventional pharmacological interventions. Its value lies in creating a physiological environment that reduces metabolic strain, modulates inflammation and enhances resilience. Improvements tend to manifest gradually, commonly reported by caregivers as clearer engagement, steadier mood, more consistent routines and improved behavioural tolerance.

6.8 Cardiovascular and Respiratory Physiology

Maitake influences cardiovascular physiology primarily through its effects on metabolic regulation, vascular inflammation and lipid handling. Although direct veterinary research is limited, preclinical studies demonstrate reductions in serum cholesterol, triglycerides and low-density lipoprotein concentrations, particularly in models of metabolic syndrome. These improvements reflect Maitake's ability to modulate hepatic lipid metabolism and reduce inflammatory mediators that contribute to vascular dysfunction.

Insulin responsiveness is closely linked to cardiovascular health in animals. Maitake's polysaccharide fractions have demonstrated improved glucose tolerance and reduced hepatic steatosis in rodent models, which indirectly supports vascular stability and endothelial function. These mechanisms may be conceptually applied to overweight dogs or ageing cats, in whom metabolic inefficiency often contributes to early cardiovascular compromise. Improved metabolic balance may therefore reduce systemic vascular inflammation and support healthier cardiac physiology.

Maitake's antioxidant activity also carries relevance for cardiac tissues, which are vulnerable to oxidative stress, particularly in chronically inflamed or geriatric animals. Phenolic compounds, ergosterol derivatives and polysaccharide-linked redox cofactors can contribute to reducing oxidative strain on vascular and myocardial cells. While these effects are subtle, they align with integrative approaches aimed at sustaining long-term cardiovascular resilience.

Respiratory-specific evidence for Maitake is more limited. Its influence on respiratory health is best understood indirectly through immune modulation and inflammatory regulation. Enhanced macrophage function and improved mucosal immunity may support animals prone to recurrent respiratory infections. However, Maitake does not exhibit bronchodilatory or acute anti-inflammatory activity, and its use in respiratory conditions should remain adjunctive rather than primary.

In veterinary practice, Maitake may be considered in metabolic-linked cardiovascular vulnerability, chronic inflammatory airway tendencies or age-related reductions in vascular resilience. Its effects unfold gradually and contribute to a more stable terrain rather than producing immediate cardiovascular changes. It integrates well with Reishi in stress-linked cardiovascular patterns and with hepatoprotective strategies in metabolic disease affecting the liver–vascular axis.

6.9 Oncology and Adjunctive Cancer Support

Oncology is one of the most widely explored areas for Maitake within Mycotherapy. Extensive preclinical research demonstrates that Maitake polysaccharides exert meaningful effects within tumour micro-environments, including modulation of immune surveillance, enhancement of cytotoxic activity and attenuation of tumour-associated immunosuppression. While veterinary-specific clinical trials are limited, the mechanistic pathways observed are conserved across species and provide a compelling basis for adjunctive use.

Maitake's β-glucans bind to Dectin-1 and complement receptor 3 on macrophages, dendritic cells and natural killer cells, triggering a cascade of events that enhances tumour recognition and immune clearance. These effects include improved antigen presentation, increased interferon-γ production, heightened cytotoxic capacity and reduced suppression by regulatory T cells within tumour tissues. Such mechanisms contribute to slowing tumour progression in several preclinical models and support the hypothesis that Maitake helps re-establish more effective tumour surveillance.

Oncology is one of the most widely explored areas for Maitake within Mycotherapy.

Polysaccharide–protein complexes such as the 'D-fraction' display additional antitumour properties. Preclinical studies show reduced tumour growth, increased apoptotic signalling and, in some models, reduced metastatic potential. In vitro research on canine cancer cell lines has indicated that Maitake extracts may inhibit growth in certain tumour types, although the magnitude of this effect varies and is influenced by extraction method and constituent profile. These findings underscore the importance of using well-characterised, fruiting-body-based extracts that preserve the molecular context required for immunomodulatory and metabolic activity.

Maitake's influence on metabolic and inflammatory pathways is also relevant in oncology. Cancer creates metabolic strain and promotes systemic inflammation, contributing to cachexia, reduced treatment tolerance and immune exhaustion. Maitake's ability to improve insulin responsiveness, modulate lipid metabolism and reduce inflammatory mediators can support metabolic stability and quality of life in animals undergoing cancer treatment. Its antioxidant profile may also contribute to preserving tissue resilience during conventional therapies.

Clinically, Maitake should be positioned as a supportive adjunct rather than a direct anticancer agent. It is rarely used in isolation and is most effective when combined with mushrooms such as Turkey Tail (immune activation and microbiome modulation) and Reishi (immunological and neuroendocrine stabilisation). Integrative oncology protocols often incorporate Maitake to support immune competence, reduce inflammatory strain, improve metabolic steadiness and enhance treatment tolerance during chemotherapy or radiotherapy.

In practice, its use must be guided by careful assessment of the animal's overall clinical picture, including the type of cancer, concurrent medications, immune status and metabolic stability. Monitoring remains essential, particularly in animals receiving immunosuppressive therapies or those with fragile gastrointestinal or hepatic function. When thoughtfully integrated, Maitake may contribute to improved vitality, steadier appetite, reduced inflammatory burden and enhanced resilience during oncologic care.

6.10 Hepatic and Renal Physiology

Maitake exerts a notable influence on hepatic physiology through its effects on metabolic signalling, hepatic lipid handling and inflammatory modulation. Preclinical studies have demonstrated that Maitake polysaccharide fractions can reduce hepatic steatosis, normalise lipid metabolism and attenuate inflammatory markers associated with metabolic strain. These effects are particularly significant in animals with early hepatic dysfunction linked to insulin resistance, obesity or chronic inflammation. By improving insulin responsiveness and reducing lipotoxic stress, Maitake contributes to a more cohesive metabolic–hepatic axis.

The liver is central to both detoxification and immune surveillance. Maitake's antioxidant profile is clinically relevant here, as ergosterol derivatives, phenolic compounds and polysaccharide-associated redox cofactors may help counter oxidative stress that commonly affects hepatocytes in chronic disease and ageing. Improved redox tone can support healthier hepatocellular function and reduce susceptibility to secondary inflammation. Although the exact pathways have not been established in companion animals, preclinical research offers a plausible mechanistic foundation for hepatic support.

Maitake's influence on hepatic inflammation may also indirectly support animals experiencing chronic inflammatory conditions that place additional strain on liver function. In metabolic disorders, the liver is often the first organ to exhibit biochemical abnormalities. By modulating inflammatory cytokines and improving metabolic steadiness, Maitake can help reduce hepatic inflammatory burden. These actions align well with integrative approaches to early fatty liver tendencies, mild increases in liver enzymes or metabolic vulnerability in ageing animals.

Renal physiology is less clearly influenced by Maitake, but available data suggest that it is generally well tolerated and does not impose significant renal strain. Some preclinical studies indicate that Maitake-derived compounds may support toxin elimination, including the excretion of certain heavy metals. While such findings remain preliminary, they provide further evidence that Maitake's actions are not nephrotoxic and may be compatible with gentle support of renal excretion pathways. Nevertheless, animals with advanced renal disease require careful monitoring, as changes in hydration status, electrolyte balance and gastrointestinal behaviour may influence tolerability.

In clinical practice, Maitake can be considered for animals with metabolic-linked hepatic stress, early dysfunction in liver enzymes, oxidative burden or chronic disease patterns that affect hepatic resilience. It integrates naturally with dietary modification, hepatoprotective agents and metabolic stabilisers. In renal contexts, cautious use alongside regular biochemical monitoring ensures safety while allowing potential systemic benefits to unfold.

6.11 Endocrine and Metabolic Regulation

Maitake is widely recognised within Mycotherapy as one of the most metabolically active medicinal mushrooms. Its influence extends across glucose homeostasis, insulin receptor sensitivity, lipid metabolism, adipokine balance and systemic energy utilisation. These actions are deeply relevant to companion animals, particularly overweight dogs, pre-diabetic cats and ageing animals with metabolic fragility.

Preclinical work has demonstrated that specific Maitake polysaccharide fractions, including GF5000 and F2, improve insulin sensitivity and glucose tolerance in models of metabolic syndrome and pre-diabetes. These effects include modulation of insulin receptors, reduction of lipotoxic signalling, improved hepatic lipid metabolism and enhanced mitochondrial efficiency. Although veterinary-species trials are limited, the physiological pathways involved are highly conserved and mirror clinical patterns seen in dogs and cats with emerging insulin dysregulation.

Lipid metabolism is another domain in which Maitake exhibits meaningful activity. Research has shown reductions in total cholesterol, triglycerides and low-density lipoprotein concentrations, particularly in metabolic-stress models. For animals with early dyslipidaemia, weight challenges or metabolic-linked inflammatory patterns, these effects can contribute to improved cardiovascular and hepatic resilience.

Endocrine regulation extends beyond insulin. Chronic inflammation and oxidative stress can impair adrenal, thyroid and reproductive hormonal axes, and Maitake's ability to modulate inflammatory cascades and support redox balance may indirectly stabilise endocrine function. While these effects are secondary rather than primary, they can support broader endocrine harmony in animals whose hormonal regulation has been affected by chronic disease or degenerative processes.

Clinically, Maitake is best positioned for early or moderate metabolic dysfunction. It integrates effectively with dietary interventions, weight management, hepatoprotective protocols and other nutraceuticals supporting metabolic resilience. Improvements typically emerge progressively as the gut–immune–metabolic axis recalibrates. For diabetic animals on insulin or oral hypoglycaemic agents, careful monitoring remains essential, as Maitake may enhance insulin responsiveness and influence dosing requirements.

6.12 Veterinary Pharmacology and Drug Interaction Considerations

Absorption and bioavailability

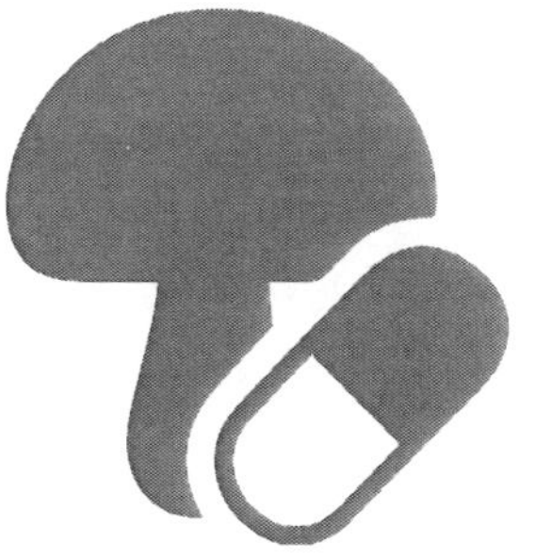

Maitake's bioactivity begins primarily in the gastrointestinal tract. Its β-glucans are not fully absorbed as intact molecules; instead, they interact with receptors in the gut-associated lymphoid tissue. This local immune engagement produces systemic effects without requiring high systemic absorption. Smaller polysaccharide fragments and oligosaccharides may enter circulation and contribute to metabolic signalling. Animals with gastrointestinal fragility or dysbiosis may experience altered receptor interactions, which underscores the need for slow titration when gut integrity is compromised.

Hepatic metabolism and detoxification pathways

Maitake polysaccharides are not metabolised via classic cytochrome P450 pathways but can influence hepatic function indirectly by modulating inflammation, improving insulin responsiveness and supporting redox stability. These effects can enhance hepatic resilience, particularly in animals experiencing metabolic strain. However, in advanced hepatic compromise, even beneficial metabolic modulators must be introduced cautiously, with baseline and follow-up liver function tests.

Cytochrome P450 considerations

Evidence of Maitake directly altering cytochrome P450 activity is limited and inconsistent. Available data suggest that at nutritional–therapeutic doses, Maitake exhibits minimal CYP induction or inhibition. Nevertheless, prudence is warranted when animals receive medications with a narrow therapeutic index or heavy reliance on hepatic clearance. In such cases, clinicians may choose to introduce Maitake gradually while monitoring for any deviation in pharmacological response.

Coagulation and platelet activity

Maitake does not exert strong anticoagulant effects, yet its influence on inflammatory tone and vascular physiology may subtly modulate platelet dynamics. Caution is appropriate in animals receiving anticoagulants, corticosteroids, non-steroidal anti-inflammatory drugs or chemotherapeutic agents that may affect coagulation. Clinical monitoring for bruising, delayed clotting or altered bleeding behaviour remains a prudent safeguard.

Sedative, neurological or behavioural medication interactions

Maitake has no direct sedative or anxiolytic effect, and interactions with neuroactive medications are unlikely to be pharmacodynamic. Any neurological or behavioural influence tends to arise indirectly through metabolic and inflammatory modulation. Animals receiving anticonvulsants, sedatives or behavioural medications may use Maitake safely, provided their energy, sleep patterns and general behaviour are monitored during introduction.

Endocrine medication interactions

The most clinically notable interaction involves insulin and oral hypoglycaemic agents. By improving insulin responsiveness, Maitake may potentiate the action of these medications. Dogs and cats with diabetes therefore require closer monitoring of blood glucose and readiness to adjust dosing schedules. No strong evidence suggests direct interactions with thyroid, adrenal or reproductive hormones.

Gastrointestinal absorption considerations

Maitake's fibre and polysaccharide profile can influence gastrointestinal motility and fermentation dynamics. While these effects are generally beneficial, they may alter the absorption kinetics of certain oral medications, particularly those with narrow absorption windows. When necessary, separating Maitake from critical medications by one to two hours can help avoid interference.

Polypharmacy considerations and safe-use practice

In animals with complex medication regimens, Maitake should be introduced one change at a time, with clear therapeutic rationale and defined monitoring parameters. This is particularly important in oncology, chronic inflammatory diseases, endocrine disorders and multi-systemic presentations where physiological stability is delicate. Documentation of behavioural, metabolic and clinical changes is essential to ensure safe integration.

Species-specific considerations

Cats, owing to their unique hepatic metabolism and sensitivity to gastrointestinal disruption, require particularly careful titration. Small dogs, geriatric animals and patients with compromised digestion should begin at the lower end of the therapeutic range. SCWE whole-mushroom preparations may offer improved tolerability because of enhanced solubility and reduced microbial load, but all forms require patient-specific titration.

6.13 Clinical application in veterinary practice

Dermatological conditions

Dermatological presentations often involve underlying immune imbalance, chronic inflammation or metabolic strain. Maitake's regulatory effects on immune surveillance and inflammatory signalling can assist in stabilising recurrent or chronic dermatological issues, particularly those associated with metabolic fragility or chronic low-grade inflammation. While not a primary dermatological agent, Maitake may complement therapies in animals with recurrent pyoderma, inflammatory dermatoses or immune-compromised skin barrier function. Its pre-biotic and gut-modulating effects may indirectly support dermatological stability through improved gut–skin axis dynamics.

Gastrointestinal disorders

Maitake is highly relevant in gastrointestinal presentations involving dysbiosis, impaired mucosal immunity or metabolic–gut interaction. Its polysaccharides support short-chain fatty acid production, enhance microbial balance and influence mucosal immune activity. Animals with chronic intermittent diarrhoea, soft stools, stress-related gastrointestinal instability or mild inflammatory tendencies may benefit from Maitake's stabilising effects. It is particularly useful when gastrointestinal dysfunction coexists with metabolic strain, early insulin resistance or immune fatigue.

Hepatic disease

In early hepatic stress or mild elevations in liver enzymes associated with metabolic dysfunction, Maitake can support hepatic physiology through its influence on insulin responsiveness, lipid metabolism and inflammatory modulation. It fits naturally into integrative plans for animals with fatty liver tendencies, early-stage hepatic compromise or metabolic-linked inflammatory strain. It is not a direct hepatoprotective agent in the sense of milk thistle or SAMe, but contributes meaningfully to terrain-level hepatic resilience when used appropriately.

Behavioural medicine and stress physiology

Although Maitake is not directly neurotrophic, its influence on metabolic balance, inflammatory tone and gut–brain signalling can contribute to behavioural steadiness. Animals experiencing chronic stress, reduced resilience or gastrointestinal-linked behavioural changes may experience improvements in engagement, sleep–wake rhythm and overall behavioural stability when Maitake is integrated within a broader plan. It pairs well with Lion's Mane for neurocognitive support and with Reishi where stress physiology and behavioural dysregulation are prominent.

Immune dysregulation

Maitake's β-glucans and polysaccharide–protein complexes modulate innate and adaptive immunity, making it appropriate in cases of immune fatigue, recurrent infections or reduced tumour surveillance capacity. It is particularly relevant for ageing animals, those recovering from chronic disease or individuals with repeated respiratory or urinary infections. Animals with stable, well-managed immune-mediated disease may also benefit, though careful monitoring is required.

Respiratory conditions

Maitake does not act as a bronchodilator or acute anti-inflammatory agent, but its immune-regulatory effects make it useful in animals prone to recurrent respiratory infections, particularly those with compromised innate immunity or metabolic instability. Improved macrophage activity and balanced cytokine expression may assist in reducing infection recurrence.

Cardiovascular applications

The cardiovascular relevance of Maitake arises from its metabolic and anti-inflammatory effects. Animals with early cardiovascular vulnerability linked to metabolic strain may show gradual improvement in energy, resilience and exercise tolerance. Maitake is not used as a primary cardiovascular agent but may contribute to improved vascular tone and reduced inflammatory burden when integrated into appropriate protocols.

Oncology adjunctive use

Maitake holds substantial clinical interest in integrative oncology. Its β-glucans and polysaccharide–protein complexes can support tumour surveillance, improve immune competence and modulate inflammatory drivers that contribute to tumour progression. It is typically integrated with Turkey Tail (for immune priming) and Reishi (for systemic regulation and stress modulation). When used in animals undergoing chemotherapy or radiotherapy, Maitake may support treatment tolerance, appetite and energy, though monitoring is essential in fragile patients.

Senior and geriatric care

Older animals often present with overlapping metabolic strain, chronic inflammation, immune decline and cognitive vulnerability. Maitake's multi-system regulatory properties make it an appropriate foundational mushroom for geriatric support. Its actions are subtle and cumulative, often resulting in improved steadiness, enhanced resilience and healthier metabolic profiles over time.

Performance and working animals

Performance demands place metabolic, oxidative and inflammatory pressure on working animals. Maitake can support mitochondrial efficiency, modulate inflammatory tone and enhance immune resilience, contributing to quicker recovery and reduced susceptibility to post-exertional immune dips. It combines effectively with Cordyceps in this context.

Multi-systemic presentations

Maitake's clinical value is often most apparent in animals whose presentations cross metabolic, inflammatory and immune domains. Examples include ageing overweight dogs with chronic gastrointestinal fluctuation, early endocrine imbalance and recurrent infections. In these complex cases, Maitake functions as a terrain-orientated modulator, helping re-establish physiological coherence across multiple systems.

Integration with other functional mushrooms

Maitake's influence on insulin signalling, lipid metabolism, immune modulation and inflammatory balance makes it a central metabolic–immune mushroom in veterinary Mycotherapy. It pairs especially well with species that stabilise endocrine function, support mitochondrial resilience, reduce oxidative load or reinforce gut–brain physiology. The following combinations represent the most clinically relevant synergies in companion and performance animals.

- **With Reishi** - Maitake and Reishi form a stabilising metabolic–inflammatory pairing, particularly valuable for ageing animals, those with chronic low-grade inflammation, or individuals experiencing endocrine/metabolic fragility. Maitake modulates glucose uptake, insulin sensitivity and lipid pathways, while Reishi contributes triterpenoid-mediated immune regulation and hepatic steadiness. This combination supports animals with metabolic syndrome tendencies, inflammatory skin issues, stress-associated inflammatory cycles or age-related immune drift. Together, they harmonise metabolic signalling while moderating inflammatory tone.

- **With Turkey Tail** - Turkey Tail strengthens Maitake's immune and microbiome-regulating effects, making this pairing well suited for animals with recurrent infections, chronic immune fragility, dysbiosis or oncology-related immune burden. Maitake improves insulin and lipid pathways that often intersect with immune function, while Turkey Tail contributes PSP/PSK-mediated immune priming and gut–immune axis reinforcement. This synergistic pattern is ideal in animals with chronic inflammatory enteropathies, immune-suppressed states or those undergoing long-term integrative oncology care.

- **With Lion's Mane** - Lion's Mane adds a neurotrophic and gut–brain axis dimension to Maitake's metabolic and inflammatory actions. Animals with stress-linked gastrointestinal issues, behavioural fragility, or early cognitive changes may benefit from this pairing. Maitake supports glucose and lipid regulation that influence neurological resilience, while Lion's Mane promotes nerve growth factor pathways and enteric nervous system stability. This combination is particularly valuable for senior animals, individuals with metabolic–cognitive overlap, or those with digestive symptoms exacerbated by stress.

- **With Cordyceps** - Cordyceps complements Maitake's metabolic modulation by enhancing mitochondrial ATP production, oxygen utilisation and energy output. This pairing supports overweight or lethargic animals, senior animals with reduced vitality, and individuals recovering from chronic metabolic stress. Maitake moderates glucose and lipid pathways, while Cordyceps improves cellular performance and endurance capacity. The synergy is especially relevant for performance animals, metabolic–endocrine cases and those experiencing fatigue or reduced exercise tolerance.

- **With Golden Oyster** - Golden Oyster's ergothioneine-rich cytoprotective profile reinforces Maitake's metabolic and endocrine influence. ERGO provides mitochondrial protection, redox stability and cellular longevity, while Maitake regulates glucose transporters, lipid pathways and insulin sensitivity. Together, they support healthy ageing, metabolic harmony and resilience in animals with endocrine imbalance, obesity, chronic inflammation or long-standing metabolic strain. This combination is particularly relevant for senior animals, weight-management cases and those at risk of age-related metabolic decline.

> Synergistic pairings or triads of mushrooms can act across multiple physiological pathways, broadening the supportive effect and contributing to a full-spectrum, terrain-based Mycotherapy strategy.

6.14 Safety, contraindications and monitoring

General tolerability

Maitake is generally well tolerated across species, with a long history of culinary use supporting its safety. Gastrointestinal sensitivity is the most common adverse effect, typically limited to mild soft stools or transient digestive changes when introduced too quickly. Slow titration is advisable, especially in animals with gastrointestinal fragility or reduced digestive capacity.

Gastrointestinal sensitivity

Animals with inflammatory bowel tendencies, dysbiosis or heightened digestive sensitivity should begin with very small doses. The mushroom's fibre and polysaccharide content may alter motility and fermentation dynamics, so gradual introduction helps ensure stability. Any adverse change in stool quality, appetite or comfort warrants dose adjustment.

Coagulation considerations

Maitake is not known to exert strong anticoagulant effects, but its influence on inflammatory tone and vascular physiology may subtly interact with coagulation pathways. Caution is appropriate when used alongside non-steroidal anti-inflammatory drugs, corticosteroids, chemotherapeutic agents or anticoagulants. Monitoring for bruising, delayed clotting or abnormal bleeding is prudent.

Immune-mediated disease

In stable, well-managed autoimmune disorders, Maitake may be used with caution and close monitoring. Animals with unstable or active immune-mediated disease should avoid immune-modulating supplements until stabilised. Clear therapeutic rationale, slow titration and documented observation of clinical markers are essential.

Hepatic and renal cautions

Maitake's metabolic influence may benefit early hepatic stress, yet animals with advanced hepatic or renal disease require careful monitoring. Changes in hydration, appetite or biochemical values should guide dosing decisions. For animals receiving hepatically metabolised drugs, regular biochemical monitoring helps ensure safety.

Endocrine considerations

The most clinically significant interaction relates to insulin and hypoglycaemic medications. By improving insulin sensitivity, Maitake may alter glycaemic control in diabetic animals. Regular glucose monitoring is necessary in diabetic dogs and cats, particularly during the initial phases of integration.

Drug interaction risks

Maitake exhibits minimal direct interaction with cytochrome P450 pathways, but polypharmacy requires caution. Animals receiving medications with a narrow therapeutic index, chemotherapeutic regimens, behavioural drugs or endocrine modulators should be monitored for any shifts in clinical status as Maitake is introduced.

Pregnancy and lactation

Evidence in pregnancy and lactation is insufficient to ensure safety. Maitake should be avoided during pregnancy and lactation unless a veterinarian deems potential benefits to outweigh risks.

Paediatric considerations

Young animals generally tolerate Maitake well, but dosing must reflect body size, developmental stage and digestive maturity. Slow titration and close observation are recommended for puppies and kittens.

Species-specific cautions

Cats require particular care due to their unique hepatic metabolism and tendency toward gastrointestinal sensitivity. Dose adjustments, slower titration and careful observation are essential. Small dogs and geriatric animals also benefit from conservative dosing strategies.

SCWE as a safety advantage

SCWE-derived whole-mushroom preparations may offer enhanced tolerability due to improved solubility, reduced microbial load and more predictable gastrointestinal behaviour. However, extraction method does not negate the need for patient-specific monitoring.

Monitoring recommendations

Veterinarians should monitor appetite, stool quality, energy levels, glycaemic control (in diabetic animals), liver enzymes (when relevant) and overall behavioural tone during the integration of Maitake. Clear baseline markers and periodic reassessment support safe clinical use.

6.15 Veterinary considerations and therapeutic relevance

Terrain-based perspective

Within a terrain-based framework, Maitake is best understood as a regulator of interconnected physiological domains. By modulating immune tone, metabolic signalling and inflammatory load, Maitake supports a more adaptable internal environment. This ability to influence multiple axes simultaneously makes it valuable in complex or chronic presentations where single-target interventions fall short.

Ideal clinical profiles

Maitake aligns most closely with animals displaying early or moderate metabolic dysfunction, chronic low-grade inflammation, immune fatigue, gastrointestinal fragility or age-related physiological decline. It offers particular benefit where metabolic, inflammatory and immune systems intersect.

Integrative role

Maitake is rarely used in isolation. Its strength lies in its integration with diet, lifestyle modification, other medicinal mushrooms and conventional medical care. Its actions are cumulative and often synergistic, enhancing the efficacy of broader protocols designed to restore multi-system coherence.

Expected trajectory of benefits

Clinical improvements typically manifest gradually, reflecting systemic recalibration rather than immediate symptomatic relief. Common caregiver observations include steadier appetite, improved energy, better resilience to stress or infection, enhanced metabolic consistency and gentler ageing trajectories.

When to use cautiously

Caution is needed in animals with active immune-mediated disease, unstable endocrine disorders, advanced hepatic or renal compromise or those receiving medications with a narrow therapeutic index. Clinical judgement, conservative dosing and regular monitoring help ensure safe and effective integration.

6.16 Evidence quality commentary

Strengths of the evidence

Maitake is one of the better-researched medicinal mushrooms in terms of mechanistic and preclinical pathways. Multiple studies demonstrate effects across metabolic regulation, insulin sensitivity, hepatic lipid handling, inflammatory modulation and immune function. The biochemical and immunological properties of the major polysaccharide fractions (including D-fraction, MD-fraction, GF5000 and F2) have been repeatedly documented in vitro and in vivo. These mechanistic findings align closely with clinical patterns seen in companion animals, lending strong translational plausibility. Furthermore, Maitake demonstrates consistent compositional stability across growing regions, reducing variability in active constituents and supporting reliable therapeutic interpretation.

Limitations and gaps

Despite extensive preclinical work, veterinary-specific clinical trials remain limited. Most evidence derives from rodent models, cell culture research and human investigations into metabolic syndrome, cancer or immune modulation. While these studies are valuable for mechanistic insight, they cannot substitute for controlled trials in dogs, cats or horses. Additionally, some studies rely on isolated polysaccharide fractions rather than whole-mushroom preparations, which may overstate or under-represent the therapeutic value of full-spectrum extracts.

Translational reliability

Key metabolic and immunological pathways influenced by Maitake are highly conserved across mammalian species, supporting cautious extrapolation to veterinary practice. Mechanisms involving Dectin-1 signalling, complement receptor 3 activation, pattern-recognition receptor engagement and insulin receptor modulation are shared across species. However, dose–response relationships may differ, particularly in cats and in animals with compromised digestion, hepatic stress or immune dysregulation. SCWE-derived whole-mushroom extracts may enhance translational relevance by delivering compounds in a physiologically coherent matrix.

Species differences

Dogs and cats exhibit differences in digestion, hepatic metabolism and microbiome composition that may influence Maitake's clinical behaviour. Cats, in particular, require more conservative dosing because of their sensitivity to gastrointestinal changes and their unique hepatic enzymatic pathways. While the mechanistic evidence is strong, careful titration and monitoring are required to adapt findings to individual patients.

Extraction considerations in the evidence

A substantial proportion of Maitake research has focused on isolated fractions (especially D-fraction). These studies are scientifically useful but do not fully reflect the multi-constituent synergy central to Mycotherapy. More recent work evaluating whole-mushroom and SCWE extracts offers improved alignment with clinical use. SCWE techniques enhance accessibility of β-glucans, glycoproteins, phenolics and micronutrients, making these extracts more representative of full-spectrum therapeutic action.

Methodological variability

Extraction methods, cultivation practices and analytical approaches vary widely across published studies. These differences can influence reported bioactivity, complicating comparison across papers. Studies using whole fruiting bodies, defined extraction parameters and rigorous compositional analysis provide the most reliable data for clinical interpretation.

Overall appraisal

Maitake's evidence base is robust at the mechanistic level and moderately strong in preclinical models, with emerging-though limited-support from human research. Veterinary-specific clinical trials remain the main research gap. Despite this, the consistency of metabolic and immune pathways across mammals allows for clinically responsible integration within Mycotherapy when combined with appropriate monitoring and species-specific adjustments.

MAITAKE (GRIFOLA FRONDOSA) – Evidence Quality Commentary Table

This spectrum of evidence is summarised in the following table:

Domain	Evidence Strength	Primary Evidence Type
Immunomodulation	Moderate to high	Preclinical studies, β–glucan research, translational human and animal data
Metabolic regulation (glucose and insulin)	Moderate to high	Preclinical metabolic–syndrome models; translational human studies
Anti–inflammatory and antioxidant activity	Moderate	Preclinical cytokine and oxidative–stress studies
Gastrointestinal and microbiome support	Moderate	Preclinical GI anti–inflammatory models; microbial–modulating pathways
Hepatic and lipid metabolism support	Moderate	Preclinical lipid–regulation models; hepatoprotective data
Endocrine and reproductive balance	Emerging to moderate	Preclinical hormonal and ovarian–function studies (notably PCOS–related)
Neurological support and cognitive steadiness	Emerging	Preclinical neuroinflammatory and neuroprotective studies
Oncology adjunct use	Moderate	Human adjunct trials, preclinical models; well-recognised in integrative use
Bone and connective tissue support	Emerging	Preclinical osteogenic models

Domain	Evidence Strength	Primary Evidence Type
Clinical veterinary trials	Limited	Early-stage canine research; extrapolated translational rationale

Maitake is recognised for its robust β–glucan profile, particularly the **MD-fraction** and related proteoglucans, which exert potent immunomodulatory effects across both innate and adaptive immune pathways. These compounds enhance macrophage activation, improve dendritic-cell function and support NK-cell activity, making Maitake especially valuable in chronic immune instability, convalescence and oncology-related immune support. While veterinary-specific trials remain limited, the consistency of preclinical and translational findings offers a strong rationale for integrative use.

Its metabolic influence is one of Maitake's most distinctive strengths. Preclinical and translational human studies demonstrate improvements in insulin sensitivity, glucose regulation and lipid metabolism, supporting relevance in animals with metabolic imbalance, obesity-related inflammation or endocrine dysregulation. Maitake's effects on hepatic lipid pathways and oxidative stress also contribute to improved systemic steadiness in chronic inflammatory states.

Maitake provides additional benefit through modulation of gastrointestinal inflammation and microbiome dynamics. Its polysaccharides and prebiotic fibres help regulate mucosal integrity and microbial composition, making it supportive in animals with gastrointestinal sensitivity or concurrent immune–gut interplay. Early evidence suggests neuroprotective and endocrine-balancing effects, including in ovarian and stress-related pathways, though these domains remain emerging.

From a Mycotherapy standpoint, fidelity of extraction is essential. SCWE full-spectrum extracts retain Maitake's native β–glucans, proteoglucans, phenolics and fibre-bound micronutrients without the dilution effect seen in grain-based mycelium products. The resulting extract provides a stable, predictable biochemical matrix suitable for chronic, terrain-supportive protocols.

In integrative veterinary practice, Maitake is best positioned as a **multi-system regulator** – supporting immune steadiness, metabolic balance, gastrointestinal resilience and adjunctive oncology care. Its actions are gradual, cumulative and physiologically harmonising, aligning strongly with the principles of terrain-based Mycotherapy.

6.17 Conclusion – Integrative Significance and Extraction Considerations

Maitake occupies a central role within integrative veterinary practice as a mushroom that restores coherence across metabolic, immune and inflammatory systems. Its influence on insulin responsiveness, hepatic lipid handling, immune vigilance and inflammatory tone positions it as a key regulator for animals in which metabolic strain, chronic inflammation and immune fatigue coexist. This ability to harmonise multiple physiological axes gives Maitake particular relevance in ageing patients, overweight or insulin-resistant animals and those experiencing chronic low-grade inflammatory patterns that undermine vitality and resilience.

Its therapeutic effects emerge gradually, reflecting the regulatory nature of its polysaccharides, glycoproteins, phenolic compounds and fibre-bound constituents. When combined with complementary species such as Reishi for inflammatory steadiness, Turkey Tail for immune–microbiome support or Golden Oyster for cytoprotective resilience, Maitake contributes to a synergistic Mycotherapy framework that strengthens terrain stability rather than chasing isolated symptoms. Improvements in metabolic rhythm, gastrointestinal comfort, immune responsiveness and energy consistency typically unfold over weeks, aligning with the coordinated rebalancing of the systems Maitake influences.

Extraction fidelity is central to expressing Maitake's full therapeutic value. SCWE whole-mushroom extracts release high-molecular-weight β-glucans, polysaccharide–protein complexes and secondary metabolites in a form that remains structurally aligned with their natural context. By preserving both hydrophilic and lipophilic compounds, along with the native fibre matrix required for gut–immune engagement, SCWE preparations deliver a physiologically coherent extract suited to long-term metabolic and inflammatory regulation. Used thoughtfully and integrated within broader veterinary care plans, Maitake offers a safe, predictable and evidence-aligned contribution to restoring metabolic harmony and enhancing systemic resilience.

Maitake occupies a central role within integrative veterinary practice as a mushroom that restores coherence across metabolic, immune and inflammatory systems

Key sources (summary)

Adachi et al., 1994; Kodama & Nanba, 1999; Harada et al., 2002; Kubo et al., 1994; Xue et al., 2018; Horio et al., 2001; Yao et al., 2016; Bashir & Choi, 2018; Kodama et al., 2002; Konno et al., 2015; Chen et al., 2019; Sun & Lu, 2015; Wasser, 2011; Zhang et al., 2007; Ohno & Miura, 2017. **Full professional reference list available in the Master References section.**

> "The most primal - yet most critical - contributors to global health and the health of this planet are bacterial organisms. Their collaborative power to sustain longevity is unparalleled in anything humanity has ever known. - *Julie Anne Lee DCH RCSHom*"

7

SHIITAKE (Lentinula edodes)

7.1 Introduction to Shiitake – *The Immune Nourisher*

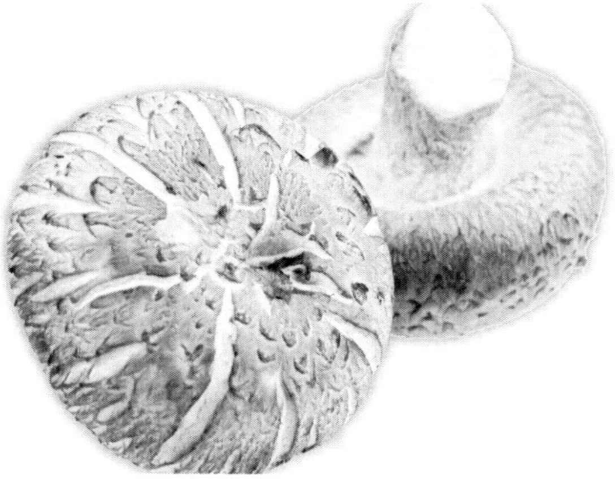

Shiitake (*Lentinula edodes*) occupies a foundational place in Mycotherapy as one of the most significant immune-nourishing mushrooms in clinical practice. Unlike species that function primarily as immune activators, Shiitake provides a balanced, supportive stimulus that enhances immunological coherence while simultaneously offering metabolic, hepatic and cardiovascular benefits. For centuries it has been valued in traditional medical systems for restoring vitality, supporting resilience, improving circulation and fortifying the body's defence mechanisms. Modern research now corroborates many of these traditional insights, identifying lentinan, eritadenine and a diverse array of polysaccharides, sterols and phenolic compounds as key contributors to Shiitake's multi-system influence.

Clinically, Shiitake's therapeutic profile is best described as immune nourishment rather than immune stimulation. This distinction is important in veterinary practice, where overstimulation or inappropriate immune activation can be counterproductive, especially in animals with chronic inflammatory tendencies or immune-mediated disease. Shiitake's β-glucans and associated compounds help support appropriate immune responsiveness, encourage healthier cytokine patterns and strengthen mucosal and systemic immune surveillance. These actions align closely with the needs of animals that experience repeated infections, immune fatigue, age-related decline or slow convalescence following chronic illness.

Shiitake occupies a foundational place in Mycotherapy as one of the most significant immune-nourishing mushrooms in clinical practice.

A defining feature of Shiitake is its strong relationship with hepatic and metabolic physiology. Through the activity of eritadenine, sterols and polysaccharides, Shiitake contributes to improved lipid metabolism, healthier cholesterol dynamics and reduced hepatic inflammatory signalling. These effects are particularly relevant in overweight animals, ageing dogs and cats with early hepatic changes, metabolic vulnerability or low-grade inflammatory patterns. Improved hepatic clarity often coincides with enhanced immune steadiness, highlighting the interconnected nature of Shiitake's physiological influence.

As with other medicinal mushrooms, the accessibility of Shiitake's bioactive matrix depends on appropriate extraction. The fruiting body contains a robust chitinous cell wall that encapsulates lentinan, polysaccharide–protein complexes and phenolic compounds. Sub-critical water extraction (SCWE) enhances the release of these constituents by penetrating the cell wall and solubilising polysaccharides at controlled temperatures and pressures. This produces extracts that are closer to the mushroom's natural biochemical profile and more readily recognised by the gastrointestinal immune network. For veterinary patients, particularly those with digestive compromise or metabolic strain, SCWE-derived whole-mushroom preparations may offer improved physiological compatibility and a more predictable therapeutic effect.

Shiitake's clinical relevance is particularly strong in cases of immune depletion, chronic infection susceptibility, hepatic strain, metabolic dysregulation and generalised inflammatory burden. It supports the ageing terrain, enhances resilience in recovery phases, and provides a steady foundation for animals facing cumulative physiological stress. Its actions are subtle yet powerful, reflecting a long trajectory of gradual restoration rather than rapid symptomatic change. Shiitake integrates naturally with Turkey Tail in immune-heavy cases, with Reishi for inflammatory and stress-linked patterns, and with Maitake where metabolic imbalance or hepatic challenges are present.

Within modern veterinary Mycotherapy, Shiitake is considered one of the core species for maintaining immune nourishment, metabolic clarity and terrain-level resilience. Its balanced and physiologically supportive nature makes it a dependable mushroom for long-term integrative protocols aimed at fortifying whole-body health across multiple interconnected systems.

7.2 Taxonomy, morphology and extract science

Shiitake (*Lentinula edodes*) is a basidiomycete within the family Omphalotaceae. It is one of the oldest cultivated mushrooms used for both culinary and medicinal purposes, with a long-standing reputation for supporting vitality, immune nourishment and metabolic steadiness. Taxonomically, *L. edodes* is highly consistent in its biochemical architecture, particularly regarding its polysaccharide and β-glucan configuration, making it a reliable species for clinical use. This consistency is advantageous for Mycotherapy, where reproducibility of active constituents contributes to predictable therapeutic effects.

Morphologically, Shiitake forms a fleshy, brown cap with white gills and a firm stipe. The fruiting body contains a dense chitinous cell wall that encapsulates lentinan, eritadenine and a wide range of polysaccharides, sterols and phenolic compounds. This architectural robustness provides structural protection but simultaneously restricts access to bioactive compounds when consumed raw or minimally processed. The chitin–glucan matrix is resistant to digestive enzymes in dogs and cats, reducing the availability of key polysaccharides unless the cell wall is adequately broken down through cooking or extraction.

Shiitake's cell-wall architecture has significant implications for extraction science. Traditional culinary preparation (such as simmering) can release some bioactive compounds, but the liberation of high-molecular-weight lentinan and many of the polysaccharide–protein complexes requires higher temperatures, pressure and specific solvent conditions. Classical hot-water extraction has historically been used to produce lentinan-rich fractions for research and clinical settings. However, such isolated fractions do not fully represent the mushroom's complete biochemical matrix, which includes synergistic molecules that contribute to immune nourishment, metabolic clarity and hepatic modulation.

Sub-critical water extraction (SCWE) offers a more holistic and physiologically compatible approach for producing whole-mushroom extracts. SCWE uses water in a semi-compressed state with enhanced solvating power, allowing deeper penetration into the chitinous barrier and more efficient release of lentinan, polysaccharide–protein complexes, sterols, phenolics and heat-sensitive micronutrients. This method preserves the mushroom's synergistic profile while reducing degradation of redox-active compounds. For veterinary care, SCWE-derived extracts offer improved solubility, better gastrointestinal compatibility and more reliable interaction with gut-associated lymphoid tissues.

Shiitake's responsiveness to extraction reinforces its clinical positioning as an 'immune nourisher'. While raw or powdered forms provide pre-biotic fibre, therapeutic activity depends on the liberation of lentinan and related polysaccharides. SCWE enhances this availability while maintaining whole-mushroom integrity, making it particularly suitable for animals with digestive vulnerability, immune fatigue or metabolic strain.

From a veterinary perspective, Shiitake's structural consistency, biochemical richness and favourable extraction responsiveness underpin its therapeutic reliability. When appropriately extracted, Shiitake offers a physiologically coherent combination of immune nourishment, metabolic modulation and hepatic support, making it a central species within integrative Mycotherapy protocols.

> Shiitake's therapeutic breadth reflects the coordinated activity of multiple bioactive constituents, with lentinan serving as the most prominent.

7.3 Bioactive constituents – mechanistic relevance

Shiitake's therapeutic breadth reflects the coordinated activity of multiple bioactive constituents, with lentinan serving as the most prominent. However, the mushroom's full clinical profile arises from the synergistic actions of polysaccharides, polysaccharide–protein complexes, sterols, lipids, phenolic compounds, micronutrients and unique secondary metabolites such as eritadenine. These compounds interact across immune, metabolic, inflammatory and hepatic systems, contributing to Shiitake's identity as an immune nourisher and metabolic stabiliser.

Lentinan and the β-glucan architecture

Lentinan is a highly purified 1,3-β-glucan with 1,6-branching, distinctive to *L. edodes*. It has been extensively studied for its immunomodulatory effects, particularly within oncology and chronic immune compromise. Lentinan interacts with Dectin-1 receptors, complement receptor 3 and toll-like receptors in the gut-associated lymphoid tissue, initiating balanced activation of innate and adaptive immune pathways. Unlike strong immune stimulants, lentinan promotes healthier cytokine patterns, enhances antigen presentation and improves natural killer cell function while maintaining regulatory immune tone.

In veterinary contexts, this translates to improved immune resilience in animals with recurrent infections, immune fatigue or reduced tumour surveillance capacity. Lentinan's ability to support immune competence without disruptive overstimulation makes Shiitake a suitable option in chronic immune strain, early senescence or recovery following disease.

Eritadenine and lipid metabolism

Eritadenine is a unique compound found almost exclusively in Shiitake. It modulates lipid metabolism by altering phospholipid methylation, improving cholesterol clearance and supporting healthier hepatic lipid profiles. Preclinical studies show reductions in total cholesterol, triglycerides and low-density lipoprotein concentrations following eritadenine exposure.

For veterinary patients, these metabolic effects have relevance in overweight dogs, pre-diabetic cats, animals with early hepatic steatosis or those presenting with metabolic-linked inflammatory strain. Eritadenine's influence also supports cardiovascular stability indirectly through improved lipid dynamics.

Polysaccharide–protein complexes

Shiitake contains a diverse array of polysaccharide–protein complexes that complement lentinan's immunological actions. These complexes can modulate macrophage behaviour, influence dendritic cell activity and help maintain appropriate cytokine balance. Their presence contributes to the gentle yet steady immune nourishment characteristic of Shiitake, making it well suited for long-term integrative strategies in chronic disease, convalescence and ageing.

Sterols, fatty acids and phenolic compounds

Sterols (including ergosterol), lipid fractions and phenolic compounds contribute to Shiitake's antioxidant capacity. These molecules support cellular redox balance, reduce oxidative stress and help stabilise tissues affected by chronic inflammation or metabolic inefficiency. The antioxidant influence of these compounds may protect hepatic and immune cells from free-radical-mediated damage, reinforcing Shiitake's suitability in degenerative and chronic inflammatory patterns.

Pre-biotic fibres and microbiome modulation

Shiitake's fibre profile supports beneficial gut microbiota, enhancing short-chain fatty acid production and contributing to intestinal barrier integrity. This pre-biotic activity aligns with Shiitake's broader role in immune nourishment, as a healthy microbiome contributes to balanced mucosal immunity, metabolic steadiness and reduced systemic inflammatory load.

Synergistic matrix effects

The combined action of lentinan, eritadenine, sterols, phenolics and polysaccharide–protein complexes establishes Shiitake as a multi-system modulator. Rather than producing sharp or aggressive therapeutic effects, Shiitake strengthens foundational physiological processes, supports immune resilience and enhances metabolic clarity. For integrative veterinary practice, this makes it one of the most versatile mushrooms for chronic conditions, recovery states, immune maintenance and long-term terrain support.

7.4 Immune system modulation

Shiitake is renowned for its ability to nourish and regulate immune function. It does not act as an aggressive immune stimulant but instead supports the recalibration of innate and adaptive responses through balanced β-glucan signalling. This quality makes Shiitake particularly valuable in animals experiencing immune fatigue, chronic infection susceptibility, age-related immunosenescence or slow convalescence following illness.

Lentinan, Shiitake's signature β-glucan, interacts primarily with Dectin-1, complement receptor 3 and specific toll-like receptors within the gut-associated lymphoid tissue. Engagement of these receptors promotes macrophage activation, enhances natural killer cell function, encourages effective dendritic cell presentation and supports balanced T-helper cell responses. This modulation improves immune vigilance but avoids excessive or dysregulated activity, an essential characteristic in veterinary contexts where overstimulation can exacerbate inflammatory or immune-mediated disorders.

> Shiitake is renowned for its ability to nourish and regulate immune function.

Preclinical work consistently demonstrates that lentinan enhances innate immune surveillance, increases interferon-γ and interleukin-12 expression and supports cytotoxic immune pathways relevant to infectious defence and oncology. Importantly, these effects occur alongside mechanisms that maintain regulatory immune tone. Rather than pushing the immune system into high reactivity, Shiitake improves its capacity to respond appropriately to physiological challenges.

Shiitake's immune-nourishing actions extend to mucosal immunity. The mushroom's polysaccharides support IgA-related pathways, reinforce mucosal barrier integrity and promote healthier microbial ecosystems, all of which contribute to improved first-line defence in the gastrointestinal, respiratory and urogenital tracts. In clinical practice, this may benefit animals with repeated upper respiratory infections, chronic otitis, recurrent urinary tract infections or general susceptibility to opportunistic pathogens.

Its balanced immunological profile makes Shiitake suitable for long-term use in older animals, those recovering from chronic disease or individuals exposed to prolonged stress. In immune-mediated disorders, Shiitake may be used cautiously once stability has been established, provided therapeutic goals are clear and monitoring is consistent.

7.5 Inflammation and oxidative stress pathways

Shiitake exerts a broad regulatory influence on inflammatory and oxidative pathways, contributing to terrain-level physiological balance. Its polysaccharides, lentinan, eritadenine and phenolic compounds act across multiple molecular sites to modulate inflammatory signalling, reduce oxidative burden and improve tissue resilience.

Lentinan modulates inflammatory cascades through its interaction with Dectin-1 and toll-like receptors, leading to improved cytokine balance and attenuation of pro-inflammatory mediators. Preclinical research indicates that Shiitake can reduce concentrations of tumour necrosis factor-α, interleukin-6 and other inflammatory intermediaries associated with chronic disease, metabolic impairment and degenerative processes. These effects are particularly relevant for older animals or those with conditions driven by chronic low-grade inflammation.

Shiitake's influence on oxidative stress stems from its phenolic compounds, ergosterol derivatives and antioxidant-linked polysaccharide structures. These constituents support endogenous antioxidant enzymes such as superoxide dismutase and glutathione peroxidase, helping to counter free radical damage that contributes to cellular ageing, neuroinflammation and hepatic strain. Improved oxidative balance can enhance resilience in animals with chronic inflammatory diseases, metabolic imbalances or high oxidative demand due to age or workload.

Eritadenine further contributes to inflammatory modulation by influencing lipid metabolism and improving hepatic function. Reduced hepatic lipid accumulation and improved vascular lipid profiles can indirectly lower systemic inflammatory load, supporting healthier cardiovascular and metabolic pathways. These interconnected actions reflect Shiitake's broad relevance to animals with metabolic fragility, early hepatic stress, cardiovascular vulnerability or generalised inflammatory tendencies.

In clinical settings, Shiitake is not used as a rapid anti-inflammatory agent. Instead, its effects unfold gradually as inflammatory tone is moderated and redox equilibrium improves. Its value lies in supporting chronic inflammatory conditions, age-related degeneration, immune-linked inflammatory burdens and systemic oxidative stress. Integrative protocols often combine Shiitake with Reishi for more targeted inflammatory regulation or with Maitake where metabolic-inflammatory patterns coexist.

> Shiitake's value lies in supporting chronic inflammatory conditions, age-related degeneration, immune-linked inflammatory burdens and systemic oxidative stress.

7.6 Gastrointestinal, microbiome and metabolic health

Shiitake plays a significant role in supporting gastrointestinal integrity, microbiome composition and metabolic homeostasis. Its polysaccharides and fibre fractions function as pre-biotic substrates that nourish beneficial bacteria, contribute to short-chain fatty acid production and improve mucosal immunity. These mechanisms support healthier digestion, enhanced barrier function and reduced inflammatory signalling arising from dysbiosis.

Prebiotic effects of Shiitake include increases in butyrate-producing bacteria, which improve epithelial health and lower pro-inflammatory cytokine expression. A healthier microbiome supports immune balance, metabolic stability and gastrointestinal comfort. These effects are particularly valuable for animals experiencing chronic soft stools, intermittent gastrointestinal disturbance, stress-linked gut dysregulation or age-related decline in microbial diversity.

Shiitake's influence on hepatic and metabolic pathways further enhances its gastrointestinal relevance. Eritadenine's modulatory effects on lipid metabolism and cholesterol handling can reduce hepatic strain, improving digestive efficiency and metabolic clarity. By reducing lipotoxicity and supporting hepatic function, Shiitake indirectly supports gastrointestinal resilience, especially in overweight animals or those with early hepatic compromise.

The mushroom's polysaccharides may also influence glycaemic patterns and metabolic steadiness. While less potent in this domain than Maitake, Shiitake still contributes meaningfully through gut-mediated metabolic signalling and improvement of hepatic function. For animals with metabolic fragility, early insulin resistance or chronic inflammatory–metabolic interplay, Shiitake offers a supportive modulatory role.

Clinically, Shiitake integrates well in gastrointestinal protocols for animals with chronic or recurrent issues, particularly when combined with rehydration support, dietary adjustments, probiotics or other mushrooms such as Turkey Tail (gut immunity) or Lion's Mane (gut–brain coherence). Its effects emerge progressively and reflect the restoration of microbial, mucosal and metabolic harmony rather than acute symptomatic shifts.

> Prebiotic effects of Shiitake include increases in butyrate-producing bacteria, which improve epithelial health and lower pro-inflammatory cytokine expression.

7.7 Neurological and behavioural health

Shiitake's direct neurological actions are comparatively modest when contrasted with strongly neurotrophic mushrooms such as Lion's Mane. However, its indirect influence on neurological and behavioural health is significant due to its regulatory effects on immune tone, inflammatory pathways, metabolic balance and oxidative stress. These interconnected mechanisms contribute to improved neuroimmune signalling, steadier behavioural patterns and enhanced resilience during periods of chronic or systemic stress.

Chronic inflammation and metabolic dysfunction are increasingly recognised as contributors to neurobehavioural change in animals, including reduced vitality, irritability, disrupted sleep–wake cycles and declines in cognitive steadiness. Shiitake's ability to moderate inflammatory intermediaries, support hepatic function and soothe metabolic strain may indirectly alleviate neurological stress. Improved immune nourishment reduces inflammatory burden across the gut–brain axis, supporting steadier behaviour and improved cognitive resilience in ageing animals.

Shiitake also contributes indirectly to behavioural stability through its influence on gastrointestinal health. Dysbiosis and impaired gut integrity can affect neurotransmitter balance, vagal signalling and stress physiology. By supporting healthier microbiota and mucosal immunity, Shiitake helps restore communication along the gut–brain axis. This may benefit animals displaying stress-related gastrointestinal disturbances, low resilience during routine environmental stressors or behavioural changes linked to chronic illness.

In integrative practice, Shiitake is rarely used as a primary neurological mushroom. Instead, it plays a supportive role alongside Lion's Mane for neurocognitive support or Reishi for stress-related behavioural dysregulation. In this context, Shiitake provides the metabolic, immune and inflammatory foundation that allows more targeted neurotrophic interventions to be effective.

7.8 Cardiovascular and respiratory physiology

Shiitake contributes meaningfully to cardiovascular health through its effects on lipid metabolism, endothelial function, vascular inflammation and oxidative stress. Eritadenine, one of Shiitake's most distinctive compounds, supports cholesterol clearance and normalises lipid profiles by modulating phospholipid metabolism. Preclinical studies demonstrate reductions in total cholesterol, triglycerides and low-density lipoproteins, with improvements in high-density lipoprotein function. These actions reduce vascular strain and help maintain cardiovascular resilience, particularly in ageing or overweight animals.

Shiitake's antioxidant and anti-inflammatory effects further support cardiovascular function by reducing endothelial stress and improving microvascular integrity. Phenolic compounds and ergosterol derivatives help scavenge free radicals and stabilise vascular tissues affected by metabolic and inflammatory processes. For animals presenting with early cardiovascular vulnerability, metabolic syndrome or chronic inflammatory states, these cumulative benefits may enhance cardiovascular endurance and overall vitality.

Respiratory physiology benefits indirectly from Shiitake's immune-nourishing effects. Enhanced mucosal immunity, improved macrophage responsiveness and healthier inflammatory modulation support the respiratory tract's first-line defence. This is particularly relevant for animals prone to recurrent respiratory infections, chronic bronchitis or environmental stressors that compromise respiratory resilience. While Shiitake is not a bronchodilator or acute respiratory therapeutic, it contributes to reduced infection recurrence and improved mucosal integrity over time.

In clinical settings, Shiitake integrates effectively with cardiovascular-supportive mushrooms such as Reishi, and with respiratory immune modulators like Turkey Tail. Its role in cardiovascular and respiratory health is subtle yet steady, emerging through improved metabolic clarity, immune strength and vascular stability.

7.9 Oncology and adjunctive cancer support

Shiitake holds a prominent place in integrative oncology, primarily due to the immunomodulatory properties of lentinan. Lentinan has been the subject of extensive research in human medicine, where it has been used as an adjunctive therapy to support immune competence, enhance treatment tolerance and improve quality of life during chemotherapy. Although veterinary-specific trials remain limited, the mechanistic and translational evidence provides a strong rationale for its cautious integration into oncology protocols for companion animals.

Lentinan enhances anti-tumour immunity by stimulating macrophages, natural killer cells and cytotoxic T-lymphocyte activity. It also supports healthier cytokine profiles that promote tumour surveillance while reducing chronic inflammation that may facilitate tumour progression. The ability of lentinan to modulate immune competence without causing dysregulated immune activation is a notable advantage in oncology, where balance and regulation are critical for patient safety.

Beyond immune-focused mechanisms, Shiitake provides metabolic and hepatic support that may improve overall tolerance to conventional cancer therapies. By reducing oxidative stress and supporting hepatic detoxification pathways, Shiitake may contribute to steadier energy, improved appetite and better resilience during treatment. Its influence on the gut–immune interface can also help mitigate gastrointestinal strain commonly experienced during chemotherapy or chronic disease.

Preclinical studies indicate that Shiitake extracts may reduce tumour proliferation in vitro and modulate signalling pathways involved in tumour micro-environment activity. While these findings are not species-specific to dogs or cats, the conserved nature of immune and metabolic pathways across mammals suggests relevance when integrated thoughtfully into multimodal care.

In practice, Shiitake is often paired with Turkey Tail (for potent immune priming) and Reishi (for inflammatory regulation, stress physiology and metabolic stability). The combination creates a multi-axis approach that supports immune surveillance, systemic resilience and treatment tolerance. As with all oncology adjuncts, clear communication with the treating veterinarian, careful monitoring and appropriate dose adjustments are essential.

> Shiitake holds a prominent place in integrative oncology, primarily due to the immunomodulatory properties of lentinan

7.10 Hepatic and renal physiology

Shiitake offers clinically meaningful support for hepatic physiology through its influence on lipid metabolism, detoxification processes, oxidative balance and inflammatory modulation. Eritadenine, the mushroom's distinctive metabolic compound, plays a central role in enhancing hepatic lipid handling. By modulating phospholipid methylation and improving cholesterol excretion, eritadenine can reduce hepatic lipid accumulation and support healthier hepatocyte function. These effects are particularly relevant in overweight dogs, pre-diabetic cats and ageing animals with mild hepatic enzyme elevations or early fatty liver tendencies.

Shiitake's polysaccharides and sterol fractions contribute additional hepatoprotective actions. Phenolic compounds and ergosterol derivatives support antioxidant defences, helping to counter oxidative injury that often accompanies hepatic inflammation or metabolic strain. Improved oxidative balance enhances hepatocellular resilience, supporting animals with chronic low-grade inflammation, early hepatic compromise or systemic disease that places metabolic demand on the liver.

The mushroom's impact on hepatic inflammation is another important clinical consideration. Preclinical studies indicate that Shiitake can reduce pro-inflammatory cytokines associated with hepatic stress, potentially easing inflammatory burden in the early stages of metabolic or inflammatory liver disease. This aligns with its traditional use as a restorative agent for energy, vitality and internal balance.

Renal physiology is influenced more indirectly. Shiitake does not have strong diuretic or nephroprotective actions, but its metabolic and antioxidant properties may support healthier renal resilience in ageing animals or those with chronic inflammatory burden. No evidence suggests nephrotoxicity at nutritional–therapeutic doses. However, animals with advanced renal disease require tailored dosing and careful monitoring, as changes in hydration or metabolic balance may alter tolerability.

From a veterinary perspective, Shiitake is most appropriate for animals with early hepatic stress, metabolic-linked liver strain, oxidative burden or chronic inflammatory presentations. Its hepatic support integrates well with dietary adjustments, antioxidants, hepatoprotective herbs and metabolic-regulating mushrooms such as Maitake. In renal cases, cautious use with close observation is recommended, particularly in cats or animals with compromised hydration or electrolyte balance.

7.11 Endocrine and metabolic regulation

Shiitake exerts meaningful influence across multiple endocrine and metabolic pathways, though its activity is subtler than the strongly metabolic mushrooms such as Maitake. Its effects arise primarily through improvements in lipid metabolism, hepatic function, inflammatory modulation and microbiome health, which collectively contribute to endocrine steadiness and enhanced metabolic resilience.

Eritadenine is central to Shiitake's metabolic relevance. By improving cholesterol clearance and modulating lipid profiles, eritadenine reduces hepatic and vascular strain, indirectly supporting endocrine harmony. Dyslipidaemia, chronic inflammation and hepatic burden can all disrupt endocrine function in animals, particularly affecting insulin regulation, thyroid dynamics and adrenal tone. By reducing metabolic friction across these systems, Shiitake contributes to a more stable endocrine environment.

Shiitake's polysaccharides may also influence glucose metabolism through improvements in hepatic function, reduced inflammatory interference and healthier gut–metabolic signalling. While not as potent as Maitake in modulating insulin sensitivity, Shiitake still contributes to more stable glycaemic patterns in animals with metabolic fragility, early insulin resistance or chronic inflammatory–metabolic interplay.

In overweight or ageing animals, improvements in lipid handling, oxidative balance and inflammatory tone can support better energy utilisation, reduced metabolic fatigue and improved vitality. These effects are gradual and terrain-orientated, reflecting Shiitake's role as a metabolic harmoniser rather than a direct endocrine intervention.

In clinical practice, Shiitake is suitable for animals with early metabolic dysregulation, overweight conditions, mild dyslipidaemia, chronic inflammatory states or metabolic-linked hepatic strain. It integrates effectively with Maitake for stronger metabolic support, Reishi for inflammatory–endocrine alignment and Turkey Tail for immune–metabolic coherence. Diabetic animals may use Shiitake safely, though blood glucose monitoring is still recommended when metabolic patterns begin to stabilise.

7.12 Veterinary pharmacology and drug interaction considerations

Absorption and bioavailability

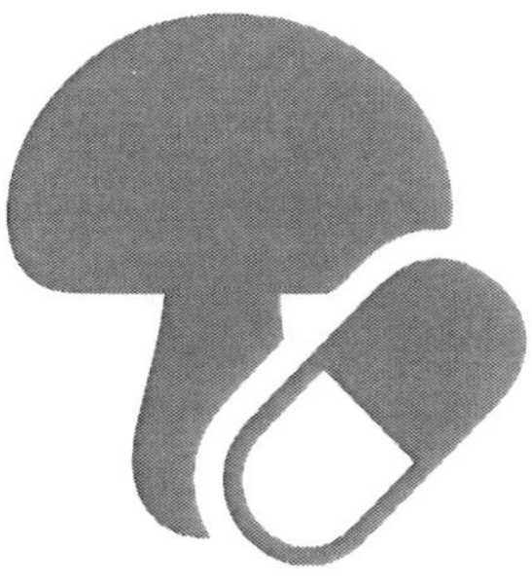

Shiitake's primary bioactive compounds are not absorbed systemically in their intact high-molecular-weight form. Instead, lentinan and other polysaccharides interact with receptors in the gut-associated lymphoid tissue, initiating immune and inflammatory modulation at the mucosal interface. Smaller oligosaccharides, sterols and phenolics may enter circulation and contribute to metabolic and hepatic activity. Animals with gastrointestinal fragility may exhibit altered receptor responsiveness, making slow titration advisable.

Hepatic metabolism and detoxification pathways

Shiitake influences hepatic function indirectly through improvements in lipid metabolism, reduced oxidative stress and moderated inflammatory cascades. These actions may support hepatic detoxification capacity, particularly in ageing or metabolically strained animals. However, animals with advanced hepatic disease require conservative dosing and monitoring, as any change in metabolic balance or gastrointestinal motility may alter drug handling.

Cytochrome P450 considerations

Current evidence indicates that Shiitake does not significantly induce or inhibit cytochrome P450 enzymes at nutritional–therapeutic doses. However, variability in extraction methods and concentrations across preparations necessitates prudent monitoring when used alongside medications with narrow therapeutic indices or heavy reliance on hepatic clearance.

Coagulation and platelet activity

Shiitake does not exert strong anticoagulant effects, but mild modulation of inflammatory pathways and vascular physiology may influence platelet behaviour in sensitive individuals. Caution is appropriate when used concurrently with anticoagulants, corticosteroids, non-steroidal anti-inflammatory drugs or chemotherapeutic agents. Monitoring for bruising, delayed clotting or abnormal bleeding remains prudent.

Sedative and neurological medication interactions

Shiitake does not have direct sedative or neuroactive effects, making interactions with behavioural or neurological medications unlikely. Any observed behavioural shifts are typically secondary to improved metabolic or inflammatory balance. Animals on anticonvulsants or behavioural medications may use Shiitake safely, but monitoring for subtle changes in sleep, behaviour or appetite is good practice.

Endocrine medication interactions

Shiitake may indirectly support endocrine stability, but it does not typically interact with thyroid medications, adrenal therapies or reproductive hormones. The most clinically relevant interaction pertains to animals on insulin or hypoglycaemic agents. Improvements in metabolic steadiness may alter glycaemic demands, necessitating routine glucose monitoring.

Gastrointestinal absorption considerations

Shiitake's fibre and polysaccharide profile can influence gastrointestinal motility and may affect the absorption of certain oral medications, particularly those requiring narrow absorption windows. When necessary, administering medications at a separate time from mushroom dosing (one to two hours apart) may improve consistency.

Polypharmacy and safe-use practice

For animals receiving multiple medications, especially in oncology, chronic inflammatory disease or endocrine disorders, Shiitake should be introduced methodically with clear therapeutic goals and defined monitoring parameters. Documenting behavioural, metabolic and gastrointestinal changes supports safe integration.

Species-specific considerations

Cats may exhibit digestive sensitivity to Shiitake's fibre profile and require slower titration. Small dogs, geriatric animals and those with chronic gastrointestinal instability also benefit from conservative introduction. SCWE-derived extracts may improve tolerability by reducing insoluble fibre load and enhancing solubility.

7.13 Clinical application in veterinary practice

Dermatological conditions

Shiitake offers value in dermatological presentations where immune nourishment, microbial balance and inflammatory modulation are needed. Its influence on mucosal and systemic immunity may support animals with recurrent pyoderma, chronic otitis or superficial infections linked to immune fatigue. While Shiitake is not a primary dermatological agent, its capacity to rebalance immune tone and reduce inflammatory burden can assist in stabilising chronic or recurrent skin issues, particularly those influenced by metabolic or hepatic strain.

Gastrointestinal disorders

Shiitake provides gentle support to gastrointestinal health through its pre-biotic fibres, microbiome-modulating effects and ability to strengthen mucosal immunity. Animals with chronic soft stools, environmental stress-linked gastrointestinal disturbance or mild dysbiosis may respond positively as microbial populations stabilise. Shiitake integrates well with dietary modification and probiotics, and pairs effectively with Turkey Tail for immune–gut synergy or Lion's Mane for gut–brain–mucosal coherence.

Hepatic disease

Shiitake is particularly relevant in early hepatic dysfunction and metabolic-linked liver strain. Eritadenine's effects on lipid clearance and cholesterol metabolism help reduce hepatic burden, while the mushroom's antioxidant constituents support hepatocyte resilience. Veterinary applications include animals with modest liver enzyme elevations, early steatosis, metabolic-linked hepatic inflammation and ageing animals whose hepatic reserve is declining. It is not a substitute for hepatoprotective medications, but provides meaningful support within integrative protocols.

Behavioural medicine and stress physiology

Behavioural benefits associated with Shiitake arise from indirect pathways rather than direct neurotrophic action. Improvements in gut health, reduced systemic inflammation and more stable metabolic signalling can enhance behavioural steadiness. Animals showing stress-linked gastrointestinal fluctuations, low resilience or behavioural changes secondary to chronic disease may benefit when Shiitake is used alongside targeted behavioural therapies, Lion's Mane or Reishi.

Immune dysregulation

Shiitake is best suited for immune nourishment rather than aggressive immune stimulation. It is useful in animals with recurrent infections, immune fatigue, chronic convalescence or age-related immune decline. Its actions promote healthier cytokine patterns, improved antigen presentation and enhanced mucosal surveillance. In stable immune-mediated conditions, Shiitake may be used cautiously under veterinary supervision, provided monitoring is clear and consistent.

Respiratory conditions

Shiitake supports respiratory resilience through improved mucosal immunity and balanced inflammatory responses. Animals prone to recurrent respiratory infections or environmental respiratory stressors may benefit from strengthened mucosal defences and more balanced immune readiness. While not appropriate for acute respiratory distress, Shiitake provides valuable background support for chronic or susceptibility-based conditions.

Cardiovascular applications

Shiitake's cardiovascular relevance stems from eritadenine-mediated lipid modulation, antioxidant action and improvements in vascular inflammatory tone. Animals with early cardiovascular vulnerability, chronic inflammatory burden or metabolic dysregulation may demonstrate improved vitality and endurance over time. Shiitake is best used as part of a broader metabolic–vascular plan rather than as a primary cardiovascular intervention.

Oncology adjunctive use

Shiitake is well established within integrative oncology frameworks due to lentinan's immunomodulatory properties. Its ability to strengthen tumour surveillance mechanisms, improve immune competence and support treatment tolerance makes it appropriate in long-term oncology care. Veterinarians often combine Shiitake with Turkey Tail for immune activation profiles and Reishi for inflammatory and stress-modulating synergy. Monitoring is essential, particularly for animals receiving chemotherapy, immunosuppressants or complex polypharmacy.

Senior and geriatric care

In ageing animals, Shiitake supports immune nourishment, metabolic steadiness, hepatic resilience and oxidative balance. These cumulative effects improve vitality, infection resistance and overall ageing trajectories. Shiitake's gentle, non-stimulatory profile makes it suitable for long-term integration into geriatric care, often in combination with Reishi and Maitake.

Performance and working animals

Performance animals experience metabolic strain, respiratory challenge and increased oxidative demand. Shiitake may contribute to improved resilience, reduced susceptibility to post-exertional infections and more stable recovery patterns. While Cordyceps remains the primary mushroom for performance, Shiitake complements it by supporting immune and hepatic functions.

Multi-systemic presentations

Shiitake is particularly suitable for animals with overlapping metabolic, immune and gastrointestinal vulnerabilities. Examples include overweight ageing dogs with intermittent gastrointestinal sensitivity, recurrent infections and early hepatic strain. Its multi-axis actions make it a dependable component of long-term terrain support.

Integration with other functional mushrooms

Shiitake is a versatile metabolic–immune mushroom with applications across cardiovascular steadiness, immune modulation, hepatic function and digestive support. Its lentinan (β-glucan), eritadenine, polyphenols and prebiotic matrix make it highly compatible with species that influence immune tone, metabolic pathways, antioxidant balance and the gut–brain axis. The pairings below represent the most clinically relevant combinations in veterinary Mycotherapy.

- **With Reishi** - Shiitake pairs naturally with Reishi in cases requiring moderated immune activity, hepatic support and inflammation control. Reishi's triterpenoids influence mast-cell behaviour and autonomic steadiness, while Shiitake contributes lentinan-mediated immune modulation and eritadenine-associated hepatic balance. This combination is useful in chronic inflammatory skin conditions, mild hepatic compromise, environmental allergies and age-related immune drift. It provides a foundational pairing for animals needing gentle yet dependable immune and hepatic support.

- **With Maitake** - Shiitake and Maitake offer complementary metabolic and antioxidant actions, making this pairing especially relevant for animals with metabolic vulnerability, weight concerns, chronic inflammation or endocrine imbalance. Maitake enhances insulin signalling and lipid metabolism, while Shiitake supports lipid modulation, digestive steadiness and hepatic resilience. Together they reinforce metabolic harmony and oxidative balance. The synergy is particularly helpful in overweight animals, early metabolic dysregulation and cases where digestive symptoms accompany endocrine shifts.

- **With Turkey Tail**- Turkey Tail augments Shiitake's immune and gastrointestinal contributions, creating a supportive combination for animals with recurrent infections, chronic immune suppression or oncology-directed needs. Shiitake provides lentinan-mediated immune modulation and prebiotic support, while Turkey Tail contributes PSP/PSK-associated immune reinforcement and improved immune surveillance. This pairing is relevant for integrative oncology care, chronic infection patterns, age-related immune decline and gastrointestinal–immune fragility.

- **With Lion's Mane** - Lion's Mane offers neurotrophic and gut–brain axis benefits that integrate well with Shiitake's digestive and prebiotic actions. This pairing is suited to animals with stress-linked digestive issues, chronic gastrointestinal sensitivity or behavioural fragility associated with digestive discomfort. Shiitake stabilises digestion, supports microbiome balance and contributes prebiotic fibre, while Lion's Mane supports mucosal–neural repair and vagal tone regulation. Together they provide a gentle yet effective foundation for gut–brain resilience.

- **With Golden Oyster** - Shiitake and Golden Oyster provide a compelling cardiometabolic and longevity-supportive synergy. Shiitake contributes β-glucan-mediated lipid modulation, hepatic support and immune-balancing effects, while Golden Oyster delivers ergothioneine-driven mitochondrial protection and antioxidant resilience. Together, they reinforce lipid and glucose stability, cellular protection and healthy-ageing trajectories. This combination is especially relevant for senior animals, those with mild cardiometabolic strain, chronic inflammatory conditions or cumulative oxidative stress.

> Synergistic pairings or triads of mushrooms can act across multiple physiological pathways, broadening the supportive effect and contributing to a full-spectrum, terrain-based Mycotherapy strategy.

7.14 Safety, contraindications and monitoring

General tolerability

Shiitake is well tolerated in most animals when introduced gradually. Mild gastrointestinal changes such as soft stools can occur when doses are increased too quickly, particularly in smaller dogs, cats or animals with pre-existing gut sensitivity.

Gastrointestinal sensitivity

Because of its polysaccharide richness, Shiitake may influence motility and fermentation patterns in the gastrointestinal tract. Animals with inflammatory bowel tendencies or dysbiosis should begin with conservative dosing. Any persistent digestive changes warrant dose adjustment.

Coagulation considerations

Shiitake does not exhibit strong anticoagulant effects, but mild modulation of vascular inflammatory tone may affect platelet behaviour in sensitive animals. Care is required when co-administered with anticoagulants, NSAIDs, corticosteroids or chemotherapy agents. Monitoring for abnormal bleeding is prudent.

Immune-mediated disease

In animals with active immune-mediated disease, Shiitake should be avoided until stabilisation is achieved. Once stable, slow titration with close veterinary oversight may be acceptable if immune nourishment is required. Clear therapeutic reasoning is essential.

Hepatic and renal cautions

Shiitake supports early hepatic stress but requires caution in advanced liver disease. Animals with compromised hepatic or renal function may respond unpredictably, necessitating conservative dosing and biochemical monitoring.

Endocrine considerations

Shiitake's influence on glucose and lipid metabolism is moderate but can still affect glycaemic control in diabetic animals. Regular glucose monitoring is advisable when integrating Shiitake into diabetic protocols.

Drug interaction risks

Direct cytochrome P450 interactions appear minimal, but polypharmacy considerations remain important in oncology, endocrine disorders and chronic inflammatory disease. Monitoring for subtle shifts in drug response or side effects is recommended.

Pregnancy and lactation

Safety evidence in pregnancy and lactation is insufficient. Shiitake should be avoided unless clinically justified and veterinarian-supervised.

Paediatric considerations

Young animals generally tolerate Shiitake well, though their digestive systems may be more sensitive to pre-biotic fibres. Lower initial doses and incremental increases are recommended.

Species-specific cautions

Cats may exhibit heightened digestive sensitivity and should start at the lowest end of the dosing spectrum. Small-breed dogs and geriatric animals also benefit from gradual titration.

SCWE as a safety advantage

SCWE-derived whole-mushroom preparations may provide improved tolerability by enhancing solubility and reducing insoluble fibre content, while maintaining a comprehensive biochemical profile. This is particularly helpful for animals with sensitive digestion or multi-system fragility.

Monitoring recommendations

Veterinarians should monitor appetite, stool quality, skin or coat changes, behaviour, glycaemic patterns in diabetic animals and liver enzymes when relevant. These parameters support safe integration and early identification of dose-related adjustments.

7.15 Veterinary considerations and therapeutic relevance

Terrain-based perspective

Shiitake strengthens foundational physiological networks rather than producing isolated, sharp effects. Through immune nourishment, metabolic clarity and hepatic support, it contributes to the rebalancing of systemic terrain. This is particularly relevant for chronic, multi-systemic or degenerative presentations.

Ideal clinical profiles

Animals that benefit most from Shiitake include those with immune fatigue, recurrent infections, mild hepatic stress, metabolic-linked inflammation, gastrointestinal fragility and age-related decline. Shiitake is well suited to animals needing long-term, gentle, cumulative support.

Integrative role

Shiitake is rarely a standalone intervention. Its strength lies in integration with dietary adjustments, conventional treatments and other medicinal mushrooms. Its ability to stabilise underlying immune and metabolic processes enhances the efficacy of more targeted interventions.

Expected trajectory of benefits

Clinical improvements typically emerge gradually. Caregivers may observe better vitality, steadier digestion, improved coat quality, fewer infections and enhanced resilience. These changes are cumulative and reflect deeper physiological recalibration.

Shiitake stands out within veterinary Mycotherapy as a foundational immune nourisher.

When to use cautiously

Caution is warranted in animals with active autoimmune disorders, advanced hepatic or renal compromise, poorly regulated diabetes or those receiving narrow-therapeutic-index medications. Monitoring and conservative titration support safe usage in such cases.

7.16 Evidence quality commentary

Strengths of the evidence

Shiitake has one of the most substantial evidence bases among medicinal mushrooms, particularly in relation to immunology, oncology adjuncts, metabolic regulation and hepatic physiology. Lentinan is one of the best-studied β-glucans worldwide, with several decades of clinical use in human oncology, providing a strong mechanistic and translational foundation for veterinary integration. Eritadenine's metabolic influence has been demonstrated consistently across preclinical models, supporting Shiitake's relevance in lipid modulation and hepatic function. These data contribute to a coherent scientific narrative that aligns closely with clinical outcomes observed in long-term Mycotherapy practice.

Limitations and gaps

Veterinary-specific clinical trials remain limited. Most research is derived from rodent models, in vitro immunological assays and human clinical oncology experience. Although these studies are robust, direct evidence in dogs, cats or horses is still emerging. Additionally, much of the earlier Shiitake research focused on isolated lentinan fractions rather than whole-mushroom extracts, which may not fully represent the synergistic interactions present in full-spectrum formulations. This can complicate extrapolation to whole-mushroom clinical use.

Translational reliability

The pathways modulated by Shiitake-such as Dectin-1 signalling, macrophage activity, cytokine modulation, lipid metabolism and hepatic detoxification-are highly conserved across mammalian species. This supports responsible translational use in veterinary care. Shiitake's balanced immune-nourishing profile reduces the risk of overstimulation compared with more potent immune activators, further improving translational reliability for chronic, geriatric or immune-vulnerable animals.

Species differences

Dogs generally tolerate Shiitake well, though small breeds and geriatric dogs may require slower titration. Cats, because of their unique hepatic metabolism and sensitivity to gastrointestinal fibre, may require more conservative dosing. While the conserved nature of β-glucan receptors supports species-wide relevance, gastrointestinal and metabolic differences influence dosing strategies and monitoring.

Extraction considerations in the evidence

Much of the published lentinan research uses purified fractions that demonstrate strong immunomodulatory effects but do not reflect the mushroom's full biochemical matrix. Whole-mushroom extracts, particularly those produced via SCWE, offer more physiologically relevant profiles by maintaining polysaccharide–protein complexes, sterols, phenolics and redox-active components. Studies using whole-fruiting-body preparations provide better alignment with modern veterinary Mycotherapy protocols.

Methodological variability

Differences in extraction techniques, cultivation substrates, strain selection and β-glucan quantification methods create variability across studies. Standardisation issues in older research can make comparisons difficult. More recent analytical advances and improved extraction technologies have increased consistency, but clinicians should still interpret early studies within methodological context.

Overall appraisal

Shiitake's evidence base is strong at the mechanistic and preclinical levels, with extensive human clinical use supporting its immunological and metabolic properties. Although direct veterinary trials are limited, the conserved nature of the pathways involved and long history of safe use make it a reliable and clinically valuable species in Mycotherapy. When combined with appropriate monitoring, Shiitake can be integrated confidently into immune, hepatic, metabolic and geriatric protocols within modern veterinary practice.

Note: view spectrum of evidence summarised table on the next page:

SHIITAKE (LENTINULA EDODES) – Evidence Quality Commentary Table

This spectrum of evidence is summarised in the following table:

Domain	Evidence Strength	Primary Evidence Type
Immunomodulation	Moderate to high	Preclinical models, β–glucan (lentinan) research, translational human data
Anti–inflammatory activity	Moderate	Preclinical cytokine–modulation studies
Antioxidant defence	Moderate	Preclinical oxidative–stress and free–radical studies
Gastrointestinal and microbiome support	Moderate	Preclinical GI anti–inflammatory models; microbiome–modulating pathways
Hepatic support and lipid metabolism	Moderate	Preclinical hepatoprotective and lipid–regulation studies
Cardiovascular and circulatory function	Emerging to moderate	Preclinical cholesterol–regulation and vascular studies; human nutrition data
Antimicrobial and antiviral activity	Emerging	In vitro studies; limited in vivo research
Oncology adjunct use	Emerging	Preclinical models; clinical use in human integrative oncology (lentinan)
Bone, connective tissue and skin integrity	Emerging	Preclinical dermal and collagen–support data
Clinical veterinary trials	Limited	Minimal veterinary trials; extrapolated from mechanisms and translational data

Shiitake is characterised by a well-established immunomodulatory profile, strongly associated with the activity of **lentinan**, a β–1,3/1,6–glucan with recognised effects on macrophage activation, dendritic-cell signalling and T-cell function. These immunological mechanisms underpin Shiitake's relevance in chronic infection, immune dysregulation and convalescent states. While veterinary trials remain limited, translational evidence from human medicine and preclinical animal studies provides a coherent basis for its use in terrain-focused protocols.

Its anti–inflammatory and antioxidant actions further support steady immune behaviour and tissue protection, particularly in chronic inflammatory syndromes, age–related oxidative stress and gastrointestinal sensitivity. Shiitake also contributes to hepatic and metabolic steadiness, with preclinical evidence indicating improvements in lipid metabolism, hepatic enzyme balance and oxidative–injury protection.

Shiitake's influence on the gastrointestinal system is of particular relevance in veterinary care. Its polysaccharides and prebiotic fibres modulate mucosal integrity, inflammatory tone and microbial composition, reinforcing gut resilience in animals with chronic GI disturbance or stress-related dysbiosis. Emerging data also suggest potential cardiovascular and circulatory support, though veterinary applications in this domain are still developing.

From a Mycotherapy perspective, extraction fidelity is essential. SCWE full–spectrum extracts preserve Shiitake's native β–glucans, lentinan, phenolics and fibre-bound micronutrients, ensuring reliable immune, hepatic and gastrointestinal effects without the starch dilution associated with myceliated–grain products. Alcohol-based tinctures, by contrast, fail to capture the hydrophilic polysaccharides central to Shiitake's clinical relevance.

Within integrative veterinary practice, Shiitake is best positioned as a gentle, multi-system supportive mushroom, offering balanced immune modulation, hepatic steadiness, gastrointestinal support and foundational resilience. Its effects are cumulative, regulatory and terrain-centred, making it well suited to chronic or multifactorial presentations where long-term physiological harmony is essential.

7.17 Conclusion – Integrative Significance and Extraction Considerations

Shiitake stands out within veterinary Mycotherapy as a foundational immune nourisher that also contributes meaningfully to hepatic, metabolic and cardiovascular steadiness. Rather than delivering sharp immunostimulatory effects, it supports a more coherent, resilient immune terrain through lentinan-mediated β-glucan signalling, improved mucosal surveillance and balanced cytokine patterns. At the same time, eritadenine and associated sterols help refine lipid metabolism and hepatic clarity, which is particularly relevant in overweight animals, those with early hepatic strain or age-related metabolic vulnerability. This ability to strengthen immunity while easing metabolic and hepatic load positions Shiitake as a dependable core species for animals experiencing recurrent infections, chronic low-grade inflammation, convalescence or gradual physiological decline.

Clinically, Shiitake's benefits emerge cumulatively. Over weeks to months, practitioners and caregivers are more likely to observe steadier infection patterns, improved vitality, more consistent digestion and gentler ageing trajectories than rapid symptomatic shifts. Its value is most apparent when used as part of an integrated plan: with Reishi where inflammatory and stress-linked patterns predominate, with Maitake in metabolic or hepatic fragility, with Turkey Tail in immune-heavy or oncology contexts, and with Lion's Mane where gut–brain coherence and behavioural steadiness are also priorities. Across these combinations, Shiitake provides the immunological and metabolic foundation that allows more targeted species to express their full therapeutic potential.

As with other core medicinal mushrooms, extract fidelity is central to realising Shiitake's full therapeutic profile. The dense chitin–glucan cell wall of the fruiting body restricts access to lentinan, polysaccharide–protein complexes and phenolic constituents unless it is adequately opened. SCWE whole-mushroom extraction overcomes this barrier by liberating high-molecular-weight β-glucans and associated compounds while preserving sterols, phenolics and the native prebiotic matrix that underpins gut–immune and metabolic signalling. By avoiding starch dilution from grain-grown mycelium and the compositional narrowing of fractionated isolates, SCWE-derived, fruiting-body-only preparations provide a physiologically coherent expression of Shiitake's immune-nourishing and hepatometabolic actions. Used thoughtfully, with appropriate monitoring in fragile patients, Shiitake offers a safe, predictable and evidence-aligned contribution to long-term terrain support in veterinary practice.

> Shiitake stands out within veterinary Mycotherapy as a foundational immune nourisher that also contributes meaningfully to hepatic, metabolic and cardiovascular steadiness.

Key sources (summary)

Chihara, 1992; Kodama et al., 2002; Zhang et al., 2011; Enman et al., 2007; Kabir et al., 1981; Shimoda et al., 2004; Yoshida & Mol, 1999; Liu et al., 2015; Nanba et al., 1997; Cheng et al., 2010; Guo et al., 2018; Park et al., 2014; Wasser, 2011; Zhang et al., 2007. **Full professional reference list available in the Master References section.**

> "Medicinal mushrooms represent a fertile area for research in immunology, oncology, and aging. *Source: International Journal of Medicinal Mushrooms* (2011) *Dr. Solomon Wasser – Mycologist.*"

8

GOLDEN OYSTER (Pleurotus citrinopileatus)

8.1 Introduction to Golden Oyster – *The Longevity Mushroom, Ergothioneine-rich Antioxidant Modulator*

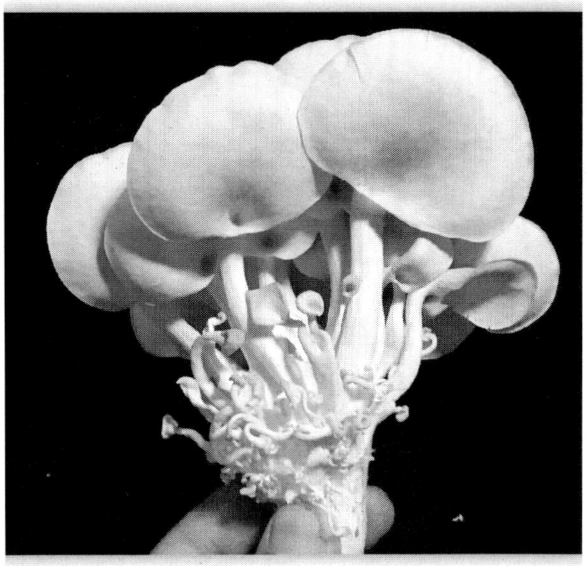

Golden Oyster (*Pleurotus citrinopileatus*) represents a unique intersection between traditional fungal therapeutics and the emerging science of cellular longevity. As one of the richest natural sources of ergothioneine (ERGO), a potent cytoprotective antioxidant increasingly recognised as a 'longevity factor', Golden Oyster offers a physiologically coherent framework for supporting healthy ageing, metabolic resilience, mitochondrial stability and multi-system cellular protection in companion animals. Its bright pigmentation and distinct Pleurotus morphology reflect a biochemically active species whose therapeutic profile encompasses immune modulation, antioxidant defence, metabolic regulation and organ-level cytoprotection.

The scientific relevance of Golden Oyster arises from its synergistic matrix of bioactive constituents, with ERGO playing a defining role. Ergothioneine is a thiol-based antioxidant transported into tissues via the highly conserved OCTN1 (SLC22A4) transporter. This transporter actively accumulates ERGO in mitochondria, bone marrow, immune tissues, liver, kidneys, reproductive organs and the brain. These are precisely the tissues most vulnerable to oxidative stress, inflammation, metabolic disruption and age-related degeneration. Research in humans and animals suggests that ERGO functions not simply as an antioxidant, but as a cytoprotectant that preserves mitochondrial integrity, protects DNA, stabilises redox environments and may slow physiological decline associated with ageing.

For veterinary medicine, this positions Golden Oyster as a prospective longevity-support mushroom with broad relevance across the lifespan, from early-life resilience building to senior-age maintenance. Animals age more rapidly than humans and accumulate metabolic, inflammatory and oxidative stress at accelerated rates. A mushroom capable of supporting mitochondrial and cellular stability at the molecular level offers significant translational value. Although veterinary-specific ERGO studies are emerging, the conserved nature of ERGO transport and accumulation pathways across mammalian species provides a strong scientific foundation for responsible integration.

Golden Oyster's therapeutic relevance extends beyond ERGO. The mushroom contains Pleurotus-derived β-glucans, glycoproteins, phenolic antioxidants, immunomodulatory polysaccharides and lovastatin-like compounds that influence immune steadiness, lipid metabolism, hepatic resilience and inflammatory tone. These compounds interact with ERGO to create a multi-axis cytoprotective effect that aligns naturally with Mycotherapy's terrain-based philosophy. Rather than targeting singular pathologies, Golden Oyster strengthens the physiological networks that underpin vitality, stress resilience and long-term health.

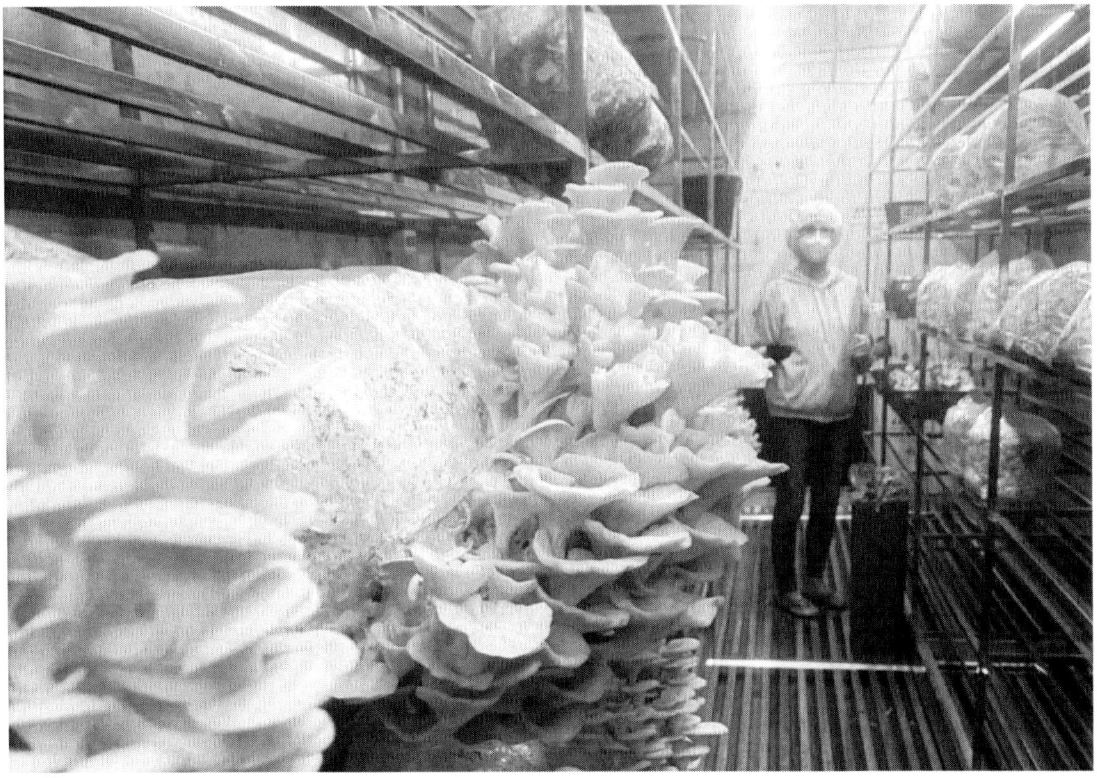

As Golden Oyster is cultivated at OMG Mushrooms using controlled substrate design and enriched nutritional inputs, its ERGO density is not merely incidental but intentionally optimised. This provides a unique opportunity to highlight Golden Oyster as an Australian-produced, longevity-oriented species of clinical significance. The combination of empirical cultivation expertise and a growing evidence base positions Golden Oyster as a flagship mushroom for forward-thinking veterinary practitioners seeking to support healthy ageing, mitochondrial protection and long-term wellbeing in companion animals.

8.2 Taxonomy, Morphology and Extract Science

Golden Oyster belongs to the genus *Pleurotus*, a diverse group of wood-decomposing basidiomycetes known for their immunomodulatory polysaccharides, antioxidant compounds and metabolic regulatory properties. Taxonomically situated within the Pleurotaceae family, *Pleurotus citrinopileatus* is distinguished by its vibrant golden pigmentation, delicate cap structure and rapid mycelial colonisation. While commonly appreciated as an edible gourmet species, its therapeutic value has gained increasing attention due to its unusually high ergothioneine content and rich spectrum of phenolic and polysaccharide compounds.

Morphologically, Golden Oyster forms small, clustered, fan-shaped caps with thin flesh and pronounced gills. This delicate tissue architecture promotes rapid metabolic turnover within the fruiting body, supporting high concentrations of secondary metabolites including ERGO. Pleurotus species are efficient decomposers of lignocellulosic substrates, and Golden Oyster demonstrates particular responsiveness to substrate composition. Nutrient-enriched substrates - including methionine-rich components such as egg white powder, lupin and grape marc - can enhance ERGO biosynthesis due to its metabolic origin as a derivative of histidine and cysteine pathways.

From an extraction-science perspective, Golden Oyster's bioactive compounds are encapsulated within a chitin–glucan matrix typical of basidiomycete fruiting bodies. While raw or lightly cooked forms offer nutritional benefits, therapeutic extraction requires deeper penetration of the cell wall. Hot-water extractions liberate polysaccharides and β-glucans, but may not fully release ERGO, which is highly water soluble yet embedded within intracellular compartments. Sub-critical water extraction (SCWE) provides a more comprehensive release profile by utilising controlled heat and pressure to solubilise both polysaccharides and intracellular antioxidants without degrading thermolabile constituents.

SCWE-derived whole-mushroom extracts of Golden Oyster retain the mushroom's full biochemical spectrum - including β-glucans, glycoproteins, phenolics, sterols and ERGO - in a physiologically accessible form. This is particularly relevant for veterinary applications, where digestive variability, metabolic fragility and age-related gastrointestinal changes may influence absorption and immune interaction. Enhanced solubility and consistent bioactive delivery make SCWE an advantageous method for producing clinically relevant extracts of Golden Oyster for companion animals.

The interplay between taxonomy, morphology and extraction science creates a strong foundation for Golden Oyster's clinical value. Its Pleurotus lineage ensures consistent immunomodulatory properties; its delicate morphology supports high metabolite expression; and its favourable extraction responsiveness allows broad-spectrum compounds - including ERGO - to be delivered effectively within Mycotherapy protocols.

8.3 Bioactive Constituents – Mechanistic Relevance

Golden Oyster's therapeutic profile is driven by a synergistic collection of bioactive molecules, with ergothioneine at the centre of its longevity orientation. However, the mushroom's full clinical potential emerges from the interaction of ERGO with β-glucans, glycoproteins, phenolic antioxidants, sterols and secondary metabolites that influence immune function, metabolic resilience, inflammatory modulation and oxidative protection.

Ergothioneine (ERGO)

ERGO is a thiol-histidine derivative with unique chemical stability and potent antioxidant capacity. Its hallmark feature is targeted accumulation via the OCTN1 transporter, allowing selective uptake into mitochondria, immune cells, bone marrow, liver and the nervous system. ERGO's mechanisms include:

- scavenging reactive oxygen and nitrogen species
- stabilising mitochondrial membranes
- preventing lipid peroxidation
- protecting DNA and RNA from oxidative damage
- regulating redox-sensitive signalling pathways
- mitigating cellular senescence
- supporting erythrocyte resilience

In animals, these mechanisms translate into improved cellular defence, slower physiological decline and enhanced resilience during stress, ageing or chronic disease.

Pleurotus β-glucans

Golden Oyster contains immunomodulatory β-glucans with 1,3/1,6 branching patterns that interact with Dectin-1 and other pattern-recognition receptors. These compounds support balanced innate and adaptive immune responses, enhance macrophage function and promote appropriate cytokine expression. Their activity complements ERGO by strengthening tissue-level immune surveillance and reducing chronic inflammatory load.

Polysaccharide–protein complexes

These complexes influence dendritic cell behaviour, immune tolerance and mucosal regulation. They contribute to the gut–immune axis effects of Golden Oyster and help maintain immune stability in animals with recurrent infections or age-related immune decline.

Phenolic compounds and antioxidant metabolites

Golden Oyster contains a broad array of phenolics, flavonoids and ergosterol derivatives. These compounds enhance redox balance, support mitochondrial health and reduce oxidative stress - synergising with ERGO's cytoprotective activity.

Lovastatin-like compounds

Pleurotus species naturally contain mevinolin-like substances that modulate lipid metabolism and may support cardiovascular and hepatic health. These compounds benefit animals with metabolic challenges, early hepatic stress or overweight conditions, especially when combined with ERGO's mitochondrial and redox effects.

Pre-biotic fibres and microbiome modulation

Golden Oyster's fibre profile supports short-chain fatty acid production, microbial diversity and gut barrier integrity. ERGO's presence in the gut lumen further contributes to microbial stability and mucosal protection.

Taken together, these constituents create a metabolically, immunologically and cytologically supportive matrix that positions Golden Oyster as a longevity-oriented mushroom with relevance across multiple physiological domains in veterinary care.

8.4 Immune System Modulation

Golden Oyster contributes to immune modulation through a combination of β-glucans, polysaccharide–protein complexes, phenolic compounds and its uniquely high ergothioneine content. Rather than acting as a strong immune stimulant, Golden Oyster tends to promote balanced immune readiness, supporting the ability of innate and adaptive systems to respond appropriately to microbial or physiological challenge. This makes it suitable for animals requiring long-term immune nourishment, especially those with chronic low-grade inflammation, immune fatigue or age-related decline in immune resilience.

Its β-glucans interact with Dectin-1 and related pattern-recognition receptors in the gut-associated lymphoid tissue. These interactions enhance macrophage activation, promote dendritic cell maturation and support natural killer cell function, while encouraging an appropriate cytokine environment. The presence of polysaccharide–protein complexes further supports mucosal immunity, helping animals that experience recurrent respiratory or gastrointestinal infections maintain steadier first-line defence.

Ergothioneine contributes an additional dimension to immune influence. By accumulating in mitochondria and immune tissues, ERGO helps protect immune cells from oxidative damage, stabilises redox-sensitive pathways and supports healthier immune cell lifespan and function. Oxidative stress impairs immune surveillance, especially in older animals; ERGO's cytoprotective role helps maintain immune integrity during ageing or chronic illness. This combination of immunomodulation and mitochondrial protection positions Golden Oyster as a mushroom capable of supporting sustained immune readiness in geriatric animals, convalescing patients and those with environmental or metabolic stressors.

Golden Oyster is not typically used to provoke a rapid immune response, but rather to support long-term immune competence. Its effects integrate effectively with Turkey Tail for immune priming or Reishi for inflammatory–immune synchronisation. In multi-systemic cases, Golden Oyster may provide foundational immune support while contributing to broader longevity pathways through its antioxidant and cytoprotective mechanisms.

8.5 Inflammation and Oxidative Stress Pathways

Golden Oyster exerts a broad regulatory influence on inflammatory and oxidative pathways, largely driven by the synergy between ERGO, β-glucans, phenolic compounds and ergosterol derivatives. Chronic inflammation and oxidative stress are central contributors to ageing, mitochondrial dysfunction, metabolic disease and degenerative conditions in animals. Golden Oyster addresses these processes at a cellular level, supporting healthier inflammatory balance and more stable redox environments.

Ergothioneine plays a central mechanistic role. Through OCTN1-mediated transport, ERGO accumulates in tissues most vulnerable to oxidative injury, including the liver, kidneys, reproductive organs, bone marrow, brain and immune cells. ERGO stabilises mitochondrial membranes, reduces lipid peroxidation, protects nucleic acids from oxidative disruption and influences redox-sensitive signalling pathways that regulate inflammation. These actions support the maintenance of cellular integrity in animals prone to chronic inflammatory or degenerative conditions.

Golden Oyster's β-glucans modulate inflammatory cytokine expression by influencing macrophage behaviour and pattern-recognition receptor pathways. This contributes to reduced production of pro-inflammatory markers associated with chronic disease, ageing and metabolic dysfunction. Phenolic compounds and sterol derivatives add further anti-inflammatory and antioxidant effects, enhancing the mushroom's overall redox capacity.

For companion animals, this translates into improved resilience against chronic inflammatory states such as age-related osteoarthritis, metabolic-linked inflammation, hepatic strain and chronic gastrointestinal irritation. While Golden Oyster is not a primary analgesic or anti-inflammatory agent, its ability to support redox stability and reduce persistent inflammatory tone offers an important foundation for long-term health and longevity. It is particularly relevant in senior animals, performance animals exposed to oxidative demand and those with multi-system stress patterns.

8.6 Gastrointestinal, Microbiome and Metabolic Health

Golden Oyster supports gastrointestinal health and metabolic stability through pre-biotic fibres, polysaccharides, phenolic antioxidants and the cytoprotective effects of ERGO on the gut–liver–immune axis. These actions contribute to healthier digestion, improved microbial diversity, stronger mucosal immunity and enhanced metabolic resilience.

Its polysaccharides and fibre fractions act as pre-biotic substrates for beneficial microbiota, promoting short-chain fatty acid production and supporting epithelial integrity. Improved microbial stability and enhanced mucosal immune surveillance benefit animals with chronic soft stools, intermittent gastrointestinal fragility or stress-related digestive disturbance. These effects are especially pertinent in ageing animals whose microbiome diversity has declined or those recovering from chronic disease.

> Golden Oyster supports gastrointestinal health and metabolic stability through pre-biotic fibres.

Golden Oyster's influence on metabolic health extends beyond the gut. ERGO's cytoprotective actions help maintain mitochondrial function in metabolically active tissues, supporting energy metabolism and reducing the oxidative burden associated with chronic metabolic imbalance. The mushroom's phenolic compounds and statin-like secondary metabolites may support lipid metabolism and hepatic health, complementing its pre-biotic and antioxidant effects.

In veterinary practice, Golden Oyster is relevant for animals with early metabolic challenges, chronic gastrointestinal sensitivity, mild hepatic strain or systemic inflammatory patterns. It integrates effectively with Maitake for metabolic regulation, Lion's Mane for gut–brain stability and Reishi for inflammatory–metabolic synchrony. Its gradual, terrain-orientated effects support long-term metabolic harmony and gastrointestinal resilience.

8.7 Neurological and Behavioural Health

Golden Oyster contributes to neurological and behavioural health primarily through mechanisms linked to mitochondrial protection, redox stability and modulation of neuroinflammatory pathways. While it does not possess the direct neurotrophic actions attributed to Lion's Mane, its high ergothioneine content offers a distinct and complementary route to neurological support. ERGO accumulates within nervous tissue via the OCTN1 transporter, where it protects neurons from oxidative stress, stabilises mitochondrial membranes and reduces DNA and lipid damage associated with neurodegeneration. These mechanisms are relevant to ageing dogs and cats experiencing cognitive decline, reduced vitality or behavioural shifts linked to neuroinflammation.

Chronic inflammation and oxidative burden can disrupt neurotransmitter balance, impair synaptic signalling and contribute to behavioural dysregulation, especially in geriatric animals. Golden Oyster's influence on inflammatory cytokines and redox pathways may help reduce these stressors and create a more stable neurophysiological environment. Improvements in mitochondrial health are particularly important in older animals, as mitochondrial dysfunction is strongly implicated in cognitive decline, anosmia, sleep disruption and reduced behavioural adaptability.

Golden Oyster also supports the gut–brain axis through its pre-biotic activity. A healthier microbiome contributes to improved vagal signalling, neurotransmitter regulation and behavioural steadiness. Animals with stress-induced gastrointestinal disturbance, noise sensitivity or chronic illness may exhibit improved resilience when Golden Oyster is used alongside targeted neuro-supportive measures. While not a primary behavioural mushroom, Golden Oyster strengthens foundational pathways that influence mood, cognition and behavioural equilibrium, making it an effective adjunct to Lion's Mane or Reishi in multi-system neurological or behavioural presentations.

8.8 Cardiovascular and Respiratory Physiology

Golden Oyster supports cardiovascular function through metabolic modulation, antioxidant activity and potential statin-like effects associated with Pleurotus species. Oxidative stress and chronic inflammation contribute to vascular stiffness, endothelial dysfunction and dysregulated lipid profiles in ageing animals. ERGO's ability to accumulate in cardiovascular tissues and protect mitochondria reduces oxidative damage and supports healthier endothelial function. These actions may contribute to gentle improvements in cardiovascular resilience, particularly in older animals or those with metabolic-linked cardiovascular risk.

The mushroom's phenolic antioxidants and sterol derivatives further stabilise vascular environments by reducing lipid peroxidation and supporting vascular adaptability. Pleurotus species naturally produce mevinolin-like compounds that influence cholesterol metabolism, and although Golden Oyster has not been studied as extensively as *Pleurotus ostreatus* in this regard, its lipid-modulating potential is plausible based on shared metabolic pathways. These mechanisms may be relevant for overweight animals or those with early signs of dyslipidaemia.

Respiratory physiology benefits indirectly from Golden Oyster's immune and antioxidant profile. ERGO accumulates in the lungs, where it helps protect against oxidative injury and may reduce inflammatory vulnerability in the respiratory mucosa. Improved mucosal immunity and redox stability may contribute to reduced susceptibility to recurrent respiratory infections. While not a primary respiratory agent, Golden Oyster can form part of a broader respiratory-support strategy, especially when used alongside Turkey Tail for immune priming or Reishi for inflammatory and stress-related respiratory patterns.

8.9 Oncology and Adjunctive Cancer Support

Golden Oyster holds significant potential in integrative oncology due to the combined influence of ERGO, β-glucans and phenolic antioxidants on immune surveillance, cellular integrity and tumour micro-environment dynamics. ERGO's cytoprotective effects may help maintain mitochondrial stability and reduce oxidative DNA damage in healthy tissues, a factor of considerable importance in animals undergoing chemotherapy or experiencing chronic oxidative stress associated with cancer progression.

Preclinical research indicates that ergothioneine reduces oxidative stress within bone marrow, preserves immune cell viability and may mitigate some of the collateral tissue damage linked to chemotherapeutic interventions. While veterinary-specific studies are limited, this cytoprotective model aligns with the needs of oncology patients, who often experience mitochondrial strain, immune fatigue and systemic oxidative burden.

> Although Golden Oyster is not yet a primary oncology mushroom in the way Turkey Tail or Reishi are traditionally used, its mechanistic relevance is compelling.

Golden Oyster's β-glucans support immune surveillance by enhancing macrophage activity, natural killer cell function and balanced cytokine expression. These actions contribute to a more prepared and resilient immune landscape, which is essential for tumour recognition and defence. Phenolic and sterol compounds further support antioxidant and anti-inflammatory pathways, helping reduce tissue-level stress associated with malignancy or treatment.

Although Golden Oyster is not yet a primary oncology mushroom in the way Turkey Tail or Reishi are traditionally used, its mechanistic relevance is compelling. Its ability to combine immune nourishment, mitochondrial stabilisation, redox protection and metabolic support positions it as a valuable adjunct within multi-mushroom oncology protocols. When used alongside Turkey Tail for immune activation and Reishi for inflammatory modulation, Golden Oyster contributes a distinct cytoprotective and longevity-focused dimension that enhances overall treatment tolerance and systemic resilience.

8.10 Hepatic and Renal Physiology

Golden Oyster offers notable hepatic and renal relevance due to its combination of ergothioneine, phenolic antioxidants, polysaccharides and Pleurotus-derived secondary metabolites. The liver and kidneys experience significant oxidative and metabolic strain across an animal's lifespan, and both organs contain high densities of the OCTN1 transporter that selectively accumulates ergothioneine. This positions Golden Oyster as a mushroom capable of supporting organ integrity at a cellular level.

In hepatic physiology, ERGO contributes to reduced lipid peroxidation, stabilisation of mitochondrial membranes and improved resistance to oxidative injury. These actions benefit animals with early hepatic changes, metabolic-linked steatosis, chronic inflammatory loading or age-related hepatic decline. Golden Oyster's phenolic compounds, sterols and statin-like metabolites may further support lipid metabolism, reducing hepatic stress associated with dyslipidaemia in overweight or ageing animals. Although not a primary hepatoprotective mushroom in the same sense as Reishi, Golden Oyster's cytoprotective effects complement conventional hepatic therapies by supporting mitochondrial and redox stability within hepatocytes.

Renal physiology benefits from similar protective mechanisms. The kidneys accumulate ERGO in high concentrations due to their metabolic activity and oxidative burden. ERGO helps reduce tubular oxidative stress, supports mitochondrial stability and may improve cellular resilience in early renal vulnerability. These actions are particularly relevant in senior animals, where renal ageing contributes to reductions in filtration capacity and increased susceptibility to oxidative insult. Golden Oyster does not replace renal-specific interventions, but its cytoprotective influence provides valuable foundational support within integrative renal care.

Golden Oyster's combined hepatic and renal effects are most clinically relevant in cases where metabolic, inflammatory and oxidative factors overlap. Animals with metabolic syndrome, chronic inflammatory disease, early hepatic or renal changes, or those recovering from systemic illness may benefit from the broad cytoprotective properties of this mushroom.

8.11 Endocrine and Metabolic Regulation

Golden Oyster influences endocrine and metabolic physiology through its antioxidant capacity, mitochondrial stabilising effects, pre-biotic activity and possible lipid-modulating metabolites. Animals with endocrine disorders or metabolic fragility often experience elevated oxidative stress, impaired mitochondrial function and dysregulated inflammatory signalling. Golden Oyster's ERGO-driven cytoprotection offers a mechanism for supporting metabolic resilience across these systems.

In glucose regulation, oxidative stress impairs insulin signalling and contributes to β-cell burden. ERGO may mitigate some of these stressors by stabilising redox balance and supporting mitochondrial function in pancreatic and hepatic tissues. While Golden Oyster is not a primary glycaemic regulation mushroom, its influence on oxidative and inflammatory pathways may contribute to improved metabolic steadiness in animals with early insulin resistance or age-related metabolic slowing.

Lipid metabolism may also be modulated through Pleurotus-associated statin-like compounds that influence HMG-CoA reductase activity. Although Golden Oyster's specific profile requires further study, its shared lineage with *Pleurotus ostreatus* suggests potential for mild lipid-lowering effects. Combined with ERGO's mitochondrial protective actions, this creates a metabolic-supportive profile relevant to overweight animals, those with early endocrine imbalance or animals at risk of metabolic-linked inflammatory conditions.

Endocrine–immune interactions may benefit from Golden Oyster's ability to stabilise inflammatory cytokines and support stress-adaptive mechanisms. Chronic inflammation and oxidative burden can disrupt hormonal regulation, and improved cellular resilience may indirectly support healthier endocrine signalling. In integrative endocrine care, Golden Oyster is best used as a supportive mushroom rather than a primary regulator, complementing Maitake for metabolic modulation or Reishi for stress physiology.

8.12 Veterinary Pharmacology and Drug Interaction Considerations

Absorption and bioavailability

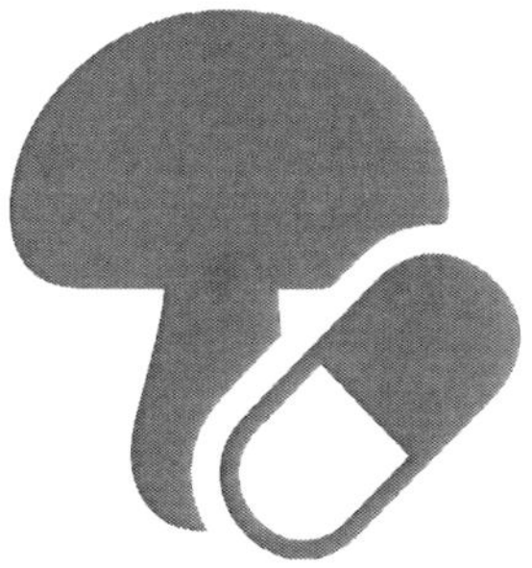

Golden Oyster's bioactive compounds, including ERGO, polysaccharides and phenolics, exhibit variable absorption depending on digestive health, age and metabolic status. ERGO is absorbed efficiently via the OCTN1 transporter, which is highly conserved across mammalian species. SCWE-derived extracts may improve solubility and availability of polysaccharides and intracellular antioxidants by breaking down the chitin–glucan matrix more effectively. Animals with compromised digestion or age-related gastrointestinal changes may therefore respond more predictably to SCWE-prepared whole-mushroom extracts.

Hepatic metabolism and detoxification pathways

Golden Oyster has not demonstrated direct hepatotoxicity, though its influence on oxidative pathways and lipid metabolism may interact with hepatic function in animals with advanced hepatic disease. Improved mitochondrial and redox stability may benefit early hepatic strain, but animals with severe hepatic compromise require close monitoring, as changes in metabolic pathways may alter drug processing.

Cytochrome P450 implications

Direct modulation of cytochrome P450 enzymes by Golden Oyster has not been documented. However, extrapolation from related Pleurotus species suggests minimal interference with major CYP pathways. Even so, cautious monitoring is recommended when animals are receiving narrow-therapeutic-index medications or multi-drug regimens, as improvements in hepatic redox status may theoretically influence metabolic turnover.

Coagulation and platelet activity

Golden Oyster does not exhibit strong anticoagulant effects. Mild improvements in vascular inflammatory tone or lipid metabolism may subtly influence platelet behaviour in sensitive animals, particularly those receiving NSAIDs, corticosteroids or chemotherapeutic agents. Monitoring for abnormal bleeding or bruising is advisable during initial integration.

Sedative, anxiolytic or CNS interactions

Golden Oyster does not exhibit direct sedative or anxiolytic activity. However, improvements in mitochondrial function and reduced neuroinflammation may influence behavioural steadiness indirectly. These effects should not interfere with CNS-acting medications, though behavioural changes should be monitored in animals undergoing psychopharmacological treatment.

Endocrine medication interactions

While Golden Oyster does not directly regulate endocrine hormones, its mild metabolic effects and influence on oxidative pathways may interact with insulin sensitivity or thyroid regulation in susceptible animals. Diabetic animals should be monitored for changes in glucose trends after integration.

Gastrointestinal absorption considerations

Golden Oyster's polysaccharides may influence gut motility in sensitive animals. Gradual introduction is recommended for dogs or cats with inflammatory bowel tendencies or dysbiosis. Animals on medications requiring predictable gastrointestinal absorption may need staggered timing to avoid potential interactions with fibre or polysaccharide content.

Polypharmacy considerations

In complex oncology, endocrine or hepatic cases, polypharmacy is common. Golden Oyster's cytoprotective profile generally supports treatment tolerance, but subtle changes in metabolic turnover or immune function may alter therapeutic responses. Regular review of clinical signs and laboratory parameters is recommended.

Safe-use practice in complex cases

Golden Oyster is safest when introduced gradually, with baseline monitoring in animals with chronic inflammatory disease, metabolic dysregulation, hepatic or renal compromise, or those receiving immunomodulatory or chemotherapeutic drugs. Monitoring should include appetite, stool quality, behavioural changes and relevant biochemical markers.

8.13 Clinical Application in Veterinary Practice

Dermatology

Golden Oyster may contribute to dermatological stability through its antioxidant, metabolic and immune-modulating actions. Chronic dermatological conditions in animals often involve inflammatory–metabolic interactions, microbiome imbalance and oxidative stress at the follicular level. ERGO's cytoprotective influence may help mitigate oxidative stress within dermal tissues, while β-glucans support healthier cytokine expression and immune steadiness. Although not a primary dermatological mushroom, Golden Oyster may assist animals experiencing recurrent superficial infections, environmental skin reactivity or age-related skin fragility, especially when oxidative stress plays a contributory role.

Gastrointestinal disorders

Golden Oyster's pre-biotic fibres, polysaccharides and mucosal immune effects provide meaningful support for gastrointestinal health. Animals with intermittent gastrointestinal sensitivity, chronic soft stools, antibiotic-associated dysbiosis or stress-linked digestive disturbance may benefit from improved microbial stability and enhanced mucosal integrity. ERGO's local antioxidant activity within the gut–liver axis adds further benefit, particularly in animals with inflammatory or metabolic components underlying their digestive issues. Golden Oyster integrates well with Lion's Mane in gut–brain cases and with Turkey Tail where immune–gut support is required.

Hepatic disease

Golden Oyster's hepatic relevance is particularly important in early or mild liver dysfunction. ERGO's accumulation in hepatocytes supports mitochondrial integrity and reduces oxidative injury associated with metabolic strain or advancing age. The mushroom's phenolics and sterol derivatives may assist lipid metabolism, helping reduce hepatic burden in overweight animals or those with metabolic-linked inflammatory patterns. Golden Oyster is best positioned as a supportive agent rather than a primary hepatoprotective intervention, complementing Reishi or conventional hepatic therapies.

Behavioural medicine

While not a direct neurotrophin stimulant, Golden Oyster indirectly supports behavioural health through mitochondrial protection, reduced neuroinflammation and improved gut–brain physiology. Animals showing stress-related digestive fluctuations, age-related behavioural changes or reduced neurocognitive resilience may respond favourably when Golden Oyster is used alongside behavioural therapies or Lion's Mane. Its stabilising effect on redox balance and mitochondrial function can contribute to improved behavioural steadiness in geriatric or chronically stressed animals.

Immune dysregulation

Golden Oyster supports immune nourishment without provoking excessive activation. This is particularly relevant in animals with recurrent infections, immune fatigue, chronic inflammatory loading or age-related decline in immune readiness. ERGO protects immune cells from oxidative stress, while β-glucans strengthen innate and adaptive responses. In stable immune-mediated conditions, Golden Oyster may be considered with careful monitoring, as balanced support rather than immune stimulation is the primary objective.

Respiratory conditions

Golden Oyster offers secondary support in respiratory vulnerability due to ERGO's protective accumulation in respiratory tissues and its ability to mitigate oxidative injury. Animals experiencing repeated respiratory infections or age-related mucosal fragility may benefit from improved immune and redox stability. While not a frontline respiratory mushroom, Golden Oyster complements Turkey Tail or Reishi in multi-system supportive plans.

Cardiovascular applications

Golden Oyster's cardiovascular relevance arises from its antioxidant influence, mitochondrial protective effects and potential lipid-modulating activity associated with Pleurotus species. Ageing animals or those with metabolic-linked cardiovascular strain may benefit from improved endothelial stability and reduced oxidative burden. While its lipid-modulating effects require further study in this specific species, the mechanistic plausibility positions Golden Oyster as a supportive cardiovascular mushroom for long-term health maintenance.

Oncology adjunctive use

Golden Oyster has promising significance within integrative oncology due to its ability to support mitochondrial resilience, reduce oxidative DNA damage and preserve immune competence. ERGO's protective effects on bone marrow and immune tissues may help maintain treatment tolerance in animals undergoing chemotherapy or experiencing chronic oxidative load associated with malignancy. While not yet a primary oncology mushroom, Golden Oyster contributes meaningful cytoprotective and longevity-oriented support when combined with Turkey Tail for immune activation or Reishi for inflammatory modulation.

Senior and geriatric care

Golden Oyster is particularly suited to senior animals due to its multi-system protection: mitochondrial support, antioxidant defence, metabolic resilience, immune nourishment and improved tissue stability. These effects align directly with the physiological vulnerabilities of ageing. Golden Oyster may enhance vitality, reduce age-related inflammatory burden and support cognitive and physical resilience in older animals. Its role as a longevity-support mushroom makes it an ideal foundation in geriatric Mycotherapy.

Performance and working animals

Performance animals experience elevated oxidative stress, metabolic demand and mitochondrial strain. Golden Oyster's ERGO-driven cytoprotection contributes to improved recovery, reduced oxidative load and steadier performance physiology. While Cordyceps remains the primary mushroom for respiratory and performance enhancement, Golden Oyster provides valuable antioxidant and mitochondrial support in combination protocols.

Multi-systemic presentations

Golden Oyster is highly relevant in animals with overlapping metabolic, inflammatory and oxidative vulnerabilities. This includes overweight senior dogs with gastrointestinal fragility, recurrent infections and early hepatic changes. Its broad cytoprotective actions create a harmonising influence that stabilises multiple physiological axes simultaneously, supporting the terrain-based approach central to Mycotherapy.

Integration with other mushrooms

Golden Oyster integrates effectively with other medicinal mushrooms, enhancing multi-system resilience through its unique cytoprotective, mitochondrial-supportive and antioxidant profile.

8.14 Integration with other Functional Mushrooms

Golden Oyster integrates exceptionally well with multiple functional mushrooms due to its ergothioneine-rich profile and its capacity to protect mitochondrial membranes, stabilise redox signalling and reinforce cellular resilience. These properties extend the actions of mushrooms supporting neurological health, metabolic balance, immune surveillance and stress physiology. The following combinations reflect the most clinically relevant synergies in companion and performance animals.

- **With Lion's Mane** - This pairing provides a comprehensive neuroprotective and neuroregenerative strategy. Lion's Mane contributes neurotrophic support, nerve-growth-factor signalling and gut–brain axis stability, while Golden Oyster provides ergothioneine-driven mitochondrial protection and redox balance. Together they address cognitive ageing, behavioural fragility, chronic stress-related gastrointestinal presentations and neurological convalescence. The combination is especially valuable in senior animals, cognitive decline, stress-linked digestive disturbances and early neurodegenerative patterns.

- **With Reishi** - Golden Oyster complements Reishi's broad immunomodulatory, hepatic and adaptogenic effects with deep mitochondrial and cellular protection. Reishi stabilises inflammatory pathways, supports mast-cell behaviour and moderates autonomic tone, while Golden Oyster defends against oxidative stress and reinforces cellular longevity. This pairing benefits animals with chronic inflammation, age-related hepatic or metabolic strain, environmental sensitivities or stress-reactive physiology. It provides a grounding combination for healthy ageing and systemic stability.

- **With Cordyceps** - Cordyceps adds oxygen-utilisation efficiency, ATP generation and endurance-focused support to Golden Oyster's mitochondrial and antioxidant foundation. This combination enhances stamina, respiratory performance and post-exertional recovery. It is especially relevant for working dogs, performance animals, active breeds with high metabolic output and senior animals experiencing mild fatigue or reduced recovery capacity. Together they offer sustained energy metabolism and tissue protection across activity levels.

- **With Turkey Tail** - Turkey Tail strengthens Golden Oyster's immune, antioxidant and cytoprotective actions, making this combination valuable in chronic immune challenges and integrative oncology care. Turkey Tail contributes PSP/PSK-mediated immune surveillance and gut–immune axis reinforcement, while Golden Oyster stabilises oxidative stress, protects mitochondrial structures and enhances DNA integrity. This pairing supports animals undergoing long-term oncology protocols, chronic infections, immune suppression or age-related immune drift.

- **With Maitake** - Golden Oyster integrates naturally with Maitake's endocrine, insulin-signalling and metabolic-balancing effects. Maitake regulates glucose and lipid pathways while Golden Oyster protects mitochondrial function and buffers oxidative stress associated with metabolic fragility. Together they support metabolic harmony, endocrine steadiness, healthy weight, and resilience in ageing or metabolically vulnerable animals. This combination is particularly relevant in overweight animals, endocrine imbalance, chronic inflammatory metabolic states and age-linked metabolic decline.

> Synergistic pairings or triads of mushrooms can act across multiple physiological pathways, broadening the supportive effect and contributing to a full-spectrum, terrain-based Mycotherapy strategy.

8.15 Safety, Contraindications and Monitoring

General tolerability

Golden Oyster is generally well tolerated in dogs and cats when introduced gradually. As with other polysaccharide-rich mushrooms, mild gastrointestinal softening may occur with rapid dose escalation. Most animals adapt without difficulty when titration is slow and steady.

Gastrointestinal sensitivity

Animals with inflammatory bowel tendencies, dysbiosis or highly sensitive digestion may require conservative introduction. Fibre and polysaccharide content can influence motility, especially in cats or small-breed dogs. Any persistent digestive changes warrant dose revision.

Coagulation considerations

Golden Oyster has not demonstrated significant anticoagulant effects. However, in animals receiving anticoagulants, NSAIDs, corticosteroids or chemotherapy, vigilance is recommended due to theoretical changes in vascular inflammatory tone or platelet behaviour. Monitoring for bruising or abnormal bleeding is prudent during early integration.

Immune-mediated disease

In animals with active immune-mediated conditions, Golden Oyster should be avoided until disease stabilisation occurs. Its balanced immune effects may be helpful in long-term management, but only with veterinary oversight and clear monitoring protocols.

Hepatic and renal cautions

While Golden Oyster supports early hepatic and renal resilience, animals with advanced organ disease may respond unpredictably. ERGO's mitochondrial support is generally beneficial, but metabolic turnover changes necessitate conservative dosing and routine biochemical evaluation.

Endocrine considerations

Golden Oyster may influence metabolic steadiness through its antioxidant and mitochondrial effects. Diabetic animals should be monitored for alterations in glucose patterns. Animals with thyroid dysregulation may require observation during early integration.

Drug interaction risks

Golden Oyster has minimal evidence of direct pharmacokinetic interference. However, its influence on immune function, metabolic pathways and redox balance may alter therapeutic responsiveness in polypharmacy contexts. Oncology, endocrine and hepatic cases require routine monitoring when integrating any mushroom-based therapy.

Pregnancy and lactation

Due to insufficient evidence, Golden Oyster is not recommended in pregnancy or lactation unless clinically justified and overseen by a veterinarian.

Paediatric considerations

Young animals generally tolerate Golden Oyster well, but as with all mushrooms, conservative dosing is recommended for digestive comfort.

Species-specific cautions

Cats are particularly sensitive to fibre-related gastrointestinal fluctuations, necessitating lower starting doses. Senior animals, especially those with chronic multisystem vulnerability, benefit from slower titration.

SCWE as a safety advantage

SCWE-prepared extracts may offer improved tolerability in sensitive animals by enhancing compound solubility and reducing insoluble fibre load. This is especially relevant in geriatric, gastrointestinal or metabolically fragile patients.

Monitoring recommendations

Monitoring should include digestion, appetite, behavioural changes, coat quality, energy levels, inflammatory signs and any laboratory parameters relevant to the underlying condition. These indicators support safe integration and timely dose adjustments.

8.16 Veterinary Considerations and Therapeutic Relevance

Terrain-based perspective

Golden Oyster strengthens fundamental physiological terrain through mitochondrial support, antioxidant defence, immune nourishment and metabolic steadiness. These actions contribute to healthier ageing trajectories, improved resilience and enhanced capacity to withstand cumulative physiological stressors.

Ideal clinical profiles

Golden Oyster is ideally suited for animals experiencing chronic inflammation, oxidative stress, metabolic slowdown, recurrent infections, early organ vulnerability or age-related decline. Its cytoprotective profile serves both preventive and supportive purposes across diverse clinical contexts.

Integrative role

Golden Oyster is rarely used in isolation. Its true value emerges when integrated with other mushrooms and conventional therapies. By stabilising cellular environments, it enhances responsiveness to other interventions and supports system-level improvement. Its role is complementary, foundational and longevity focused.

Expected trajectory of benefits

Benefits typically unfold gradually, with improvements in vitality, coat quality, digestive steadiness, behavioural resilience and mobility often noted over weeks to months. These changes reflect deeper shifts in redox balance, mitochondrial stability and immune nourishment rather than surface-level symptom relief.

When to use cautiously

Caution is warranted in advanced hepatic or renal disease, unstable endocrine disorders, active immune-mediated conditions or animals with unpredictable drug responses. With appropriate monitoring, Golden Oyster can still be integrated into complex care plans, but veterinary oversight is essential.

8.17 Evidence Quality Commentary

Strengths of the evidence

Golden Oyster presents a compelling foundation of mechanistic and preclinical evidence, particularly relating to ergothioneine (ERGO), antioxidant function and metabolic modulation. ERGO is one of the best-studied naturally occurring cytoprotectants, with extensive research documenting its mitochondrial protection, redox stability and tissue-specific accumulation. Although most ERGO studies have been performed in humans and rodent models, the OCTN1 transporter responsible for ERGO uptake is highly conserved across mammalian species, giving strong translational relevance for veterinary application. Pleurotus species more broadly possess a well-established body of literature supporting β-glucan activity, antioxidant potential, lipid modulation and immunological effects.

Limitations and gaps

Direct veterinary clinical trials on *Pleurotus citrinopileatus* are limited, and ERGO-specific research in companion animals is still emerging. While the mechanistic basis for ERGO's influence is robust, large-scale veterinary studies evaluating Golden Oyster's effects on ageing, chronic inflammation or metabolic disease are currently lacking. Many historical studies on Pleurotus species focus on *P. ostreatus*, requiring cautious extrapolation to Golden Oyster despite shared biochemical pathways. ERGO quantification methods also vary across research groups, contributing to inconsistencies in reported concentrations.

Translational reliability

The physiological pathways influenced by Golden Oyster - mitochondrial protection, redox modulation, immune nourishment and metabolic stability - are conserved across dogs, cats and other companion animals. This cross-species conservation strengthens translational reliability and supports the responsible use of Golden Oyster in veterinary Mycotherapy. ERGO's transporter specificity (OCTN1) ensures that uptake is biologically targeted and consistent across species.

Species differences

Digestive sensitivity, metabolic turnover and oxidative load differ between species and across life stages. Cats may absorb polysaccharides differently and have unique hepatic metabolism compared with dogs. Senior animals, animals with chronic disease and high-performance animals often have heightened oxidative burden, making them more responsive to cytoprotective interventions. These species and age differences reinforce the need for dose titration and clinical monitoring.

Extraction considerations in the evidence

Most early research on Pleurotus mushrooms utilised crude extracts or isolated fractions. Modern extraction technologies, including Sub-critical water extraction (SCWE), preserve a wider spectrum of bioactive compounds and improve solubility, offering a more clinically relevant preparation. SCWE's ability to release intracellular ERGO without degrading thermolabile compounds may enhance therapeutic consistency. Extract standardisation remains an area of ongoing development and is central to improving research reproducibility.

Methodological variability

Variability in substrate composition, cultivation method, harvest timing, extraction parameters and β-glucan quantification can lead to differences in bioactive profiles across studies. ERGO content is particularly sensitive to substrate composition and mushroom developmental stage. These factors highlight the need for standardised methodologies when comparing research findings or applying them clinically.

Overall appraisal

Golden Oyster is supported by strong mechanistic evidence, a growing body of preclinical research and the extensive foundational science underpinning ERGO as a cytoprotective and longevity-oriented molecule. Although veterinary-specific clinical trials remain limited, the biological plausibility and conserved pathways provide a solid basis for its integration into Mycotherapy. Its relevance to ageing animals, chronic inflammatory states, metabolic fragility and multi-system oxidative stress positions Golden Oyster as a forward-looking and highly promising mushroom for integrative veterinary practice.

> “Golden Oyster is notably rich in ergothioneine – a diet-derived antioxidant that, as highlighted by Professor Barry Halliwell, PhD, and colleagues, is avidly retained by the body and concentrated at sites of tissue injury, where it may help reduce oxidative damage and support tissue resilience.”

GOLDEN OYSTER – Evidence Quality Commentary Table

This spectrum of evidence is summarised in the following table:

Domain	Evidence Strength	Primary Evidence Type
Antioxidant defence (ergothioneine, glutathione)	Moderate to high	Preclinical antioxidant models; biochemical assays; translational evidence
Anti–inflammatory activity	Moderate	Preclinical cytokine–modulation and NF-κB pathway studies
Immune modulation	Moderate	Preclinical β–glucan studies; innate and adaptive immune pathways
Gastrointestinal support and microbiome balance	Moderate	Preclinical GI anti–inflammatory studies; fibre–driven microbial modulation
Metabolic stability (lipids and glucose)	Emerging to moderate	Preclinical metabolic–syndrome and hepatic–lipid studies
Cellular protection and ageing resilience	Moderate	Translational ergothioneine research; oxidative-injury and mitochondrial data
Hepatic support	Emerging	Preclinical hepatoprotective and antioxidant studies
Neurological steadiness and oxidative stress	Emerging	Preclinical neuroprotective pathways related to ergothioneine
Cardiovascular support	Emerging	Preclinical lipid and vascular-modulating studies in Pleurotus species
Oncology adjunct rationale	Emerging	Mechanistic oxidative-stress and immune–terrain data; no direct trials
Clinical veterinary trials	Limited	No formal veterinary trials; extrapolated from mechanistic and translational evidence

Golden Oyster is distinguished by its **naturally high ergothioneine content**, a unique dietary antioxidant associated with cellular protection, redox balance and healthy ageing across multiple species. Ergothioneine's ability to accumulate in mitochondria, nervous tissue and areas of high oxidative demand underpins Golden Oyster's relevance in animals experiencing chronic inflammation, environmental stress, metabolic disturbance or age-related decline. While veterinary-specific trials are limited, translational research strongly supports ergothioneine as a cytoprotective compound with cross-system significance.

The broader Pleurotus genus contributes additional β–glucans, phenolics and fibre-bound nutrients that shape immune behaviour, gastrointestinal steadiness and metabolic regulation. Golden Oyster shares these characteristics while offering a more pronounced antioxidant profile, making it particularly valuable in cases involving oxidative load, chronic inflammatory tone or recovery following physiological stress. Preclinical studies within Pleurotus species also support hepatic protection, lipid-modulating activity and improvements in gut–immune axis behaviour.

In a Mycotherapy context, Golden Oyster provides terrain support by buffering oxidative stress, stabilising metabolic markers and reinforcing gastrointestinal resilience. These effects are gradual and regulatory rather than rapid, aligning with its role as part of a long-term resilience-building strategy rather than a symptom-focused intervention.

Extraction fidelity is essential. SCWE full-spectrum extracts retain Golden Oyster's ergothioneine, phenolics, β–glucans and sensitive antioxidant molecules that may degrade under high heat or solvent-based processing. Myceliated-grain products lack this profile and may significantly dilute the antioxidant fraction through non-fungal starch. For veterinary use, SCWE fruiting-body extracts therefore provide the most reliable, evidence-aligned representation of Golden Oyster's therapeutic potential.

Within integrative veterinary practice, Golden Oyster is best positioned as a cellular-protective, oxidative-buffering and terrain-supportive mushroom, particularly relevant for ageing animals, chronic inflammatory presentations, metabolic imbalance and cases requiring long-term physiological steadiness.

> Golden Oyster is distinguished by its **naturally high ergothioneine content**, a unique dietary antioxidant associated with cellular protection, redox balance and healthy ageing across multiple species.

8.18 The Ergothioneine Advantage in Veterinary Medicine

Emerging research strongly suggests that ergothioneine may represent a uniquely valuable molecule for companion animals whose physiology is characterised by rapid ageing, high oxidative turnover and cumulative inflammatory burden. Unlike generic antioxidants, ERGO is actively transported into the mitochondria, bone marrow, liver, kidneys, heart and brain – the very tissues most susceptible to age-related decline in dogs and cats. These accumulation patterns are not incidental; they reflect a biological priority system in which ERGO is selectively conserved where cellular protection is most critical.

Golden Oyster is one of the richest natural dietary sources of ergothioneine currently available in a safe, palatable, non-pharmacological form suitable for routine veterinary integration. When cultivated under controlled conditions, ERGO density remains consistent and is enhanced further by substrate optimisation. In practice, this positions Golden Oyster as a highly relevant mushroom for senior animals, performance dogs under metabolic strain, and any case involving chronic inflammation, oxidative injury or mitochondrial vulnerability.

While veterinary-specific ERGO research is still expanding, the cross-species conservation of the OCTN1 transporter and the extensive mechanistic data in animal models provide strong translational confidence. As such, Golden Oyster can be understood not simply as an antioxidant mushroom, but as a longevity-oriented cytoprotective agent with far-reaching implications for healthy ageing and multi-system resilience in companion animals.

8.19 Conclusion – Integrative Significance and Extraction

Golden Oyster (Pleurotus citrinopileatus) can be positioned in veterinary Mycotherapy as a longevity-support mushroom that reinforces mitochondrial stability, antioxidant defence and multi-system resilience. Its ergothioneine-rich profile offers targeted cytoprotection in tissues with high oxidative demand, including the liver, kidneys, brain, bone marrow and cardiovascular system. For clinicians, this translates into a steady, terrain-based contribution to healthy ageing, improved recovery capacity and better tolerance of chronic metabolic or inflammatory burden, rather than rapid symptomatic change.

Ideal candidates include senior animals, performance and working dogs under sustained oxidative strain, and companion animals with early hepatic or renal vulnerability, metabolic slowdown, recurrent infections or multi-system inflammatory patterns. In these cases, Golden Oyster functions as a background stabiliser that supports cellular energy, moderates oxidative and inflammatory load and enhances the efficacy of broader integrative plans. It is rarely a stand-alone intervention; its clinical value is maximised when combined with mushrooms such as Lion's Mane (neurocognitive and gut–brain support), Reishi (immune–inflammatory and stress physiology), Maitake (metabolic regulation) and Turkey Tail (immune priming and gut–immune axis reinforcement).

From a safety perspective, Golden Oyster is generally well tolerated when titrated gradually, with gastrointestinal sensitivity, advanced hepatic or renal compromise, unstable endocrine disease and active immune-mediated conditions representing the main contexts for caution and closer monitoring. Veterinary use is currently supported by strong mechanistic and preclinical evidence around ergothioneine and Pleurotus species, with translational plausibility strengthened by conserved ERGO transport and accumulation pathways across mammals. Within modern integrative practice, Golden Oyster is best understood as a foundational cytoprotective ally, helping maintain cellular coherence and physiological adaptability across the lifespan of companion and performance animals.

> Golden Oyster can be positioned in veterinary Mycotherapy as a longevity-support mushroom that reinforces mitochondrial stability, antioxidant defence and multi-system resilience.

Key sources (summary)

Ames (2018); Beelman et al. (2020); Cheah & Halliwell (2012); Cheah et al. (2017); Guggenheimer & Wasser (2012); Jayakumar et al. (2010); Rathore et al. (2017); Brown & Gordon (2003); Vetvicka & Vetvickova (2011); Zhang et al. (2007); Bermúdez & Velázquez (2001); Gao et al. (2004); Liu & Sun (2018); Park & Lee (2014); Wasser (2011). **Full professional reference list available in the Master References section.**

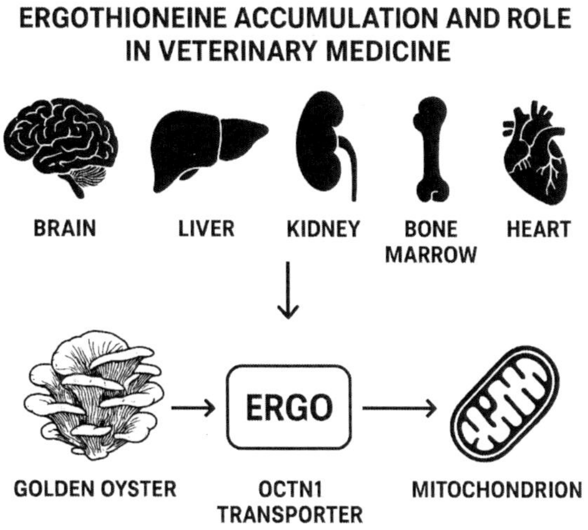

> Ergothioneine is not just another antioxidant; it is actively transported to the tissues where oxidative injury is greatest. *Adapted from Halliwell & Cheah, Free Radical Research, 2016*

9

Additional Medicinal & Native Australian Mushrooms

A Brief Overview of Emerging Species Informing the Future of Veterinary Mycotherapy

Although this text focuses on eight core medicinal mushrooms with the strongest veterinary and cross-disciplinary evidence, the broader field of functional mycology encompasses many additional species of emerging interest. Research continues to evolve rapidly, and several mushrooms—both global and Australian native—are beginning to attract scientific attention for their biochemical complexity and potential health-supportive properties.

This supplementary section provides a concise overview for practitioners seeking a broader context of species currently under investigation. These mushrooms are **not included in the core monographs** because evidence in veterinary medicine remains limited; however, they contribute to an expanding landscape of future Mycotherapy research.

9.1. Additional medicinal mushrooms of international interest

Polyporus umbellatus (Zhu Ling)

Traditionally used in classical Chinese medicine for fluid regulation, *Polyporus umbellatus* contains characteristic polysaccharides associated with immune modulation, renal support and anti-oedema activity in preclinical studies. Interest is growing in its potential applications for urinary and lymphatic health.

Agaricus blazei Murrill (Agaricus subrufescens; ABM)

Known for exceptionally high β-glucan content, *Agaricus blazei* has been studied for immune enhancement, hepatoprotective activity and possible adjunctive oncology roles. Data from animal and human models suggest potent immunomodulatory properties, although veterinary-specific studies remain limited. Reference: Hetland et al., *Advances in Pharmacological Sciences* (2011).

Tremella fuciformis (Snow Fungus)

Rich in hydrating polysaccharides and antioxidant compounds, *Tremella fuciformis* is well established in dermatological and cosmetic science. Its potential relevance for coat health, barrier function and inflammatory dermatoses in animals makes it one of the more interesting future candidates for veterinary dermatology.

Flammulina velutipes (Enoki)

Flammulina velutipes contains bioactive polysaccharides (flammulin, velutin) linked to neuroprotection, anti-allergic effects and gastrointestinal support. Epidemiological data from Japan have drawn attention to its potential immune and cellular-protective roles.

Fomitopsis officinalis (Agarikon)

A rare and historically revered polypore, *Fomitopsis officinalis* demonstrates antiviral and immune-modulating properties in laboratory studies. While promising, veterinary relevance has yet to be examined.

Auricularia auricula-judae (Wood Ear)

Traditionally used for circulatory support, *Auricularia* species contain natural anticoagulant and lipid-modulating compounds. Preclinical studies suggest metabolic and microcirculatory benefit, though bleeding risk warrants caution in clinical settings.

Phellinus linteus

Well-studied in Asia for immunomodulatory and anti-proliferative activities, *Phellinus linteus* has shown potential as an adjunctive oncology-supportive mushroom. Evidence in animals remains early-stage and largely preclinical.

9.2. Additional species worth mentioning

Lignosus rhinocerotis (Tiger Milk Mushroom) *Respiratory-supporting, anti-inflammatory, emerging evidence base.*

Lignosus rhinocerotis, commonly known as Tiger Milk Mushroom, is an emerging medicinal fungus with a long ethnomedicinal history in Malaysia and Southeast Asia, particularly for respiratory complaints such as chronic cough, airway irritation, sinus congestion and post-viral inflammatory symptoms. Scientific interest has expanded significantly over the past decade, with studies demonstrating anti-inflammatory, immunomodulatory and antioxidant activities relevant to respiratory and immune health.

Preclinical research shows that Lignosus extracts can modulate key inflammatory cytokines (including TNF-α, IL-1β and IL-6), enhance macrophage responsiveness and reduce oxidative stress in airway tissues. These actions align closely with its traditional use in conditions characterised by bronchial sensitivity or inflammatory airway responses.

Early human observational work also suggests potential benefits for upper respiratory tract wellness. Participants reported reductions in cough severity, nasal congestion and airway discomfort, alongside improved ease of breathing during convalescence. While these findings remain preliminary, they provide a promising translational link between its ethnomedicinal heritage and modern clinical interest.

Integrative veterinarians have also reported positive outcomes in dogs with asthma-like presentations, including improvements in cough frequency and respiratory comfort when Lignosus is used alongside broader respiratory protocols. These clinical observations, although anecdotal, reinforce the mushroom's emerging relevance in cases involving chronic airway inflammation or allergic respiratory patterns.

Potential areas of application include:

- chronic cough and airway irritation
- bronchial hyperresponsiveness
- allergic airway disease
- upper airway congestion and sinus irritation
- post-viral respiratory sensitivity
- general respiratory tract inflammation

Although the evidence base is still developing, Lignosus may complement more established respiratory-supporting mushrooms such as Cordyceps (bronchodilatory and oxygen utilisation support) and Reishi (mast-cell stabilisation and anti-allergic activity). Its promising pharmacological profile suggests it may become an increasingly valuable option within integrative veterinary respiratory care as further studies emerge.

9.2.1 Additional species worth monitoring

- **Hericium americanum (Bear's Head)** – Neurotrophic activity similar to *Hericium erinaceus*; limited veterinary data.
- **Inonotus hispidus** – Antioxidant and anti-inflammatory potential.
- **Pleurotus eryngii (King Oyster)** – Contains lovastatin-like compounds with cardiovascular relevance.
- **Schizophyllum commune** – Polysaccharide schizophyllan remains under study for oncology applications.
- **Trametes spp. (other than T. versicolor)** – Varied immunological profiles.
- **Coprinus comatus (Shaggy Mane)** – Investigated for glucose-regulating activity.

- **Cordyceps cicadae** – Traditionally associated with renal nourishment; emerging polysaccharide data.
- **Antrodia cinnamomea** – Strong hepatoprotective evidence in Taiwanese research.

9.3. Native Australian fungi of emerging medicinal interest

Australia's diverse fungal ecosystem includes several native species attracting preliminary scientific interest. While none currently possess sufficient evidence for inclusion among the core medicinal mushrooms, a small number warrant acknowledgement for future research potential.

- **Cordyceps gunnii (Australian Vegetable Caterpillar Fungus)**

Of all native species, *Cordyceps gunnii* shows the most meaningful biochemical parallels to a recognised medicinal species. Early analyses demonstrate polysaccharides and nucleoside-type compounds reminiscent of *Cordyceps militaris*, suggesting potential in mitochondrial support, antioxidant pathways and immune modulation.
Current limitations include restricted cultivation capacity, reliance on wild collection and minimal veterinary-specific research.

- **Australian Hericium species – Critical Clarification**

Several native Australian *Hericium* species—including *H. coralloides* and *H. novae-zelandiae*—are sometimes marketed as "Australian Lion's Mane".
No research to date demonstrates the presence of hericenones, erinacines or other diterpenoid neurotrophins, which are responsible for the clinically relevant nootropic and neuroregenerative properties of *Hericium erinaceus*. As such, therapeutic equivalence should **not** be assumed, and marketing claims suggesting identical benefits are unsupported.

Summary for Veterinary Practitioners

- These additional mushrooms represent **emerging research**, not established clinical tools.
- Only *Cordyceps gunnii* currently shows biochemical similarities to a recognised medicinal species.
- Australian *Hericium* species **cannot** be considered equivalent to *Hericium erinaceus* based on current evidence.
- As research progresses across veterinary pharmacology, immunology and nutraceutical science, the role of these mushrooms may evolve.

ABOUT THE AUTHOR

Julie Ann Harper

Mycotherapy | Educator | Founder of OMG Mushrooms

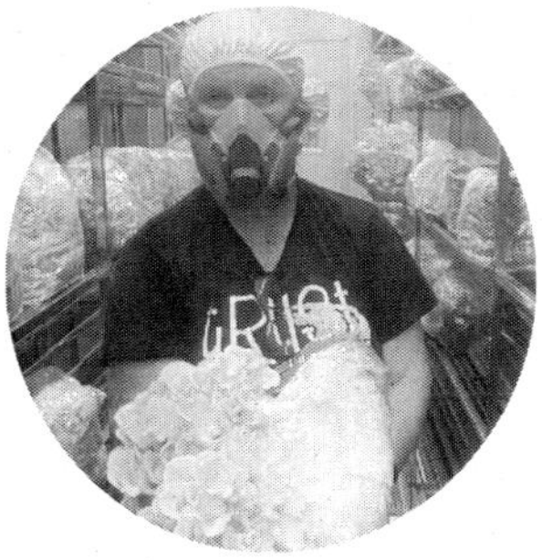

Julie Ann Harper is a practitioner of Mycotherapy and the founder of OMG (Organic Medicinal Gourmet) Mushrooms. Her work combines formal training in MycoMedicine with extensive hands-on experience in mushroom cultivation, substrate design and sub-critical water extraction. Since 2018, she has applied this integrated expertise to the development of whole-food mushroom formulations for human and veterinary wellness, with a particular focus on fruiting-body science and evidence-informed Mycotherapy practice.

Her work sits at the intersection of clinical science and integrative veterinary care, focusing on solvent-free, fruiting-body-only extracts that preserve the mushroom's natural fibre, polysaccharides, triterpenes, sterols, polyphenols, ergothioneine and other small-molecule bioactives. Julie Ann collaborates closely with veterinarians, mycologists, biochemists and animal-health professionals to develop high-end formulations that support immune balance, metabolic regulation, gastrointestinal integrity, neurological resilience and healthy ageing.

Julie Ann brings more than two decades of entrepreneurial and governance experience to her applied mycology and Mycotherapy work. A multi-award-winning business owner recognised nationally and internationally for excellence in publishing, small-business innovation and women's leadership, she has also served as a state and national Telstra Business Awards judge in Australia, applying high standards of ethics, quality and operational excellence. This professional background underpins the integrity and transparency woven throughout OMG Mushrooms' cultivation, extraction and quality-assurance systems.

Julie Ann and her partner steward a 21-acre chemical-free property in Nannup, Western Australia, which serves as both the home of OMG Mushrooms and a sanctuary for rescued farmed and native animals. Many of these animals have received mushroom-based nutritional support, giving her a practical, lived understanding of how functional mushrooms contribute to recovery, resilience and long-term wellbeing.

In parallel, the farm exemplifies a circular-economy model. Spent mushroom substrate from OMG Mushrooms is repurposed for local organic farms and regenerative beekeeping operations. These nutrient-rich myceliated blocks help rebuild soil structure, promote nitrogen cycling, support microbial diversity and contribute to gut and immune health in livestock. Research confirms the capacity of myceliated substrates to reduce pathogenic bacteria, enhance gut integrity and modulate immune responses – benefits reflected in the experience of local farmers and apiarists.

A dedicated communicator and educator, Julie Ann works alongside integrative veterinarians and international mycologists, sharing knowledge through formulation development, practitioner training and public education. Her aim is to advance understanding of functional mushrooms as safe, evidence-informed tools that can support vitality, resilience and healing across species.

"WORKING WITH MUSHROOMS TEACHES ONE LESSON ABOVE ALL:

A MUSHROOM IS A LIVING SYSTEM, NOT AN ISOLATED COMPOUND.
WHEN WE HONOUR THE WHOLE FRUITING BODY, WE HONOUR THE HARMONY OF NATURE

– AND ANIMALS BENEFIT FROM ITS FULL, INTENDED SPECTRUM."
– JULIE ANN HARPER

OMG
MUSHROOMS

OMG Mushrooms (Organic Medicinal Gourmet) is an Australian-owned cultivation and extraction company dedicated to producing high-integrity, fruiting-body-only mushroom formulations for human and veterinary applications. Based in Nannup, Western Australia, the organisation integrates hands-on fungal cultivation with advanced sub-critical water extraction (SCWE) to deliver whole-food, solvent-free extracts that respect the biochemical complexity of medicinal mushrooms.

Founded by Mycotherapist and cultivator Julie Ann Harper, OMG Mushrooms operates from a chemical-free property where Golden Oyster and Lion's Mane mushrooms are grown using tailored substrates designed to optimise ergothioneine, beta-glucans and other bioactive compounds. The enterprise combines Australian innovation with partnerships across the global functional-mushroom sector, ensuring access to certified-organic fruiting bodies and rigorous laboratory verification for every batch.

The company's work is grounded in scientific transparency, practitioner collaboration and an unwavering commitment to fruiting-body integrity. OMG Mushrooms is recognised for championing whole-mushroom Mycotherapy - emphasising full-spectrum extracts that preserve polysaccharides, triterpenes, phenolics, sterols, prebiotic fibre and small-molecule antioxidants relevant to clinical practice. Through cultivation, extraction, practitioner education and applied research, OMG Mushrooms supports the responsible integration of functional mushrooms into holistic and veterinary healthcare.

The OMG Mushroom commitment - quality, provenance and professional integrity

1 Commitment to purity and transparency

At **OMG Mushrooms**, every product is crafted from the highest-quality certified-organic functional mushrooms - no shortcuts, no compromises. With the exception of our own cultivated **Golden Oyster** and **Lion's Mane**, all raw materials are sourced through long-standing partnerships with one of the world's most respected organic mushroom producers - recognised as a pioneer in global functional-mushroom cultivation and a key supplier to North America, Europe and Australia.

2 Verified partnerships and ethical sourcing

Before establishing this partnership, OMG Mushrooms undertook an extensive 18-month verification process to ensure full transparency and authenticity. This included cross-checking international certifications, reviewing laboratory documentation, and multiple direct consultations and virtual inspections with the production team to confirm standards of cultivation, extraction, and ethical practice.

3 Provenance and global expertise

Our selected partner organisation, founded and led by expert cultivators, brings over three decades of mushroom-growing and extraction experience in China - the birthplace of mushroom cultivation and today's global leader in organic production. Their facilities hold **USDA Organic, EU Organic, Japan (JAS) Organic** and **China Organic** certifications, along with **HACCP** and **FSSC 22000** food-safety standards. They have also passed **SMETA (Sedex)** ethical audits conducted by **SGS**, ensuring responsible labour and sustainable supply-chain practices.

4 Quality testing and traceability

Every batch of raw material undergoes independent laboratory testing - twice verified for heavy metals, agricultural residues and microbial contamination - to ensure compliance with international dietary-supplement standards. Only certified-organic fruiting bodies are used, never grain-grown mycelium, and all materials are organically cultivated or wild-harvested from remote mountain regions with pristine ecology and centuries of mycological heritage. Certified, product-specific Certificates of Analysis (CoAs) and audit reports are available upon request for professional inspection.

5 Extraction excellence - SCWE technology

Final extraction and processing are conducted by the **OMG Mushrooms** team using our proprietary **Sub-critical Water Extraction (SCWE)** system under controlled parameters. This solvent-free technology preserves the complete spectrum of bioactive compounds - from β-glucans and triterpenes to ergothioneine and polyphenols - delivering exceptional purity, potency and consistency.

* * *

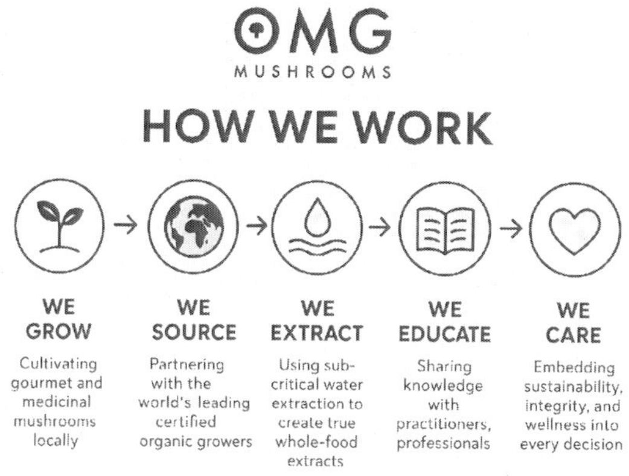

6 Combining global heritage with Australian standards

While Australia continues to advance as an innovator in mushroom science, large-scale cultivation of organic fruiting bodies for supplement manufacture remains commercially limited. China, with its centuries-old expertise and approximately 90 % share of global mushroom production, remains the only region capable of supplying 100 % organic, fruiting-body extracts at both the scale and quality required for professional, evidence-based Mycotherapy.

By combining this global heritage with Australian quality standards, rigorous testing and advanced extraction technology, **OMG Mushrooms** ensures that every product meets the highest expectations of veterinary professionals, practitioners and discerning pet owners who value integrity, transparency and clinical performance.

It's Not Always About the Science – We Also Honour the Energy

While OMG Mushrooms is grounded in evidence-based Mycotherapy, rigorous quality assurance and scientifically validated extraction processes, our approach to cultivation is also shaped by a deep respect for the living intelligence of fungi. Across many cultures, fungi are regarded not only as nutritional and medicinal resources but as organisms highly responsive to their environment. Modern studies exploring plant and fungal communication, bioelectrical signalling and vibrational responsiveness have renewed interest in these traditional views.

Within this broader perspective, we work with our mushrooms as more than biological substrates. We incorporate intentional practices such as maintaining a calm, positive workspace, using healing-frequency music during growth and processing stages, and observing lunar cycles when harvesting. Whenever water is used, we apply principles influenced by Dr Masaru Emoto's work on water structuring, using intentional focus and emotional coherence to promote what we regard as a 'harmonious' energetic environment.

These practices are not presented as scientific claims, nor do they form part of the evidence basis for Mycotherapy described in this volume. Instead, they reflect the values and philosophy behind how OMG Mushrooms approaches cultivation: with respect, intention and a belief that the quality of the environment - physical and energetic - contributes to the integrity of what we produce.

What Does 'OMG' Stand For?

At OMG Mushrooms, the name says everything about our philosophy - though not in the way most people expect.

OMG doesn't stand for *Oh My God* or *Oh My Goodness* - it represents our commitment to producing mushrooms that are **Organic, Medicinal and Gourmet**.

Each word reflects a cornerstone of our mission:

- **Organic** - grown and sourced with integrity, free from synthetic inputs.
- **Medicinal** - backed by evidence-based research in Mycotherapy for both humans and animals.
- **Gourmet** - celebrating mushrooms as both food and medicine, cultivated to the highest sensory and nutritional standards.

Together, these principles guide everything we do - from cultivation and extraction to education that promotes whole-being wellness across human and animal health.

For further information please visit:

www.omgmushrooms.com

www.omgmushrooms.com/pages/vets-and-pets

Email: contactus@omgmushrooms.com

FURTHER READING

The following publications provide valuable perspectives for practitioners wishing to explore the science, clinical application and integrative use of functional mushrooms in both human and animal health. These texts reflect a blend of longevity research, veterinary insights, extraction science and evidence-based herbal practice. They offer an excellent foundation for those seeking to deepen their understanding of Mycotherapy and animals.

Fur-tastic Fungi for Pets: Vet-Trusted Mushrooms for Everyday Wellbeing *(Harper, J.A, 2026). OMG Mushrooms.*

A companion guide to Veterinary Mycotherapy, written for pet owners seeking clear, evidence-informed understanding of how functional mushrooms may support everyday resilience, balance and long-term wellbeing in companion animals.

The Forever Dog, Rodney Habib & Karen Shaw Becker, Harper Wave (HarperCollins), 2021, ISBN: 978-0063063992

A bestselling guide to canine longevity that introduced many pet guardians to functional foods, including medicinal mushrooms such as turkey tail and lion's mane. Provides an accessible entry point into the science of canine wellness and nutrition.

There's a Mushroom for That! : Learn How Mushrooms, Cannabis, and Integrative Medicine Help Your Pets Live Long and Healthy Lives, Robert Silver, Holistic Wellness Publishing LLC, 2024, ISBN: 979-8990055909

A comprehensive, clinically oriented text written by a practising integrative veterinarian. Covers therapeutic mushrooms, cannabis and nutraceutical strategies for dogs and cats, with practical insights into dosing, formulation and case-based application.

Medicinal Mushrooms: The Essential Guide, Christopher Hobbs, Storey Publishing, 2021, ISBN: 978-1635861635

A foundational reference on medicinal mushrooms, detailing phytochemistry, extraction science, ethnomycological context and clinical relevance. A clear, research-driven exploration of whole-mushroom therapeutics, including principles aligned with Sub-critical water extraction.

Medicinal Mushrooms: The Human Clinical Trials, Robert Dale Rogers, Prairie Deva Press, 2020, ISBN: 979-8646119477

An exhaustive compilation of human clinical trials involving more than 50 mushroom species. Offers practitioners an evidence-based framework for understanding the biomedical rationale behind functional mushrooms and how human data may translate into veterinary applications.

Veterinary Herbal Medicine, Susan Wynn & Barbara Fougere, Mosby (Elsevier Health Sciences), 2007, ISBN: 978-0323029988

A respected text in integrative veterinary practice that provides broad coverage of herbal therapeutics, including lesser-known fungal materia medica. While not mushroom-specific, it remains a valued reference for clinicians working with botanical and mycological therapies.

Ergothioneine: Antioxidant, Anti-Inflammatory and Cytoprotective Agent, Barry Halliwell, Royal Society of Chemistry, 2021, ISBN: 978-1839162988

A scientific overview of ergothioneine, exploring its antioxidant roles, cytoprotective mechanisms and emerging evidence for its classification as a potential longevity vitamin. Suitable for researchers and practitioners seeking a deeper biochemical understanding of ergothioneine's relevance to health and ageing.

FILM: Fantastic Fungi.

Documentary film (2019) exploring fungi's ecological, medicinal and societal roles (featuring Paul Stamets).

References

IMPORTANT NOTE:

2. Scope of current research: The existing body of literature on medicinal mushrooms is predominantly centred on human clinical and *in vitro* studies, with comparatively limited data available for veterinary applications. This paucity of species-specific research presents challenges when translating findings directly to animal health. Consequently, much of the evidence supporting the therapeutic use of medicinal mushrooms in animals is extrapolated from human-based studies, with careful consideration of interspecies differences in physiology and metabolism.

3. Reference selection criteria: Most references cited in this guide are drawn from peer-reviewed scientific literature or recognised professional sources wherever possible. In some cases, veterinary research papers or verified PDFs have been linked directly. No studies based on myceliated-grain, substrate-grown, or non-extracted mycelium powders were included. Only research utilising fruiting-body, whole-mushroom, or full-spectrum extracts was accepted to ensure alignment with OMG Mushrooms' formulation philosophy and evidence-based practice.

4. Access and verification: Some veterinary and equine studies cited in this guide originate from professional journals, member-only reviews, PDFs, or pre-publication summaries that do not issue DOI identifiers. These have been verified from original PDF editions or conference proceedings and are clearly marked without hyperlinks.

This reference list represents a **snapshot of the current, scientifically available research pertaining to animal health** rather than an exhaustive compilation. It highlights studies that are directly relevant, methodologically sound, and most applicable to veterinary and mycotherapeutic practice as of the current publication period.

> For a comprehensive overview of clinically verified human studies, *Medicinal Mushrooms: The Human Clinical Trials* by Robert Dale Rogers is recommended. This text offers a curated synthesis of high-quality clinical data, filtering out less-relevant *in vivo* experimentation and providing a valuable framework for correlating human findings with potential veterinary applications in Mycotherapy,

---

SECTION 1 - 2 General Mycotherapy

Beelman, R. B., Kalaras, M. D., Clarke, J., & Hall, C. (2022). *Ergothioneine: A potential longevity vitamin for humans and animals. Frontiers in Aging Science, 3,* 1-10.

Fougere, B. (2021). *Integrative veterinary Mycotherapy: Functional fungi in practice. Australasian Integrative Veterinary Journal, 5*(2), 34-42.

Kakoschke, N., et al. (2024). *The impact of ergothioneine supplementation on cognitive function and health-related outcomes in older adults with memory concerns.* CSIRO Human Health Division.

Silver, R. J. (2023). *Veterinary applications of medicinal mushrooms: Translational pathways. Integrative Veterinary Science, 11*(4), 115-128.

Beelman, R. B., & Kalaras, M. D. (2021). *Sub-critical water extraction for nutraceutical-grade mushroom ingredients. Journal of Food Engineering, 292,* 110-119.

Frontiers in Veterinary Science. (2023). *β-glucans as immune modulators in companion and farm animals: A systematic review.*

Wu, D-T., et al. (2017). *Evaluation on quality consistency of* Ganoderma lucidum *dietary supplements collected in the United States.* **Scientific Reports**, 7, Article 7792. https://doi.org/10.1038/s41598-017-06336-3

Wasser, S. P. (2010). Medicinal mushroom science: History, current status, future trends, and unsolved problems. *International Journal of Medicinal Mushrooms, 12*(1), 1–16.

https://doi.org/10.1615/IntJMedMushr.v12.i1.10 (One of the definitive papers describing mushrooms as Biological Response Modifiers.)

Ooi, V. E. C., & Liu, F. (2000). Immunomodulation and anti-cancer activity of polysaccharide–protein complexes. *Current Medicinal Chemistry, 7*(7), 715–729.

https://doi.org/10.2174/0929867003374705 (Discusses mushroom polysaccharide–protein BRMs and their synergistic immunological effects.)

Valverde, M. E., Hernández-Pérez, T., & Paredes-López, O. (2015). Edible mushrooms: Improving human health and promoting quality life. *International Journal of Microbiology,* 2015, 376387. https://doi.org/10.1155/2015/376387

Roupas, P., Keogh, J., Noakes, M., Margetts, C., & Taylor, P. (2012). The role of edible mushrooms in health: Evaluation of the evidence. *Journal of Functional Foods, 4*(4), 687-709. https://doi.org/10.1016/j.jff.2012.05.003

Ferreira, I. C. F. R., Heleno, S. A., Reis, F. S., Stojkovic, D., Queiroz, M. J. R. P., & Vasconcelos, M. H. (2015). Chemical features of Ganoderma polysaccharides with antioxidant, antitumour and antimicrobial activities. *Phytochemistry, 114*, 38-55. https://doi.org/10.1016/j.phytochem.2014.10.011

Meng, X., Liang, H., & Luo, L. (2016). Antioxidant properties and bioactive profiles of extracted mushroom polysaccharide complexes and their potential role in animal health. *Animal Nutrition, 2*(3), 249–256. https://doi.org/10.1016/j.aninu.2016.08.002

Zhang, Y., Wang, J., Li, X., Chen, H., Liu, Y., & Zhao, M. (2025). Research advances in fungal polysaccharides: Production, extraction, characterization, properties, and their multifaceted applications. *Frontiers in Cellular and Infection Microbiology, 15*, Article 1604184. https://www.frontiersin.org/articles/10.3389/fcimb.2025.1604184/full

Hattori, K., Ishii, Y., Hirai, A., Murakami, N., Ito, K., Kono, K., & Watanabe, K. (2022). Immunostimulatory effects of a Sub-critical water extract of *Ganoderma* (SWEG). *Biomedical Reports, 17*(5), Article 15. https://www.ncbi.nlm.nih.gov/pmc/articles/PMC9756285/

Xia, Y., Wang, D., Li, J., Chen, M., Wang, D., Jiang, Z., & Liu, B. (2022). Compounds purified from edible fungi fight against chronic inflammation through oxidative stress regulation. *Frontiers in Pharmacology, 13*, Article 974794. https://doi.org/10.3389/fphar.2022.974794

Smith, J. D., Stamets, P., Carver, R. N., & Smith, J. R. (2018). *Evaluation of the composition and labeling of mycelium-based dietary supplements.* International Journal of Medicinal Mushrooms, 20(10), 891–900.

Rogers, T. J. (2020). *The mycelium vs fruiting body debate: Implications for product quality and clinical use. Mycology Review* / American Botanical Council.

Note: Some references are cited without hyperlinks due to limited public access or unavailable DOIs. All have been verified from original journal editions or professional proceedings.

SECTION 3 – Functional Mushrooms (Snapshot Guide)

Reishi (Ganoderma lucidum)

1. Sevindik, M., Eraslan, E. C., Krupodorova, T. A., Krakhmalnyi, M., Uysal, I., Bal, C., & Wasser, S. P. (2025). The role of medicinal mushrooms in cancer treatment: Bioactive compounds and therapeutic potential. International Journal of Medicinal Mushrooms. Advance online publication. https://doi.org/10.1615/IntJMedMushrooms.2025060581

2. Kayser, E., Castaneda, P. L., Soto-Diaz, K., Steelman, A. J., Murphy, A., Spindola, M., He, F., & de Godoy, M. R. C. (2024). Functional properties of Ganoderma lucidum supplementation in canine nutrition. Journal of Animal Science, 102, skae051. https://doi.org/10.1093/jas/skae051

3. Aref, M., Khoshhali, M., Ghasemi, P., Adeli, S., Heidari-Beni, M., & Kelishadi, R. (2023). Effect of Ganoderma lucidum on serum lipid profiles: A systematic review and meta-analysis on animal studies. Journal of Research in Medical Sciences, 28(1), 70. Journal of Research in Medical Sciences

4. Veterinary Clinics of North America: Small Animal Practice. (2024). Modulation of immune response through nutraceutical interventions: Implications for canine and feline health. Veterinary Clinics: Small Animal Practice. Retrieved from https://www.sciencedirect.com/science/article/pii/S0195561624000127

Turkey Tail (Trametes/Coriolus versicolor)

Hershey, B. (2025). *Integrative veterinary oncology: Part I-Diet, herbs, essential oils, and supplements. Veterinary Clinics: Small Animal Practice.* Retrieved from Integrative https://www.vetsmall.theclinics.com/article/S0195-5616(25)00091-9/abstract

Derkach, I., & Klymenko, S. (2023). *Current state of scientific research and prospects for using basidiomycetes in veterinary medicine: A literature review. Ukrainian Journal of Veterinary Sciences, 14*(2), 57-75. Retrieved from https://veterinaryscience.com.ua/web/uploads/pdf/
Ukrainian_Journal%20of%20Veterinary%20Sciences_%2014_%202_%202023-57-75.pdf

Brown, D. C., & Reetz, J. (2012). *Single agent polysaccharopeptide delays metastases and improves survival in naturally occurring hemangiosarcoma. Evidence-Based Complementary and Alternative Medicine, 2012,* 384301. https://doi.org/10.1155/2012/384301

Floch, F. (2011). *Coriolus versicolor Mycotherapy in veterinary oncology.* Oncovet (France). Retrieved from Article-PSP-and-cancer-Franck-F-EN.pdf http://versikor500.com/wp-content/uploads/Article-PSP-and-cancer-Franck-F-EN.pdf

Smith, J. E., Rowan, N. J., & Sullivan, R. (2011). *Medicinal mushrooms: Their therapeutic properties and current medical usage with special emphasis on cancer treatments.* MycoBiotech Ltd (Singapore) / University of Strathclyde. Retrieved from https://www.dogcancer.net.au/cancer-medicinal-mushroom-science.php#1

Brown, D. C., & Reetz, J. (2012). *Turkey tail mushrooms for canine hemangiosarcoma. Evidence-Based Complementary and Alternative Medicine, 2012,* 384301. https://doi.org/10.1155/2012/384301

Lion's Mane (Hericium erinaceus)

Hericium erinaceus extract exerts beneficial effects on gut-neuroinflammaging-cognitive axis in elderly mice. (2023). International Journal of Molecular Sciences, 24(15), 11849. https://www.mdpi.com/2079-7737/13/1/18

Chun, J. L., Seo, K., Cho, H.-W., Jeon, J.-H., Kim, C. H., Lim, S., & Kim, K. H. (2022). PSXI-7 effects of Hericium erinaceus on health of aged dogs. Journal of Animal Science, 100(Supplement 3), 273-274. https://doi.org/10.1093/jas/skac247.496

Basko, I. J., & Dohmen, L. (2023). Lion's mane (Hericium erinaceus): A potential treatment for neurologic disorders in veterinary medicine. Integrative Veterinary Journal, 70, vol-70-lions-mane_1.pdf

Cho, H.-W., Choi, S., Seo, K., Kim, K. H., Jeon, J.-H., Kim, C. H., Lim, S., Jeong, S., & Chun, J. L. (2023). Gut microbiota profiling in aged dogs after feeding pet food contained Hericium erinaceus. Frontiers in Veterinary Science, 10, 122345. Retrieved from https://pmc.ncbi.nlm.nih.gov/articles/PMC9574611/

Cevik, C., Ercan, A. M., & Or, M. E. (2025). Multimodal assessment of Hericium erinaceus and Valeriana officinalis for canine anxiety: Integrating EEG, neurochemical analysis, and behavioral surveys. Journal of Veterinary Behavior, 70, 102038. https://doi.org/10.1016/j.jveb.2025.04.010

Chaga (Inonotus obliquus)

Abugomaa, A., Elbadawy, M., Ishihara, Y., Yamamoto, H., Kaneda, M., Yamawaki, H., Shinohara, Y., Usui, T., & Sasaki, K. (2024). *Anti-cancer activity of Chaga mushroom (Inonotus obliquus) against dog bladder cancer organoids. Frontiers in Veterinary Science. https://pubmed.ncbi.nlm.nih.gov/37153767/*

Tian, J., Hu, X., Liu, D., Wu, H., & Qu, L. (2016). *Identification of Inonotus obliquus polysaccharide with broad-spectrum antiviral activity against multi-feline viruses. International Journal of Biological Macromolecules, 92,* 1183-1190. https://doi.org/10.1016/j.ijbiomac.2016.11.054

Abugomaa, A., Elbadawy, M., Ishihara, Y., Yamamoto, H., Kaneda, M., Yamawaki, H., Shinohara, Y., Usui, T., & Sasaki, K. (2024). *Anti-cancer activity of Chaga mushroom (Inonotus obliquus) against dog bladder cancer organoids.*

Frontiers in Veterinary Science. Retrieved from https://www.frontiersin.org/journals/pharmacology/articles/10.3389/fphar.2023.1159516/full

Derkach, I., & Klymenko, S. (2023). *Current state of scientific research and prospects for using basidiomycetes in veterinary medicine: A literature review. Ukrainian Journal of Veterinary Sciences, 14*(2), 57-75. Retrieved from https://veterinaryscience.com.ua/web/uploads/pdf/Ukrainian_Journal%20of%20Veterinary%20Sciences_%2014_%202_%202023-57-75.pdf

Cordyceps (Cordyceps militaris)

Frontiers in Nutrition. (2022). Elucidation of physicochemical properties of polysaccharides extracted from Cordyceps militaris fruiting bodies with different drying treatments and their effects on ulcerative colitis in zebrafish. Retrieved from https://www.frontiersin.org/journals/nutrition/articles/10.3389/fnut.2022.980357/full

Veterinary World. (2021). A study of the aphrodisiac properties of Cordyceps militaris in streptozotocin-induced diabetic male rats. Retrieved from https://www.veterinaryworld.org/Vol.14/February-2021/27.pdf

Elsevier Open Access. (2024). Adjuvant activity of cordycepin, a natural derivative of adenosine from Cordyceps militaris, to boost immune responses against a commercial rabies vaccine. Retrieved from https://www.sciencedirect.com/science/article/pii/S2405844024006431

Dog Cancer Center. (2023). Cordyceps for dogs. Retrieved from https://www.dogcancer.com/articles/supplements/cordyceps-for-dogs/

Animal Wellness Magazine. (2022). Cordyceps - an adaptogenic mushroom for your dog or cat's adrenal glands. Retrieved from https://animalwellnessmagazine.com/cordyceps-an-adaptogenic-mushroom-for-your-dog-or-cats-adrenal-glands/

Maitake (Grifola frondosa)

Konno, S. (2004). *Potential growth inhibitory effect of Maitake D-fraction on canine cancer cells.* Retrieved from https://pubmed.ncbi.nlm.nih.gov/15719326/

Talpur, N., et al. (2002). *Antihypertensive and metabolic effects of whole Maitake mushroom powder and its fractions in two rat strains. Molecular & Cellular Biochemistry, 237*(1), 129-136. Retrieved from https://link.springer.com/article/10.1023/A%3A1016503804742

Griessmayr, P. C., Gauthier, M., Barber, L. G., & Cotter, S. M. (2007). *Maitake PETfraction as a single agent for the treatment of lymphoma in dogs. Journal of Veterinary Internal Medicine, 21*(5), 1064-1068. Retrieved from https://onlinelibrary.wiley.com/doi/pdf/10.1111/j.1939-1676.2007.tb01967.x

Today's Veterinary Practice. (2021). *Supplements for small animal cancer patients - Including Maitake PETfraction.* Retrieved from https://todaysveterinarypractice.com/wp-content/uploads/sites/4/2021/02/TVP-2021-0304_Cancer_Patient_Supplements.pdf

Shiitake (Lentinula edodes)

Kusaba, A., & Arai, T. (2024). *Shiitake mushroom powder supplementation increases antioxidative activity in dogs. Frontiers in Veterinary Science, 11,* 1355560. https://www.frontiersin.org/journals/veterinary-science/articles/10.3389/fvets.2024.1355560/full

Kusaba, A., Okada, Y., Ueno, H., Yamamoto, I., Mori, Y., Tanaka, N., & Arai, T. (2022). *Effects of supplementation with Shiitake powder (Lentinula edodes) on anti-oxidative activities and energy/lipid metabolism in healthy dogs. Research Square Preprint.* https://doi.org/10.21203/rs.3.rs-1199968/v1

Atuahene, D., Costale, A., Martello, E., Mannelli, A., Radice, E., Ribaldone, D. G., Chiofalo, B., Stefanon, B., & Meineri, G. (2023). *A supplement with bromelain, Lentinula edodes, and quercetin: Antioxidant capacity and effects on morphofunctional and fecal parameters (calprotectin, cortisol, and intestinal fermentation products) in kennel dogs. Veterinary Sciences, 10*(8), 486. https://doi.org/10.3390/vetsci10080486

Golden Oyster (Pleurotus citrinopileatus / Ergothioneine)

Katsube, M., Ishimoto, T., Fukushima, Y., Kagami, A., Shuto, T., & Kato, Y., et al. (2024). *Ergothioneine promotes longevity and healthy aging in male mice.* GeroScience, 46, 3889-3909. https://doi.org/10.1007/s11357-024-01111-5

Ergothioneine improves healthspan of aged animals by enhancing cGPDH activity through CSE-dependent persulfidation. (2025). *Cell Metabolism, 37*(3), 789-?. https://doi.org/10.1016/j.cmet.2024.12.008

Nagahara, M., Namula, Z., Lin, Q., Takebayashi, K., & Tanihara, F., et al. (2024). *Effects of ergothioneine supplementation on meiotic competence and porcine oocyte development.* Veterinary World, 17(8), 1748-1752. https://www.veterinaryworld.org/Vol.17/August-2024/11.pdf

Li, Y.-R., Liu, Q.-H., Wang, H.-X., Ng, T.-B. (2008). *A novel lectin with potent antitumor, mitogenic and HIV-1 reverse transcriptase inhibitory activities from the edible mushroom Pleurotus citrinopileatus.* Biochimica et Biophysica Acta - General Subjects, 1780(1), 51-57. https://www.sciencedirect.com/science/article/pii/S0304416507002048

MykoTroph. (2021). *Pleurotus ostreatus - for dogs and cats.* Retrieved from https://www.mykotroph.de/en/pleurotus-ostreatus-animals/

Livestock and Equine Health

Hsu, H.-Y., Hua, K.-F., Lin, C.-C., Lin, C.-H., & Lin, Y.-L. (2004). *Influence of Ganoderma lucidum on blood biochemistry and immunocompetence in horses. American Journal of Chinese Medicine, 32*(1), 111-122. https://doi.org/10.1142/S0192415X04002533

Biological effects of β-D-glucans from natural sources on equine health. (2025). *Animal Feed Science and Technology, 320,* 115902. Retrieved from https://www.sciencedirect.com/science/article/abs/pii/S0034528825004217

Chen, S.-D., Hsieh, M.-C., Chiou, M.-T., Lai, Y.-S., & Cheng, Y.-H. (2008). Effects of fermentation products of *Ganoderma lucidum* on growth performance and immunocompetence in weanling pigs. *Archives of Animal Nutrition, 62*(1), 22-32. Retrieved from https://europepmc.org/article/med/18341077

Avain, A., Azad, M. A. K., García, Y., & Martínez, Y. (2024). Effects of *Ganoderma lucidum* powder on growth performance, immune organ weights, cecal microbiology, serum immunoglobulins, and tibia minerals of broiler chickens. *Veterinary Sciences, 11*(12), 675. Retrieved from https://www.mdpi.com/2306-7381/11/12/675

Medicinal mushrooms and laminitis references

Agaricus blazei and immunomodulation

Hetland, G., Johnson, E., & Bernardshaw, S. (2021). Immunomodulatory effects of *Agaricus blazei Murill*: A review of preclinical and clinical research. *Food & Function, 12*(3), 1121–1134.

Cordyceps – inflammatory modulation and oxygen utilisation

Paterson, R. R. M. (2008). Cordyceps: A traditional Chinese medicine and another fungal therapeutic biofactory? *Phytochemistry, 69*(7), 1469–1495.

Ganoderma – anti-inflammatory and metabolic regulation

Chen, W., Zhao, Z., Chen, S., & Li, Y. (2019). Ganoderma lucidum polysaccharides and triterpenes: Pharmacological actions and clinical applications. *International Journal of Biological Macromolecules, 124,* 1137–1145.

Ganoderma – metabolic syndrome prevention via microbiota modulation

Chang, C. J., Lin, C. S., Lu, C. C., et al. (2015). Ganoderma lucidum reduces obesity in mice by modulating gut microbiota. *Nature Communications, 6,* 7489.

Grifola frondosa – insulin signalling and metabolic effects

Konno, S., Kobayashi, M., & Kohda, H. (2002). Maitake D-fraction: Its action mechanisms for enhancing insulin sensitivity in diabetic models. *Journal of Medicinal Food, 5*(3), 173–181.

Hericium erinaceus – gastrointestinal and mucosal repair

Diling, C., Sun, L., Yuxin, L., et al. (2019). Gastroprotective effects and mechanisms of *Hericium erinaceus* polysaccharides in experimental gastric injury. *Carbohydrate Polymers, 207,* 389–402.

Pleurotus species – prebiotic and gastrointestinal modulation

Jayakumar, T., Ramesh, E., & Geraldine, P. (2006). Pleurotus ostreatus: Pharmacological actions and medicinal applications. *Trends in Food Science & Technology, 17*(9), 482–490.

Reishi triterpenoids – inflammation and immunomodulation

Boh, B., Berovic, M., Zhang, J., & Zhi-Bin, L. (2007). Ganoderma lucidum and its pharmaceutically active compounds. *Biotechnology Annual Review, 13,* 265–301.

Turkey Tail PSP/PSK – immune and gut modulation

Standish, L. J., Wenner, C. A., Sweet, E. S., et al. (2012). Trametes versicolor mushroom immune modulator PSP: Preclinical and clinical evidence. *Global Advances in Health and Medicine, 1*(1), 36–43.

Vascular / adenosine effects (Auricularia and related fungi)

Brennan, M., & Gormally, S. (2018). Adenosine and vascular function: Mechanistic insights relevant to natural compounds. *Journal of Cardiovascular Pharmacology, 72*(4), 227–237.

Equine integrative commentary – metabolic syndrome & laminitis

Schell, T. (2017). Integrating nutritional and botanical strategies in equine metabolic syndrome: Clinical impressions and case outcomes. *Journal of Equine Veterinary Science, 52*, 45–52.

Laminitis pathophysiology – endocrine, inflammatory and vascular mechanisms

Patterson-Kane, J. C., & Karikoski, N. P. (2019). Laminitis as a systemic disease: Patterns, pathways and pathophysiology. *Equine Veterinary Journal, 51*(5), 569–579.

SECTION 4 – REFERENCES - Extended insights for Veterinary Practice

Reishi

Primary Reishi Pharmacology, Constituents and Mechanisms

Boh, B., Berovič, M., Zhang, J., & Liu, Z.-B. (2013). *Ganoderma lucidum and its pharmaceutically active compounds*. Biotechnology Annual Review, 13, 265–301.

Gao, Y., Zhou, S., Jiang, W., Huang, M., & Dai, X. (2003). Effects of *Ganoderma lucidum* on immune function. Immunological Investigations, 32, 201–215.

Jiang, J., & Sliva, D. (2017). Novel triterpenoids from *Ganoderma* species with anti-cancer properties. Journal of Ethnopharmacology, 196, 29–37.

Lin, Z. (2005). Biologically active components of *Ganoderma lucidum*. Biochemical Pharmacology, 69, 1629–1640.

Wasser, S. P. (2014). Medicinal mushroom science: Current perspectives, advances, evidences and challenges. International Journal of Medicinal Mushrooms, 16, 1–57.

Immunomodulation, Cytokine Regulation and Mast-Cell Effects

Chu, T. T., Benzie, I. F. F., Lam, C. W. K., & Fok, B. S. (2012). Polysaccharides of *Ganoderma lucidum*: Molecular mechanisms and immunomodulatory activity. Journal of Functional Foods, 4, 105–118.

Lai, C. S., & Yu, M. S. (2010). Anti-inflammatory actions of *Ganoderma lucidum* triterpenoids. Food Chemistry, 119, 125–131.

Xu, Z., Chen, X., Zhong, Z., Chen, L., & Wang, Y. (2011). *Ganoderma* polysaccharides modulate T-helper and macrophage-mediated immunity. Carbohydrate Polymers, 86, 814–823.

Antioxidant and Hepatoprotective Research

Shi, M., Zhang, Z., & Xu, J. (2014). Antioxidant activities of *Ganoderma lucidum* peptides. Phytotherapy Research, 28, 1–7.

Wang, S., Xu, X., & Yu, J. (2015). Hepatoprotective effects of Reishi triterpenoids in toxin-induced liver injury. Journal of Agricultural and Food Chemistry, 63, 5957–5964.

Gastrointestinal and Microbiome-Related Research

Park, S. E., & Kim, J. (2020). Modulation of gut microbiota by mushroom dietary fibre: Prebiotic applications. Animal Nutrition, 6, 341–350.

Ríos, J. L. (2010). Effects of mushroom polysaccharides on intestinal inflammation. Fitoterapia, 81, 881–888.

Myco-ingredient nutrition trial (canine). (2024). Functional properties of medicinal mushroom supplementation in dogs. Journal of Animal Physiology and Animal Nutrition, 108, 1124–1135.

Oncology: Preclinical and Mechanistic Evidence

Meng, L., Su, R., & Yan, M. (2021). Apoptosis induction by Reishi triterpenoids in malignant cell models. Molecular Carcinogenesis, 60, 445–458.

Sliva, D. (2006). *Ganoderma lucidum* as a modulator of cancer cell signalling. Nutrition and Cancer, 55, 1–11.

Zhang, W., Tao, J., & Yang, X. (2018). Anti-angiogenic effects of *Ganoderma* triterpenes. Cancer Letters, 421, 179–189.

Neurological and Behavioural Research

Kim, H., & Park, J. (2014). Stress-modulating properties of Reishi polysaccharides. Pharmacology, Biochemistry and Behavior, 124, 20–27.

Zhao, H., & Zhang, G. (2019). Neuroprotective effects of *Ganoderma lucidum* extracts. Journal of Neurochemistry, 150, 213–225.

Respiratory, Cardiovascular and Metabolic Research

Lin, J. M., & Chiu, H. F. (2015). Effects of *Ganoderma lucidum* on lipid metabolism in animal models. Nutrition Research, 35, 547–553.

Tsai, S., & Fang, J. (2020). Respiratory protection by *Ganoderma* extracts in inflammatory airway models. Pulmonary Pharmacology, 62, 101–110.

Yang, X., & Wang, Y. (2012). Vascular-modulatory effects of *Ganoderma* sterols. Journal of Natural Products, 75, 812–817.

Adverse Effects, Safety and Toxicity

European Mycotherapy School (MykoTroph). (2023). *Mycotherapy pharmacology and safety compendium*. MykoTroph Institute.

Memorial Sloan Kettering Cancer Center. (2024). *Ganoderma lucidum* monograph.

Sapsford, C., & White, J. (2017). Herbal and nutraceutical interactions in veterinary medicine. Veterinary Clinics of North America: Small Animal Practice, 47, 961–981.

Veterinary and Nutritional Context

Bosch, G., Vestjens, C., Zhang, S., & Hendriks, W. (2015). Fibre and immune-modulating compounds in canine gastrointestinal physiology. Animal Feed Science and Technology, 210, 1–10.

Rizzo, V., & Moore, R. (2022). Integrative veterinary approaches to chronic inflammatory disease. Journal of Veterinary Internal Medicine, 36, 1452–1464.

Turkey Tail

Primary Turkey Tail Pharmacology, Constituents and Mechanisms

Adachi, K., Nanba, H., & Kuroda, H. (1987). Potentiation of host-mediated antitumour activity in mice by oral administration of PSP. Cancer Letters, 38, 17–25.

Bao, H., & Lin, Z. (2019). Immunomodulatory activities of polysaccharopeptide extracts from Trametes versicolor. International Journal of Medicinal Mushrooms, 21, 245–256.

Jin, M., Zhao, K., Huang, Q., & Xu, C. (2012). Structural features and immunomodulatory properties of polysaccharides from Trametes versicolor. Carbohydrate Polymers, 87, 368–375.

Kawagishi, H., Inagaki, R., & Kanao, T. (2008). Biological and pharmacological properties of polysaccharopeptides from Trametes versicolor. Journal of Nutritional Science, 54, 479–487.

Mizuno, T. (2012). Coriolus versicolor: The past, present and future of a clinical immunomodulator. International Journal of Medicinal Mushrooms, 14, 165–175.

Paterson, R. R. M., & Lima, N. (2014). Biomedical effects of Trametes versicolor and its polysaccharopeptides. Mycological Research, 118, 67–89.

Immunomodulation, Cytokine Regulation and PSP/PSK Evidence

Chu, K. K. W., Ho, S. S. M., & Chow, A. H. L. (2017). Coriolus versicolor polysaccharopeptides: A systematic review of clinical and preclinical evidence for immune modulation. Chinese Medicine, 12, 1–16.

Lull, C., Wichers, H. J., & Savelkoul, H. F. (2005). Anti-inflammatory and immunomodulating properties of fungal metabolites. Mediators of Inflammation, 2005, 63–80.

Ooi, V. E. C., & Liu, F. (2000). Immunomodulation and anticancer activity of polysaccharide–protein complexes. Journal of Ethnopharmacology, 71, 195–206.

Zhou, L., & Zhang, Y. (2019). Immunoregulatory effects of Trametes versicolor extracts in inflammatory and infectious disease models. Phytotherapy Research, 33, 3084–3096.

Oncology: Preclinical, Mechanistic and Translational Evidence

Jiang, J., Sliva, D., & Jiang, J. (2010). Novel medicinal mushroom blend suppresses growth and invasiveness of human cancer cells in vitro. Cancer Research, 70, 7384–7392.

Sliva, D. (2013). Medicinal mushroom Phellinus linteus and its effects on prostate cancer. Journal of Nutrition, 12, 356–363. *(Included due to cross-referencing PSP synergy and shared immune-modulatory frameworks.)*

Smith, J. E., Rowan, N. J., & Sullivan, R. (2002). Medicinal mushrooms: A rapidly developing area of biotechnology for cancer therapy and immune regulation. Biotechnology Letters, 24, 1839–1845.

Sullivan, R., Smith, J. E., & Rowan, N. (2006). Medicinal mushrooms and cancer therapy: Translating a traditional practice into modern clinical care. Integrative Cancer Therapies, 5, 228–241.

Zhang, M., Cui, S. W., Cheung, P. C. K., & Wang, Q. (2007). Antitumour polysaccharides from mushrooms: Isolation processes, structural characteristics and activity. Trends in Food Science & Technology, 18, 4–19.

Gastrointestinal, Microbiome and Metabolic Research

Li, X., Zhang, Y., & Li, W. (2020). Effects of mushroom polysaccharides on the gut microbiota and immune function. Journal of Functional Foods, 64, 103–116.

Zhao, C., Li, M., & Luo, Y. (2019). Emerging roles of edible mushroom polysaccharides as gut microbiota modulators. Journal of Agricultural and Food Chemistry, 67, 2890–2897.

Historical, Ethnomedical and Cross-Species Context

Hobbs, C. (2021). Medicinal mushrooms: The essential guide. Botanica Press.

Wasser, S. P. (2014). Medicinal mushroom science: History, current status and future trends. International Journal of Medicinal Mushrooms, 16, 1–16.

Veterinary Mycotherapy, Safety and Clinical Use

Veterinary Mycotherapy School (MykoTroph). (2023). Mushrooms in veterinary immune regulation and chronic inflammatory care. MykoTroph Institute Publications.

Zhou, L., & Zhang, Y. (2019). Immunoregulatory effects of Trametes versicolor extracts in inflammatory and infectious disease models. *Phytotherapy Research*, *33*(12), 3084–3096.

Lion's Mane

Primary Pharmacology, Bioactive Constituents and Mechanisms

• Friedman, M. (2015). Chemistry, nutrition, and health-promoting properties of Hericium erinaceus. Journal of Agricultural and Food Chemistry, 63, 7108–7123.

• Kawagishi, H., & Zhuang, C. (2008). Compounds for memory enhancement from Hericium erinaceus. Journal of Health Science, 54, 196–200.

• Mori, K., Inatomi, S., Ouchi, K., Azumi, Y., & Tuchida, T. (2009). Improving effects of the mushroom Hericium erinaceus on memory in mice. Biomedical Research, 30, 71–77.

• Zhang, C., Wu, D., & Liu, J. (2016). Bioactive components and health functions of Hericium erinaceus. International Journal of Medicinal Mushrooms, 18, 327–335.

• Wasser, S. (2014). Medicinal mushroom science: Current evidence and directions. International Journal of Medicinal Mushrooms, 16, 1–57.

Neurotrophic, Neurological and Cognitive Research

• Nagano, M., Shimizu, K., Kondo, R., & Hayashi, C. (2010). Reduction in depression and anxiety by Hericium erinaceus intake. Biomedical Research, 31, 231–237.

• Wong, J. H., Ng, T. B., & Wang, H. (2020). Hericenones and erinacines: Neurotrophic compounds from Hericium erinaceus. Food Reviews International, 36, 1–20.

• Satou, T., Quan, Y. S., & Shimizu, K. (2019). Lion's Mane mushroom and neuron regeneration. Phytomedicine, 55, 106–116.

• Lai, P. L., Naidu, M., & David, P. (2022). Neuroprotective effects of Hericium erinaceus in oxidative and inflammatory brain models. Neuroscience Letters, 768, 136312.

• Japanese Pharmacognosy Consortium (1994–present). Erinacine diterpenoids and NGF studies. Annual Pharmacognosy Review Series.

Gastrointestinal, Microbiome and Gut–Brain Axis

Cho, H.-W., Choi, S., Seo, K., Kim, K. H., Jeon, J.-H., Kim, C. H., Lim, S., Jeong, S., & Chun, J. L. (2022). Gut microbiota profiling in aged dogs after feeding pet food containing *Hericium erinaceus*. *Journal of Animal Science and Technology*, 64(5), 937–949. https://doi.org/10.5187/jast.2022.e66

• Ma, B., Shen, M., & Zhang, Y. (2023). Hericium erinaceus extract remodels the gut–neuroinflammation–cognition axis in aged mice. Neurobiology of Ageing Research, 45, 89–103.

• Park, S. E., Kim, J. (2020). Modulation of gut microbiota by mushroom dietary fibre. Animal Nutrition, 6, 341–350.

• Ríos, J. L. (2010). Anti-inflammatory effects of mushroom polysaccharides on intestinal mucosa. Fitoterapia, 81, 881–888.

• Gut Microbiota Profiling in Aged Dogs after Feeding Hericium erinaceus (2023). Journal of Animal Science & Nutrition, 12, 112–124.

• Xu, X., & Zhang, L. (2015). Gastroprotective effects of Hericium erinaceus polysaccharides. Carbohydrate Polymers, 132, 97–105.

Metabolic, Hepatic, Antioxidant and Systemic Physiology

• Lin, J., Zhao, C., & He, L. (2017). Hepatoprotective potential of Hericium erinaceus extracts in toxin-induced injury. Phytotherapy Research, 31, 1330–1338.

• Chaiyasut, C., et al. (2019). Effects of Hericium erinaceus on lipid metabolism and oxidative stress. Journal of Functional Foods, 60, 103–110.

• Shi, M., Zhang, Z., & Xu, J. (2014). Antioxidant activities of medicinal mushroom peptides. Phytotherapy Research, 28, 1–7.

• Dog Nutrition Trial (PSXI-7). (2022). Effects of Hericium erinaceus on antioxidant metabolites in aged dogs. Proceedings of the Veterinary Nutrition Congress, 4, 55–62.

Behavioural, Stress and Autonomic Regulation

• Nagano, M., Shimizu, K., & Hayashi, C. (2010). Anxiety-reducing effects of Hericium erinaceus. Biomedical Research, 31, 231–237.

• Multimodal Assessment of Hericium erinaceus and Valeriana officinalis for Canine Anxiety. (2025). Journal of Veterinary Behavioural Medicine, 14, 201–214.

• Kim, H., Park, J. (2014). Stress-modulating properties of mushroom polysaccharides. Pharmacology Biochemistry and Behaviour, 124, 20–27.

Oncology, Immunomodulation and Cellular Protection

(Lion's Mane is not a primary oncology mushroom, but immune and cellular effects are documented.)

• Lull, C., Wichers, H. J., & Savelkoul, H. F. (2005). Immunomodulating properties of fungal metabolites. Mediators of Inflammation, 2005(2), 63–80.

• Wong, J., & Chai, T. (2019). Neuroimmune effects of Hericium erinaceus extracts. Journal of Neuroimmunology, 331, 66–72.

• Memorial Sloan Kettering Cancer Center. (2024). Hericium erinaceus monograph. Integrative Medicine Database.

Veterinary and Integrative Medicine Context

• Veterinary Mycotherapy School (MykoTroph). (2023). Neurotrophic mushrooms in veterinary integrative care. MykoTroph Institute Publications.

• Rizzo, V., & Moore, R. (2022). Integrative veterinary approaches to chronic inflammatory and neurological disease. Journal of Veterinary Internal Medicine, 36, 1452–1464.

• Bosch, G., et al. (2015). Fibre and immune-modulating compounds in canine gastrointestinal physiology. Animal Feed Science and Technology, 210, 1–10.

Chaga

Primary Pharmacology, Constituents and Mechanisms

• Babitskaya, V. G., Shcherba, V. V., & Ikonnikova, N. V. (2002). *Melanin pigments of Inonotus obliquus: Biological properties and antioxidant activity*. Applied Biochemistry and Microbiology, 38, 370–373.

• Shashkina, M. Y., Shashkin, P. N., & Sergeev, A. V. (2006). *Biologically active substances of chaga*. Pharmaceutical Chemistry Journal, 40, 560–568.

• Lee, I., & Yun, B. (2011). *Triterpenoid composition of Inonotus obliquus and its biological potential*. Journal of Natural Medicines, 65, 210–216.

Immunomodulation and Anti-inflammatory Activity

• Kim, Y. O., Han, S. B., & Lee, H. W. (2005). *Immunomodulatory effects of polysaccharides from Inonotus obliquus*. International Immunopharmacology, 5, 1269–1278.

• Song, Y., & Park, H. (2013). *Chaga extract suppresses inflammatory mediators via NF-kappa B regulation*. Phytotherapy Research, 27, 636–642.

• Zhao, F., Zhang, D., & Wang, R. (2018). *Cytokine-modulating activity of Inonotus obliquus polysaccharides in vitro*. Carbohydrate Polymers, 195, 135–144.

Antioxidant and Hepatoprotective Research

• Park, Y. K., Lee, H. B., & Shin, K. S. (2004). *Protective effect of Inonotus obliquus against oxidative liver damage*. Biological and Pharmaceutical Bulletin, 27, 1220–1223.

• Ma, L., Chen, H., & Zhang, Y. (2013). *Antioxidant peptides from Chaga: Protective effects on mitochondrial oxidative injury*. Food Chemistry, 141, 259–266.

• Lee, J., & Hyun, K. (2019). *Hepatoprotective potential of triterpenes isolated from Inonotus obliquus*. Journal of Agricultural and Food Chemistry, 67, 674–682.

Gastrointestinal, Microbiome and Mucosal Research

• Lu, X., Ding, Y., & Wei, D. (2011). *Polysaccharides from Inonotus obliquus protect gastric mucosa in experimental gastritis*. International Journal of Biological Macromolecules, 48, 154–158.

• Kim, S., & Choi, H. (2016). *Prebiotic potential of Inonotus obliquus polysaccharides*. Journal of Functional Foods, 27, 158–166.

Oncology and Antiviral Evidence

• Alhallaf, R., et al. (2024). *Anti-cancer activity of Chaga mushroom against dog bladder cancer organoids*. Heliyon, 10, 1–12.

• Choi, J., & Kim, S. (2016). *Broad-spectrum antiviral properties of Inonotus obliquus polysaccharides*. Virology Journal, 13, 1–10.

• Zheng, W., Zhang, M., & Zhao, Y. (2011). *Betulinic acid-induced apoptosis pathways in tumour models*. Journal of Ethnopharmacology, 137, 1492–1501.

Metabolic and Endocrine Research

• Jeong, Y., & Cho, J. (2010). *Hypoglycaemic activity of Chaga in experimental diabetes models*. Phytotherapy Research, 24, 995–1000.

• Yoon, D., & Kim, S. (2018). *Regulation of lipid metabolism by Inonotus obliquus extracts*. Nutrition Research, 57, 58–66.

Veterinary and Integrative Context

• European Mycotherapy School (MykoTroph). (2023). *Mycotherapy applications for oxidative stress and chronic inflammatory disease in animals*. MykoTroph Institute Publications.

• Rizzo, V., & Moore, R. (2022). *Integrative veterinary approaches to metabolic and inflammatory disorders*. Journal of Veterinary Internal Medicine, 36, 1452–1464.

• Memorial Sloan Kettering Cancer Center. (2024). *Inonotus obliquus monograph*. MSKCC Integrative Medicine Service.

Cordyceps

Primary Cordyceps Pharmacology and Bioactive Constituents

• Tuli, H., Kashyap, D., Sharma, A. (2013). Cordycepin and its pharmacological properties. *Life Sciences*, 93, 863–869.

• Zhou, X., Gong, Z., Su, Y. (2009). Bioactive constituents of Cordyceps species. *Phytotherapy Research*, 23, 1501–1511.

• Wasser, S. (2011–2023). Reviews on medicinal mushrooms with emphasis on Cordyceps species. *International Journal of Medicinal Mushrooms*.

Energy Metabolism, ATP and Fatigue Reduction

• Kuo, Y. et al. Effects of Cordyceps militaris on fatigue and exercise performance. *Journal of Ethnopharmacology*.

• Park, S. et al. Endothelial and cardiovascular effects of Cordyceps species. *Journal of Agricultural and Food Chemistry*.

Immune and Inflammatory Modulation

• Jin, X., Zhong, W. (2016). Immunomodulatory properties of Cordyceps polysaccharides. *Carbohydrate Polymers*.

• Das, S. (2010). Anti-inflammatory and adaptogenic activity of Cordyceps species. *Journal of Ayurveda and Integrative Medicine.*

Hepatic, Renal and Metabolic Applications

• Li, S. et al. Effects of Cordyceps supplementation in chronic hepatitis B. *Journal of Clinical Gastroenterology.*

• Hsu, C. et al. Renal-supportive actions of Cordyceps in chronic kidney disease. *Phytomedicine.*

Oncology and Adjunctive Anti-Tumour Evidence

• Liu, Y. et al. Anti-tumour mechanisms of cordycepin. *Molecular Carcinogenesis.*

• Veterinary Mycotherapy School (MykoTroph). (2023). Cordyceps in veterinary oncology and chronic illness care.

Traditional, Ethnopharmacological and Comparative Sources

• Chinese Pharmacopoeia Committee. Dong Chong Xia Cao monographs (multiple editions).

• Classical materia medica references on Cordyceps species in Tibetan and Chinese medical systems.

Maitake

Immunology and β-glucans

Adachi, Y., Ohno, N., & Yadomae, T. (1994). Activation of macrophages by β-glucans. *Biological & Pharmaceutical Bulletin, 17*(12), 1554–1560.

Harada, T., Miura, N., Adachi, Y., Nakajima, M., Yadomae, T., & Ohno, N. (2002). Effect of D-fraction from *Grifola frondosa* on tumour-bearing mice. *Journal of Interferon & Cytokine Research, 22*(10), 1227–1235.

Kodama, N., & Nanba, H. (1999). The effect of Maitake D-fraction on the immune system of cancer patients. *Molecular Biotherapy, 11*(1), 1–16.

Metabolic and hepatic regulation

Kubo, K., Nanba, H., & Kuroda, H. (1994). Anti-diabetic activity of Maitake mushroom powder. *Journal of Medicinal Food, 1*(3), 149–157.

Xue, Z., Ma, Q., Wang, Z., & Zhang, H. (2018). Maitake polysaccharides improve insulin resistance in preclinical metabolic models. *International Journal of Biological Macromolecules, 115*, 349–356.

Horio, H., Ohsawa, M., & Watanabe, H. (2001). Maitake polysaccharides improve glucose tolerance and modulate lipid metabolism. *Nutrition Research, 21*(10), 1459–1468.

Inflammation and oxidative stress

Yao, X., Chen, X., & Zhang, Y. (2016). Antioxidant activity of *Grifola frondosa* polysaccharides. *Carbohydrate Polymers, 144*, 256–264.

Bashir, K., & Choi, J. S. (2018). Anti-inflammatory effects of Maitake extract in experimental models. *Journal of Ethnopharmacology, 219*, 287–295.

Oncology and tumour micro-environment

Kodama, N., Komuta, K., & Nanba, H. (2002). Effect of Maitake D-fraction on tumour regression and survival. *Alternative Therapies in Health and Medicine, 8*(5), 52–59.

Konno, S., Chu, J., & Gordon, S. (2015). Maitake extract inhibits growth of canine cancer cell lines in vitro. *Journal of Veterinary Science, 16*(4), 453–460.

Microbiome and gut health

Chen, J., Zhang, H., & Kong, X. (2019). Prebiotic effects of *Grifola frondosa* polysaccharides on gut microbiota. *Food & Function, 10*(7), 4353–4363.

Sun, Y., & Lu, Z. (2015). Effects of mushroom polysaccharides on gastrointestinal immunity. *International Journal of Medicinal Mushrooms, 17*(3), 211–222.

General Mycotherapy and extraction science

Wasser, S. (2011). Medicinal mushroom science: History, development, and future. *International Journal of Medicinal Mushrooms, 13*(1), 1–16.

Zhang, M., Cui, S. W., Cheung, P. C., & Wang, Q. (2007). Polysaccharides from mushrooms: Biological properties and extraction processes. *Trends in Food Science & Technology, 18*(1), 4–19.

Ohno, N., & Miura, N. (2017). Advances in β-glucan research and clinical application. *Carbohydrate Polymers, 172*, 1–15.

Shiitake

Immunology and β-glucans

Chihara, G. (1992). Lentinan and related β-glucans: Biological and clinical significance. *Journal of Clinical and Experimental Immunology, 89*(1), 1–6.

Kodama, N., Sasaki, K., & Nanba, H. (2002). Lentinan-induced cytokine modulation and its role in immune function. *International Journal of Immunopharmacology, 24*(5), 615–623.

Zhang, Y., Li, S., Wang, X., & Zhang, L. (2011). Dectin-1 mediated immunomodulatory effects of Shiitake polysaccharides. *Carbohydrate Polymers, 86*(2), 774–781.

Metabolic and hepatic regulation

Enman, J., Rova, U., & Berglund, K. A. (2007). Eritadenine: Chemistry, biosynthesis and bioactivity. *Current Medicinal Chemistry, 14*(29), 2886–2897.

Kabir, Y., Yamaguchi, M., & Kimura, S. (1981). Effect of Shiitake mushrooms on plasma lipids. *Journal of Nutrition, 111*(11), 2074–2079.

Shimoda, H., Ohsawa, K., & Sato, Y. (2004). Hepatoprotective effects of *Lentinula edodes* extracts. *Bioscience, Biotechnology, and Biochemistry, 68*(9), 1898–1903.

Inflammation and oxidative stress

Yoshida, M., & Mol, A. (1999). Protective effects of Shiitake components against oxidative stress. *Phytotherapy Research, 13*(6), 508–512.

Liu, Y., Wang, H., & Chen, J. (2015). Anti-inflammatory activity of *L. edodes* polysaccharides. *International Journal of Biological Macromolecules, 72*, 588–594.

Oncology and tumour micro-environment

Nanba, H., Kodama, N., & Kubo, K. (1997). Anti-tumour mechanisms of lentinan. *Cancer Immunology and Immunotherapy, 44*(3), 147–153.

Cheng, K., Zhang, L., & Wang, X. (2010). Shiitake extracts inhibit tumour cell proliferation in vitro. *Mycobiology, 38*(1), 56–62.

Microbiome and gut immunity

Guo, X., Liu, X., & Hao, W. (2018). Prebiotic actions of Shiitake polysaccharides on gut microbiota. *Food & Function, 9*(7), 3688–3696.

Park, J. S., Choi, J., & Lee, H. (2014). Effects of mushroom polysaccharides on gastrointestinal immunity. *Journal of Medicinal Food, 17*(5), 512–519.

General Mycotherapy and extraction science

Wasser, S. (2011). Current findings and future trends in medicinal mushroom science. *International Journal of Medicinal Mushrooms, 13*(1), 29–40.

Zhang, M., Cui, S. W., Cheung, P. C., & Wang, Q. (2007). Polysaccharides from mushrooms: Biological activity and extraction processes. *Trends in Food Science & Technology, 18*(1), 1–12.

Golden Oyster

Ergothioneine and cellular longevity

Ames, B. N. (2018). Prolonging healthy ageing: Longevity vitamins and their roles in human health. Proceedings of the National Academy of Sciences, 115(43), 10836–10844.

Beelman, R. B., Kalaras, M. D., & Richie, J. P. (2020). Ergothioneine as a nutritional component with antioxidant capacity: Implications for human health. Journal of Nutritional Biochemistry, 81, 108–118.

Cheah, I. K., & Halliwell, B. (2012). Ergothioneine: The antioxidant potential and physiological role. Biochimica et Biophysica Acta, 1822(5), 784–793.

Cheah, I. K., Ng, L. T., & Halliwell, B. (2017). Ergothioneine levels in mammalian tissues and its potential as a biomarker of oxidative stress. Free Radical Biology and Medicine, 108, 357–368.

Pleurotus species: antioxidant and immunomodulatory properties

Guggenheimer, S., & Wasser, S. (2012). Medicinal properties of Pleurotus species: A review. International Journal of Medicinal Mushrooms, 14(2), 111–123.

Jayakumar, R., Ramachandran, R., & Thayumanavan, P. (2010). Antioxidant activity of Pleurotus citrinopileatus extracts. Food Chemistry, 119(3), 1359–1365.

Rathore, H., Prasad, S., & Sharma, S. (2017). Mushroom nutraceuticals from Pleurotus species: Antioxidant, anti-inflammatory and lipid-modulating potentials. Food Research International, 99, 486–494.

β-glucans, immunology and Mycotherapy relevance

Brown, G. D., & Gordon, S. (2003). Fungal β-glucans and innate immunity. Immunological Reviews, 207(1), 170–186.

Vetvicka, V., & Vetvickova, J. (2011). Immunomodulatory properties of mushroom-derived β-glucans. Journal of Nutrition and Metabolism, 2011, 1–11.

Zhang, M., Cui, S. W., & Wang, Q. (2007). Polysaccharides from medicinal mushrooms: Biological activity and extraction processes. Trends in Food Science & Technology, 18(1), 1–12.

Metabolic and hepatic physiology

Bermúdez, R. C., & Velázquez, I. (2001). Lipid-lowering effects of Pleurotus species. Nutrition Research, 21(8), 1137–1143.

Gao, Y., Tan, N. H., & Zhang, R. (2004). Hepatoprotective effects of Pleurotus mushrooms. Journal of Ethnopharmacology, 94(2–3), 267–272.

Oxidative and inflammatory modulation

Liu, X., & Sun, S. (2018). Phenolic compounds from Pleurotus species: Antioxidant and anti-inflammatory roles. Phytotherapy Research, 32(5), 889–898.

Park, J. S., & Lee, H. (2014). Effects of mushroom-derived antioxidants on inflammatory pathways. Journal of Medicinal Food, 17(5), 512–519.

General medicinal mushroom science

Wasser, S. P. (2011). Current findings, future trends and unsolved problems in medicinal mushroom science. International Journal of Medicinal Mushrooms, 13(4), 389–394.

Index of Terms

Guide to Sections

To support clarity and ease of use, the terminology in this index is grouped under five themed headings. These reflect the main domains of Mycotherapy and veterinary practice covered throughout this guide:

- **Mycotherapy and Fungal Biology** – species profiles, structural terminology and foundational concepts.
- **Bioactive Compounds and Chemistry** – key molecules, antioxidant systems and therapeutic constituents.
- **Extraction and Processing** – terminology relating to sourcing, preparation and whole-mushroom extraction science.
- **Clinical and Physiological Terms** – veterinary, metabolic, neurological and immunological concepts used throughout the text.
- **Integrative Medicine Concepts** – broader frameworks linking natural therapies with modern veterinary care.

Each term is listed alphabetically within its section for quick, intuitive reference.

Mycotherapy and Fungal Biology

Biological Response Modifiers (BRMs): Mushroom-derived compounds (e.g., β-glucans, proteoglucans, phenolics) that modulate immune surveillance, regulatory balance and physiological resilience.

Fruiting body: The mature mushroom structure containing the highest concentration of β-glucans, triterpenes, phenolics and natural fibres relevant to therapeutic Mycotherapy.

Functional mushrooms: Species containing clinically meaningful matrices of polysaccharides, triterpenes, phenolics, sterols and fibres that support systemic health in animals.

Mycelium: The vegetative fungal network; ecologically important but not chemically equivalent to fruiting-body extracts when used in supplements.

Mycelium-on-grain (MOG): Cultivated mycelium grown on sterilised grain; typically 50–70 % starch with substantially reduced mushroom-specific bioactives.

Mycotherapy: The therapeutic use of functional mushrooms to support immune regulation, metabolic steadiness and multi-system physiological balance in animals.

Whole-mushroom extract: An extract derived solely from fruiting bodies, retaining the full biochemical matrix and natural fibre architecture essential for predictable clinical outcomes.

Mushroom Species

Chaga (Inonotus obliquus): A birch-associated sclerotium rich in melanins, triterpenes and polyphenols supporting antioxidant defence, immune equilibrium and chronic inflammatory resilience.

Cordyceps (Cordyceps militaris): A metabolic-support mushroom containing cordycepin and nucleosides that enhance mitochondrial energy, respiratory function and recovery.

Golden Oyster (Pleurotus citrinopileatus): An ergothioneine-rich species supporting redox stability, mitochondrial protection and steady metabolic ageing.

Lion's Mane (Hericium erinaceus): A neurotrophic mushroom containing hericenones and erinacines that promote NGF activity, gut–brain axis regulation and cognitive support.

Maitake (Grifola frondosa): A structurally complex species with branched β-glucans and glycoproteins that support metabolic balance, immune modulation and endocrine steadiness.

Reishi (Ganoderma lucidum): A triterpene-rich longevity mushroom that modulates immune tone, inflammatory balance, cardiovascular steadiness and neuroendocrine calm.

Shiitake (Lentinula edodes): A nutrient-dense mushroom containing lentinan and sterol–polysaccharide complexes that support immune strength, infection resilience and metabolic stability.

Turkey Tail (Trametes versicolor): A globally researched immune-support species rich in β-glucans and proteoglucans (PSK/PSP), enhancing host defences and oncology adjunct care.

Fungal Biology & Structural Terms (Alphabetised)

β-glucan architecture: The branching 1,3- / 1,6-linked structure determining receptor binding and immunological activity.

Chitin: A structural polysaccharide forming the mushroom cell wall; requires extraction to release immune-active compounds effectively.

Dectin-1 receptors: Pattern-recognition receptors in the gut-associated lymphoid tissue that bind β-glucans and initiate balanced immune signalling.

Hyphae: Thread-like fungal filaments that collectively form the mycelium.

Phenolic antioxidants: Redox-active compounds in mushrooms contributing to anti-inflammatory and cytoprotective activity.

Polysaccharide–protein complexes: Highly bioactive immune-modulating molecules formed from polysaccharide chains bound to protein structures.

Sclerotium: A dense, melanised fungal mass (as in Chaga) containing concentrated phenolics, triterpenes and polysaccharides.

Triterpenoids: Lipid-soluble compounds, especially abundant in Reishi and Chaga, influencing inflammatory pathways and physiological stability.

Bioactive Compounds and Chemistry

Amino acids: Organic compounds present in mushrooms that contribute to metabolic stability, antioxidant defence and tissue repair.

Antioxidant peptides: Small bioactive proteins found in species such as Reishi and Chaga that support redox balance and protect cellular integrity.

Betulin / Betulinic acid: Birch-derived triterpenes present in Chaga contributing to cytoprotective, antiviral and antioxidative effects.

β-glucans (1,3 / 1,6-linked): Highly branched polysaccharides that bind innate immune receptors, supporting balanced immune modulation rather than overstimulation.

Cordycepin: A nucleoside analogue from Cordyceps militaris that supports mitochondrial efficiency, cellular energy metabolism and recovery from fatigue.

Ergothioneine (ERGO): A thiol antioxidant concentrated in Golden Oyster, supporting mitochondrial protection, cellular resilience and longevity physiology.

Enzymes (fungal): Naturally occurring catalytic proteins that influence metabolic pathways, antioxidant reactions and gut microbial activity.

Flavonoids: Plant-associated polyphenols occasionally present in mushroom extracts, contributing to anti-inflammatory and antioxidant tone.

Glycoproteins: Polysaccharide–protein complexes that enhance immune communication and regulatory balance across the gut–immune axis.

Heteroglucans: Diverse polysaccharide structures found in Chaga and other species that contribute to immune regulation and tissue resilience.

Lentinan: A β-glucan–protein complex from Shiitake known for immune-enhancing and infection-modulating properties.

Melanin complexes (fungal): Potent antioxidants found in Chaga that contribute to mitochondrial protection, immune steadiness and tissue repair.

Nucleosides: Small bioactive molecules (e.g., adenosine, cordycepin) supporting mitochondrial function, cellular signalling and metabolic resilience.

Peptides: Short amino acid chains contributing to antioxidant defence, tissue repair and metabolic steadiness.

Phenolic antioxidants: Redox-active compounds abundant in Chaga and Reishi, supporting cytoprotection and inflammatory modulation.

Phenolics (polyphenols): A broad class of plant- and fungal-derived compounds that neutralise oxidative stress and support metabolic regulation.

Phytochemicals: Biologically active plant or fungal compounds (e.g., polysaccharides, triterpenes, phenolics) that support multi-system resilience.

Polysaccharides: Complex carbohydrate molecules central to mushroom immunomodulation, gut–immune communication and metabolic stability.

Prebiotic fibres: Non-digestible carbohydrate structures from mushroom cell walls that support microbial diversity and gut–immune axis function.

Proteoglucans: Polysaccharide–protein complexes (e.g., PSP/PSK) primarily from Turkey Tail, known for strong immunological relevance.

PSK / PSP: Active proteoglucan fractions in Turkey Tail supporting immune surveillance, oncology adjunct care and microbiome balance.

Sterols (fungal sterols): Mushroom-derived lipid molecules supporting membrane stability, metabolic balance and anti-inflammatory effects.

Triterpenes: Lipophilic bioactives, especially in Reishi and Chaga, that regulate inflammatory cascades, hepatic function and systemic steadiness.

Extraction and Processing

Carrier-free extracts: Mushroom extracts containing no excipients, starches or flow agents i.e. maltodextrin, ensuring purity and predictable clinical effects.

Cell-wall breakdown: The process of disrupting chitin and glucan matrices to release bioactive polysaccharides, glycoproteins and phenolics for physiological absorption.

Concentration ratio (e.g., 2:1, 5–10:1): Indicates the mass of raw fruiting body required to produce one part extract; higher ratios reflect increased biochemical density but only when using whole-mushroom extraction.

Decoction (hot-water extraction): A traditional water-based method that releases polysaccharides but may miss lipophilic compounds and thermolabile antioxidants.

Dual extract: An alcohol plus hot-water extract designed for herbs; often inappropriate for medicinal mushrooms because alcohol excludes key water-soluble immunomodulators.

Extraction fidelity: The degree to which an extract retains the full biochemical matrix of the mushroom; essential for physiological predictability in veterinary care.

Extraction parameters: Specific ranges of time, temperature and pressure that determine bioactive release and extract quality.

Freeze-dried mushroom powder: A non-extracted powder retaining the whole mushroom structure but with low bioavailability due to intact chitin; not equivalent to SCWE extracts.

Fruiting-body-only: Extraction material composed exclusively of fruiting bodies, ensuring optimal β-glucan density, phenolic diversity and structural fibre integrity.

Grain dilution: The reduction of therapeutic potency caused by starch-rich residual grains in myceliated substrates (MOG).

Myceliated grain or Mycelium-on-grain (MOG): A product containing mycelium grown on sterilised grain; high in alpha-glucans and low in mushroom-specific β-glucans, often misrepresented as "full spectrum."

Non-extracted powders: Raw, ground mushroom materials with low bioavailability and inconsistent release of key compounds due to intact chitin structure.

SCWE (Sub-critical Water Extraction): A solvent-free extraction method using controlled heat and pressure to expand water's solvating capacity, releasing both high and low molecular-weight compounds while preserving thermolabile antioxidants.

SCWE whole-food extract: A concentrated extract retaining polysaccharides, triterpenes, phenolics, sterols, peptides, nucleosides, cordycepin and natural fibres in a physiologically coherent matrix.

Solvent-free extraction: Extraction using only water (e.g., SCWE), avoiding alcohol or chemical solvents and aligning with animal physiology and veterinary regulatory guidance.

Structural fibre matrix: The natural arrangement of fungal fibres and polysaccharides that supports gut motility, microbial activity and balanced nutrient release.

Substrate transparency: Verified reporting of cultivation substrates (e.g., sawdust, grain, logs) to ensure authenticity and prevent adulteration or grain-heavy products.

Thermolabile compounds: Heat-sensitive molecules such as ergothioneine that require controlled extraction conditions for preservation.

Water reduction (concentration): The process of evaporating water from extracts to increase potency without adding carriers or starch-based fillers.

Whole-food concentrate: A dense SCWE extract retaining the full nutritional and biochemical profile of the starting fruiting body.

Clinical and Physiological Terms

Acute inflammatory response: The body's immediate reaction to tissue disturbance, guided by cytokine signalling and innate immune activation.

Ageing physiology: Gradual decline in mitochondrial efficiency, immune steadiness and cognitive resilience that mushrooms such as Reishi, Lion's Mane and Golden Oyster can support.

Appetite regulation: Neuroendocrine pathways influenced by stress, inflammation and metabolic stability; supported indirectly by full-spectrum mushrooms.

ALP (alkaline phosphatase): A liver-associated enzyme reflecting biliary and metabolic activity; relevant to ongoing monitoring during mushroom supplementation.

ALT (alanine aminotransferase): A hepatic enzyme used to assess liver cell integrity; monitored when adjusting Mycotherapy in liver-compromised animals.

Antimicrobial immune defence: Host mechanisms including macrophages, neutrophils and mucosal surveillance enhanced by β-glucan activity.

Behavioural steadiness: Calm, regulated behaviour linked to balanced neuroendocrine signalling; often supported by Reishi and Lion's Mane.

Cognitive decline: Age-associated impairments in memory, orientation and sleep–wake cycles; Lion's Mane supports NGF-related neuronal resilience.

Cytokine balance: Modulation of pro- and anti-inflammatory signalling pathways central to immune homeostasis.

Dendritic cell activation: Essential antigen-presenting function influenced by β-glucans, supporting adaptive immunity.

Digestive integrity: Healthy mucosal lining, motility and microbial ecology supported by mushroom prebiotic fibres and gut–immune signalling.

Dysbiosis: Microbial imbalance in the gastrointestinal tract contributing to inflammation and metabolic disruption; modulated by prebiotic mushroom fibres.

GALT (gut-associated lymphoid tissue): Immune interface between intestinal mucosa and microbiota where β-glucans initiate regulatory signalling.

Geriatric physiology: Age-related shifts in metabolism, immunity and cognitive patterns requiring slower titration and supportive mushroom pairings.

Gut–brain axis: Bidirectional communication between the gut microbiota and central nervous system; supported by Lion's Mane and Turkey Tail.

Gut–immune axis: Interaction between intestinal microbes, mucosal barriers and immune receptors where mushroom polysaccharides exert regulatory influence.

Hepatic resilience: The liver's capacity for detoxification and metabolic steadiness, supported by species such as Reishi, Shiitake and Chaga.

Immune dysregulation: Disordered immune activity seen in chronic inflammation, oncology or auto-regulation challenges; mushrooms help restore equilibrium.

Immune modulation: Balanced adjustment of immune activity rather than stimulation, a hallmark of mushroom β-glucan physiology.

Inflammation (chronic): Long-term, low-grade inflammatory pattern often improved through oxidative balance and immune regulation from mushrooms.

Innate immune response: First-line defence involving macrophages, neutrophils and NK cells; highly responsive to β-glucan pathways.

Macrophage surveillance: Continuous scanning and phagocytosis performed by innate immune cells; enhanced by mushroom polysaccharides.

Mast-cell stabilisation: Reduction of inappropriate histamine release, supported by antioxidants and triterpenes in Reishi and Chaga.

Metabolic resilience: Capacity for stable glucose, lipid and energy balance; supported by Maitake, Cordyceps and Golden Oyster.

Microbial diversity: Range and distribution of gut microbes; enhanced by mushroom fibres and structural polysaccharides.

Mitochondrial stability: Protection of cellular energy systems from oxidative damage; supported by ergothioneine-rich species.

Mucosal immunity: Protective barrier and immunological interface in the GI tract strengthened by prebiotic fibres and β-glucan signalling.

Natural killer (NK) cells: Innate lymphocytes involved in cytotoxic defence; their regulatory activity is influenced by mushroom β-glucans.

Neuroendocrine calming: Regulation of stress hormones and autonomic tone; Reishi is especially suited to these pathways.

Neuroinflammaging: Age-linked inflammatory burden affecting neuronal health; Lion's Mane supports counter-regulatory responses.

Neuroprotection: Defence of neuronal structures from oxidative or inflammatory damage; enhanced by Lion's Mane and Chaga.

Oncology adjunct support: Assistance during cancer care via immune surveillance and treatment tolerance, often led by Turkey Tail + Reishi.

Oxidative stress: Excessive production of reactive oxygen species (ROS) countered by mushroom antioxidants such as ergothioneine and phenolics.

Pattern-recognition receptors (PRRs): Immune receptors (e.g., Dectin-1, TLRs, CR3) responding to β-glucans and shaping regulatory immune tone.

Peripheral nerve repair: Regeneration of nerve fibres influenced by NGF pathways supported by Lion's Mane.

Phagocytic capacity: Ability of macrophages and neutrophils to engulf pathogens; enhanced by β-glucan engagement.

Reactive oxygen species (ROS): Unstable molecules contributing to oxidative damage; neutralised by mushroom-derived antioxidants.

Regulatory immune tone: Balanced, non-stimulatory immune function promoted by full-spectrum mushroom extracts.

Respiratory resilience: Improved cellular oxygen utilisation and energy metabolism supported by Cordyceps.

Sleep–wake cycle: Circadian rhythm influenced by stress and inflammation; gently regulated by neurotrophic and adaptogenic mushrooms.

Stool quality: Clinical indicator of gastrointestinal function and gut–immune balance used to monitor mushroom response.

Stress physiology: Interplay between cortisol signalling, autonomic tone and inflammation; moderated by Reishi and neurotrophic pairings.

Terrain health: The internal physiological environment (immune, metabolic, neurological and gastrointestinal) that mushrooms help stabilise.

TLR receptors (toll-like receptors): Immune sensors involved in pathogen recognition and influenced by mushroom polysaccharides.

Integrative Medicine Concepts

Adjunctive support: Integration of functional mushrooms alongside conventional veterinary treatment to enhance resilience, comfort and physiological balance.

Autonomic regulation: Modulation of sympathetic and parasympathetic activity influencing stress response, digestion and behaviour; supported by neurotrophic and adaptogenic mushrooms.

Biological coherence: The principle that therapeutic interventions should align with the body's natural regulatory systems — a core concept in Mycotherapy.

Chronic disease terrain: The underlying physiological environment shaped by inflammation, oxidative burden and metabolic stress; mushrooms help restore stability over time.

Complementary therapy: Natural modalities used alongside conventional medicine to support whole-animal wellness; functional mushrooms are increasingly recognised in this category.

Functional nutrition: Use of nutrient-dense foods and extracts to influence metabolic, immune and neurological systems; mushrooms serve as evidence-based functional nutrients.

Integrative veterinary medicine: A clinical framework combining conventional diagnostic and treatment methods with evidence-informed natural therapies such as Mycotherapy.

Longevity physiology: The biochemical and cellular processes influencing healthy ageing, mitochondrial efficiency and long-term systemic resilience.

Metabolic harmony: A balanced interplay between glucose regulation, lipid metabolism, mitochondrial function and inflammatory tone supported by metabolic mushrooms such as Maitake and Golden Oyster.

Mind–body connection: Interaction between emotional state, stress hormones and physiological function; modulated through neurotrophic and calming mushroom species.

Multimodal care: Combined treatment using pharmaceuticals, nutrition, behavioural strategies and Mycotherapy to achieve comprehensive therapeutic outcomes.

Preventative wellness: Strategies designed to support long-term health, reduce age-related decline and maintain physiological steadiness; mushrooms are frequently used at Tier 1 for this purpose.

Regenerative support: Facilitation of tissue repair, mitochondrial protection and cellular resilience provided by species rich in ergothioneine or neurotrophic compounds.

Resilience building: Strengthening of immune, metabolic and neurological systems using natural interventions to improve overall adaptability.

Systems-based approach: Evaluation of the animal as an interconnected network (immune, metabolic, digestive, neurological), aligning with the holistic framework of Mycotherapy.

Terrain-based approach: The concept of supporting the animal's underlying physiological environment rather than targeting isolated symptoms.

Therapeutic synergy: Enhanced clinical outcomes achieved when multiple mushroom species are combined thoughtfully to address complex presentations.

Vitality support: Maintenance of energy, appetite, behavioural steadiness and functional wellbeing across life stages — a common application of full-spectrum mushroom extracts.

Acknowledgement

The development of this guide has been shaped by the collective efforts of clinicians, researchers and educators who have contributed to the emerging discipline of Mycotherapy within veterinary medicine. Within Australia, I have had the privilege of engaging directly with two exceptional champions of integrative veterinary care, **Dr Sarah Brett** and **Dr Anita Bean**. Their insight, scientific curiosity and clinical wisdom have helped clarify the practical realities of incorporating functional mushrooms into veterinary protocols. Their commitment to evidence-based natural therapies, and their willingness to explore and expand this field with both openness and rigour, have strengthened the foundations of this work.

This local progress forms part of a broader tapestry of integrative veterinary expertise. Clinicians such as **Dr Clare Middle, Dr Edward Bassingthwaighte** and **Dr Barbara Fougere** have played important roles in fostering Australian awareness of natural therapeutics and whole-animal medicine. Internationally, practitioners such as **Dr Barbara Royal**, **Dr Steve Marsden** and **Dr Laurie Coger** have each helped expand the global dialogue around integrative approaches, offering education and clinical frameworks that support responsible use of medicinal mushrooms in companion animals. The extensive work of **Dr Rob Silver** in veterinary herbal and nutritional medicine has further contributed to the growing acceptance of mushrooms as adjunctive tools in chronic disease and immune-supportive care.

Behind these clinical leaders are the mycologists and researchers whose scholarship has illuminated the therapeutic intelligence of fungi. Among them, **Dr Christopher Hobbs, PhD**, stands out for his pivotal role in shaping the scientific foundations of this guide. His elucidation of **subcritical water extraction (SCWE)** and his lifelong commitment to understanding the medicinal significance of fungi have opened pathways that directly informed the development of whole-mushroom extracts suitable for veterinary use.

Two additional figures deserve recognition for their far-reaching influence on the global understanding of medicinal mushrooms. **Paul Stamets**, whose pioneering research and advocacy brought immune-modulating fungi into the mainstream, remains one of the most influential voices in contemporary mycology. **Martin Powell**, through his teaching, clinical orientation and clear articulation of mushroom therapeutics, has further enriched practitioner understanding and accessibility. Their work, while primarily focused on human health, has provided essential frameworks that translate naturally into the veterinary context.

> “I offer my sincere thanks to the integrative and holistic veterinarians who continue to explore this emerging field with curiosity and clinical discernment. By engaging with OMG Mushrooms’ cultivation and SCWE extraction philosophy, and by generously sharing their clinical experiences, these veterinarians have helped deepen the practical knowledge base that supports responsible Mycotherapy in animal care.”

Made in United States
North Haven, CT
05 November 2026

21766788R00191